Mixing Medicines

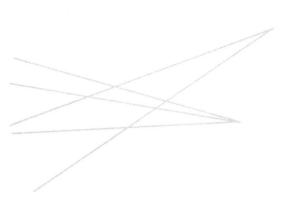

Thinking from Elsewhere

MIXING MEDICINES

Ecologies of Care in Buddhist Siberia

TATIANA CHUDAKOVA

FORDHAM UNIVERSITY PRESS
New York 2021

Visit us online at www.fordhampress.com.

Library of Congress Control Number: 2021907105

Printed in the United States of America

23 22 21   5 4 3 2 1

First edition

CONTENTS

Mixing Medicines

INTRODUCTION

THE END OF THE LINE

The Tibetan medicine hospital was at the very end of a microbus line, past other unmarked stops one had to request from the driver—a Buddhist temple, an open-air museum, a dumplings restaurant stylized as a Mongolian yurt, a bright orange entertainment complex that sprouted from the crest of a sloping hill like a cubist mushroom. Past the slowly crumbling pioneer camp with its faded sky-blue stucco, past the Soviet-era house of rest. From the stop, the clinic was another fifteen minutes by foot along the edge of a field of hard-crusted snow, following a long dirt road that is, in winter, more ice sheet than earth. The local dogs greeted the rare pedestrians with enthusiastic menace.

I took this route many times during my fieldwork in Buryatia, a multireligious ethnic minority region of the Russian Federation located in southeastern Siberia. In 2009, when I came to Buryatia for fourteen months of sustained ethnographic research on the institutionalization of traditional medicine, the *marshrutki*—the microbuses that shuttled from downtown Ulan-Ude to the regional capital's outskirts—could comfortably carry about twelve passengers, but often more crammed in, to the grumbling protests of other riders. This far from the city's main arteries, the shuttle emptied out. After the gleaming yellow silhouette of the Buddhist temple, the number of passengers dwindled to a handful, and most were not headed to the clinic: they would get off somewhere before, perhaps on the way to their *dachas*, built during the oil-fueled construction boom of the early 2000s, a period of relative prosperity even in this rural and economically poor region of

Russia. In the half-empty microbus, barreling at top speed along the surprisingly smooth highway, built especially for the Russian president's visit, as I was often told in an apocryphal explanation for many local construction projects in the city, the terminus became an object of debate. With the shuttle practically empty, the driver or a passenger might strike up a conversation. "Where are you stopping?"

To my claims that there is a hospital that specializes in Tibetan medicine, responses varied by interlocutor. Some passengers expressed puzzlement that there was a clinic nestled in the seemingly empty hills. Most had heard about the medical complex to which the hospital belonged: the East-West Medical Center figured prominently in the republic's self-presentation, mobilized by the regional government and local tourism operators to feature as one of Buryatia's regional landmarks. However, not everyone had encountered the center's infrastructural expressions. My fellow passengers frequently uttered a surprised, "Oh, *that's* where it is," and the subsequent conversations patterned into the predictable rhythms of a stable discursive genre. One wiry Russian man in his forties cautioned that Tibetan medicine might be uncomfortably close to shamanism—he was caught between interest in its potential to relieve his arthritic pain and worry over his good Russian Orthodox standing. Middle-aged Buryat women often commented that a relative underwent treatment at the clinic. Shuttle riders traded in obvious, pressing questions: How does one sign up? Isn't the waiting list terribly long? Is a referral needed? Are the treatments costly? What about pensioners, are there quotas? Do I have a phone number I could share? Do the treatments help? Is that the one where they diagnose *po pul'su* (based on the pulse)? Does the clinic offer *real* Tibetan medicine?

The terminal quality of the hospital's location, at the end of an empty field at the edge of a provincial town, with nowhere else to go, resonated with familiar discourses about traditional healing in Russia and stayed with me long after the time I spent shadowing doctors and nurses through the clinic's halls, interviewing patients, or pursuing other constellations of therapeutic practices centered on Tibetan medicine in particular and what is more broadly referred to as "traditional medicine" (Rus. *traditzionnaia meditzina*) in Buryatia and Moscow. At the beginning of my fieldwork, carried out in intervals totaling twenty months between 2006 and 2017, which brought me first to Moscow and then to Ulan-Ude, Buryatia's capital, my initial questions about Tibetan medicine's place in regional and national healthcare were met with nods of understanding. Nonbiomedical healing had become widely popular in Russia and other post-socialist countries, and since the 1990s, scholars and media commentators have speculated about the causes of this unusual therapeutic effervescence (S. Brown 2008; J. Brown and Rusinova 2002; Caldwell 2005; Jašarević 2017; Lindquist 2005; Pedersen 2011). Buryatia seemed like a good entry point into exploring Russia's budding therapeutic plurality: along with Buddhism, Sowa Rigpa, the Tibetan science of healing, which is locally glossed as Tibetan medicine (*tibetskaia meditzina*), had recently been redeployed as a feature of Buryatia's political imaginary, but its local prominence ran counter to the complex and perpetually shifting tangle of federal and regional legislation and professional frameworks charged with arbitrating medical practice in the country. Despite an absence of official legal recognition at the federal level, Tibetan medicine featured as an important element of Buryatia's cultural and religious heritage, woven into the hopeful projections for its economic future. As one of Russia's historically Buddhist regions, claimed the many promotional materials intended to present the area to travelers, potential outside investors, and central bureaucracies, Buryatia had developed its own unique tradition of Buddhist healing, one especially suited to both regional and national bodies. The East-West Center was a testament to this history, as it championed a model of medical integration that strove to incorporate Tibetan medicine into the local system of healthcare delivery, alongside both biomedical and other treatment modalities.

My early queries about Tibetan medicine's local role often seemed to arrive at an answer almost as soon as they began. To my interlocutors, it seemed quite obvious why different types of traditional medicine had become so commonplace after the collapse of the Soviet Union. A prominent local ethnographer commented, with a somewhat impatient wave of her cigarette, that all forms of traditional medicine were there simply because something had to take up the space at the end of the line—a terminal placeholder at the exhausted end of patients' desperate therapeutic trajectories. "Their [regular doctors] send them home to die, so then people start searching," she suggested.

In the first decade of the 2000s, Buryatia's local government was vocal in its promotion of Tibetan medicine as a unique regional offering. But the locations it invoked—the East-West Center, which employed biomedically trained doctors who practiced it, the regional archives and museums that documented Buryatia's contributions to its history, the local sciences center that conducted research on it—were only the more visible recent chapters in over a century of Tibetan medicine's complicated entanglement with the Russian, Soviet, and, subsequently, post-socialist states. Throughout this history, Tibetan medicine had at times basked in the favorable limelight of Russia's political elites; at other times, it found itself in the crosshairs of the state's ideological projects. Sometimes it actively eluded the state's gaze; at others it sought the state's legitimation and financial support, and frequently it seemed to operate in confusingly intersecting and overlapping variations of these different modes of engagement. Over the years, it recruited likely and unlikely allies, sometimes enthusiastic, but often no less deeply ambivalent.

Like the Tibetan medicine for which it was known, the East-West Center occupied the uncomfortable middle ground between what people in Buryatia often called official medicine, or "*ofitzial'naya meditzina*" (whether that meant state-endorsed or epistemically valid was often left productively underdetermined) and "traditional medicine," between open governmental support and administrative disavowal. Founded in 1989, two years prior to the collapse of the Soviet Union in 1991, East-West appeared to be a harbinger of things to come: at its inception an innovative example of international collaboration, interdisciplinary openness, and an experimental space for new forms of care. It was, in some accounts at least, the first state-supported medical institution of its kind—though by the late 2000s, most clinics of so-called Eastern medicine in Russia would claim the distinction of firstness. East-West promised to integrate standard biomedical care with Buryatia's Buddhist healing traditions, emphasizing the region as the place where Russia's reach extended into Asia and Asia's cultural influences stretched back into Russia.

As my social relations became less formal, the more optimistic official pronouncements about the future of Tibetan medicine in the republic and in Russia more generally were complicated by alarmingly bleak admissions—

bleak, in any case, for an ethnographer set on researching the topic: sure, it was popular, but there was no such thing as *real* Tibetan medicine in Buryatia. Don't listen to the hype. Despite the local government's rhetorical invocations of a distinctly Buryat Buddhist medical tradition, and despite the presence of a variety of infrastructural expressions that claimed it, Tibetan medicine seemed to flicker in and out of focus. During an interview with Khambo Lama Damba Ayusheev, the leader of Buryatia's Buddhist Sangha, I asked him what he thought the future of Tibetan medicine in Buryatia might be. I had come with a Buryat friend who had known Khambo Lama since before immigrating to the U.S. After some relentless teasing about his two visitors' suspicious "Americanness," Khambo Lama responded, in the brusquely ironic manner I was told characterized his style of interaction, "You know what they say, if you want to cheat people, go read the *zurkhai* (the practice of Buddhist astrology and divination), if you want to kill people, become an *emchi* (Tibetan medicine practitioner). That's why now, I build instead."

I take this disparaging evaluation of the two common professional activities that a Buddhist lama in Buryatia might undertake as at once a performance and a provocation—and an example of Ayusheev's subtle political humor. By way of clarification, he invoked his own stint with practicing Tibetan medicine. The disappointments of not being able to reliably help patients was a dense social fact: after all, such is the nature of *saṃsāra*, and, besides, few holders of "real" knowledge were available as teachers after Buryatia's Buddhist monasteries and practitioners were decimated during the Stalinist purges of the 1930s, he had intimated.[1] His statement offered a staunchly practical take on the possibilities of spiritual life in a place like Buryatia. From the perspective of an international Buddhist world, Buryatia is a periphery. Similarly, from the perspective of Russia's geopolitical imaginary, Buddhism is a state-sanctioned ethnic minority religion, mostly confined to the three "ethnically Buddhist" parts of the Russian Federation: Buryatia, Kalmykia, and Tyva. At the edges of both symbolic geographies—the political and the religious—building stupas and temples appeared to promise a more concrete expression of devotion and a more solid means of cultural and religious revival than other forms of practice, the Khambo seemed to suggest.

Although quite different in style and exposition, another comment made by a prominent local scientist, herself an authority in the field of botany, pharmaceutical research, and a well-known scholar and translator who had devoted her professional life to the study of Buryat *materia medica*, created striking interference with the Khambo's disparaging remarks. Because Tamara Anatolyevna had been conducting research on Tibetan medicine for the better part of the last forty years, and because she had a successful and prolific career as both a biologist focusing on plants used in Tibetan medicine and as a historian and translator of its canonical texts, her statement about the status of Tibetan medicine in Buryatia seemed to me especially poignant—if not outright contradictory. Tibetan medicine, she said, *"yele teplitsia"*: it is barely smoldering. Upon seeing my surprise, she quickly qualified the original statement with a cautiously optimistic interpretation: perhaps, she suggested, the ember is lying dormant, waiting for the historical winds to change and fan the fire.[2]

Articulations of doubt were not isolated incidents or, in the case of the researcher, simply an expression of displeasure at the bureaucratic tedium and low prestige of science and scholarly research in present-day Russia. I occasionally encountered similar questions at Western academic conferences on Tibetan medicine, where I was mostly met with expressions of surprise or, on occasion, deep skepticism. But is it *really* Tibetan medicine? At what point does it stop being Tibetan medicine and becomes something else? How are such cutoff points evaluated? As I sat down with the very diverse experts in Tibetan medicine in Ulan-Ude—Buryats, Tibetans, Russians, practicing in clinics, temples, private offices, or from the kitchens of their apartments, surrounded by jars of ground herbs, Buddhist paintings, and sometimes very obvious signs of financial success in a provincial Siberian city with a sluggish economy, all of them unanimously assured me that "real" practitioners were remarkably few, their number negligible, and the knowledge or practice of the rest was suspect at best. Of course, as I came to know many of these practitioners better, these narratives changed again, and skepticism was replaced by something different. They expressed a pride in their professional undertakings and commitments and of being able to treat patients who had fallen through the cracks of regular state care. They described the pleasure of finding and collecting the right ingredients and making a new batch of medicines, of completing translations of the canonical texts, and they issued cautiously optimistic speculations about the future of Tibetan medicine in the region and the possibilities of expanding and improving their own practice.

Expressions of doubt about the vitality—or, indeed, the *realness*—of Tibetan medical practice in Buryatia go against its widespread, albeit not always visible, presence. Historically, Tibetan medicine flourished in Buryatia's Buddhist temples before the Soviet revolution and continued to exist, with various degrees of visibility, during Soviet times. Tibetan medicine is currently one of the "selling points" of Buryatia's regional image. Buryatia's government officials incorporate it into what is commonly referred to in the local official and media discourses as "Buryatia's brand" in an effort to render the region attractive for investors and tourists. Two private treatment centers, claiming Tibetan medicine as their main therapeutic specialty, opened in 2009, and the East-West Medical Center, officially under the administrative responsibility of Buryatia's Ministry of Health Protection, expanded in 2012, building a brand-new in-patient hospital. Conferences on the "integration of Eastern and Western medicine" regularly take place. A majority of Buddhist temples, and some of the Buddhist communes both within city limits and outside of the city, boasted one or more practicing *emchi*. A network of *chastniki* or private practitioners, largely absent from these more public displays, received and treated patients from their apartments or privately rented offices, touring in Moscow for a portion of the year to supplement their income and sometimes to escape the harsh Siberian winter. The local affiliate of the International Academy of Traditional Tibetan Medicine, with its headquarters in Italy, provided classes for all who were interested, inviting lecturers from Tibet and India, and amassed a large and faithful public despite the steep "Moscow-style" costs of attendance. The market of herbal medicines and biologically active supplements was booming; various herbal concoctions, teas, capsules, tinctures, and powders were bought and sold at official and private pharmacies and through multi-level marketing; and "Tibetan medicine" was frequently mobilized to make these products more appealing to consumers. *Emchi* and other healers regularly gave interviews to the local newspapers and periodicals, provided advice on diet, and suggested simple home remedies for common ailments, explicated certain diseases, or tried to answer the questions of a faithfully reading public.

In 1989, a project initiated by the republic's own Ministry of Health led to the creation of a medical complex—what I refer to in this book as the East-West Medicine Center. Composed of several facilities, including a city in-patient polyclinic, an out-patient hospital, a licensed herbal pharmacy, and a health resort on the shores of Lake Baikal, East-West was known both in Buryatia and in Russia more broadly and successfully expanded its infrastructure, staff, and collaborative projects. Its principal claim to fame was the successful implementation of Tibetan medicine with the full endorsement of Buryatia's Ministry of Health Protection. The irony of its popularity consisted in the fact that the legal structure of Russia's federal medical administration does not recognize Tibetan medicine as an accredited medical specialization. Despite an absence of legal recognition, arguments for the usefulness and necessity of developing Tibetan medicine in the clinic, with an eye to its eventual integration into Russia's official healthcare, have been quite convincing to Russia's federal administration and local investors. In 2006, Buryatia's regional government successfully applied for federal financing to expand the center's infrastructure. The text of the bid, composed by the members of the administration of East-West and Buryatia's Ministry of Health Protection, seamlessly blended a critique of global biomedicine with Russia's struggles with reforming official healthcare, weaving arguments about the multinational "deep" history of the Russian state, the cultural and religious needs of the local ethnic population, the potential for scientific development and research on Tibetan medicine unique to the region, and cosmopolitan claims about Buryatia's geopolitical transnationalism. The federal grant, reported to equal around 324 million rubles (10.5 million dollars at the time), allowed the center to complete its new in-patient hospital facility, purchase equipment, and hire more specialists.

How to evaluate the current public resurgence of Tibetan medicine in Buryatia is a debated point for local scholars, and, as we will see, for practitioners and patients the stakes of these debates are different. Some local researchers actively reject the terminology of revival, insisting on the historical rupture between the late nineteenth-century institutional strength and active development of Tibetan medicine in the temples and monasteries of Buddhist Siberia and the late Soviet and post-Soviet recuperation of it, after many decades of state policies that disparaged the philosophy of Tibetan medicine as reactionary religious dogma and persecuted practitioners. These scholars describe the present phase as one of reform and integration, rather than revival, primarily because, unlike Tibetan medicine in Buryatia at the turn of the twentieth century, they see the present moment as defined by the domination of "modern" medicine (see Dulganov

2009). Others suggest a more continuous tradition, one that had certainly changed and gone underground during the years of early Soviet persecutions against religious practices, but that has survived and adapted to its new conditions (Aseeva 2008), progressively entering the region's scientific and medical mainstream.[3]

Beyond simply a cultural offering of "traditional" therapy that might augment the patchwork of Russia's multiple vision of post-socialist healthcare, Tibetan medicine is also a site of complicated geopolitical claims about the region's cultural, religious, and historical connections to the Russian state and its political neighbors. It is thus possible to interpret the skepticism voiced by my interlocutors as a commentary on the history of Buryatia's relationship with the Russian Empire and its settler colonial expansions in Siberia, and subsequently with Soviet projects of modernization. From this perspective, it is the progressive loss of tradition, political repressions, cultural standardization, the restrictions and state control over Buddhism and its institutions, the destruction of temples and the disruptions of transmission lineages, and the increased difficulty of apprenticing across the border in Mongolia, Tibet, and India during the years of Soviet isolation that come to the forefront. In other words, the suggestion that there is perhaps no "authentic" traditional medical knowledge and practice left, after decades of political upheavals, suppression, and cultural loss, serves as a critique that challenges present-day efforts of medical "integration" and revival as a belated attempt to recuperate a cultural past that is no longer fully retrievable.

Mixing Medicines is about understanding a therapeutic practice at the flickering thresholds of visibility. It asks what it means for certain forms of care to occupy this space at the cusp of uncertainty, in the marginalia of patients' imagined therapeutic itineraries, where the very existence of a culturally marked therapeutic approach is at once validated, commercialized, and put into doubt. The debates over Tibetan medicine in Buryatia patterned into an ontological conundrum that encapsulated broader questions—those of the relationship between Russia and Siberian indigenous minorities, about whose histories count, and about arguments over potency and efficacy writ large: both about what constitutes "medical work" and what might count as a "working medicine." The tensions often remained unresolved for those who made Tibetan medicine their life's calling, their means of economic subsistence (and sometimes flourishing), or their path to physical survival. Doubts persisted—when Tibetan medicine was driven out of public view by the currents of history, it seemed to reemerge in the seams, in informal practices, proliferating all manner of "private" domains. On the (relatively rarer) occasions when it became publicly endorsed, was it *still* medicine, and if so, by whose account?

THE BIOPOLITICS OF INTEGRATIVE MEDICINE

While the concept of medical "integration" is now widely used in Russia to refer to efforts at combining "traditional" and "modern" medicine, the term is a false cognate of what is implied by "integrative medicine" in Euro-American contexts. Research on the popularization of complementary and alternative medicine (CAM) and the rise of so-called "integrative medicine" in the West tends to focus either on the "domestication" of nonbiomedical therapies or on their destabilizing effects on biomedical authority (Baer 2004; Coulter and Willis 2004; Baer and Coulter 2008; Keshet and Popper-Giveon 2013; Broom and Tovey 2007). In the first instance, scholars track how the production and consumption of discourses and practices associated with "wellness" and "holism" are complicit in a biopolitical imaginary that promotes neoliberal models of self-governance and patient responsibility in the management of health (Kaptchuk and Eisenberg 1998; Fries 2008; Nichter and Thompson 2006). Alternatively, the focus is on CAM's transformative potential for a paradigm shift in biomedicine itself and for the possibilities of a more humane medical practice. Within the medical field, "integration" appears to focus on questions of patient-centered, collaborative care, informed by a more personalized view of the body, and treatment focused on improving the quality of life (Ruggie 2004).

In Russia as elsewhere, fugues from biomedical treatment are often framed through the dual specters of desperation and noncompliance. The story is a familiar one. Compromised subjects are suspected of flight toward therapeutic margins, pushed away from standard care by faltering physiologies increasingly impossible to ignore that miss the window of opportunity when established forms of treatment might have been effective, by the complexity of symptoms for which conventional medicine offers no clear promise of a cure, and by an omnivorous consumption of hopeful medical rumors and popular self-help literature and advice that does. In these framings, discontent with or rejection of the therapeutic default propels patients along more and more peripheral medical journeys. Dissatisfied patients wonder—and wander. Sufferers and seekers, even when they are not anyone's "patient" in the proper sense, reject or give up on biomedicine and look for other ways of maintaining the body. Disappointment with or distrust in conventional medical approaches and healthcare systems is assumed to power such departures. These explanatory frameworks account for patients' deviations from the biomedical ordinary through a logic of failure. Physical and emotional suffering are at the center of the physics of such models, and patients' centrifugal trajectories are powered by the self-evident needs of alleviation.

Therapeutic landscapes where biomedicine is taken to be the natural center of gravity of patients' medical lives and all other trajectories lead *away* from this unspoken center also translate easily to audiences in the Global North. Scholarly writings, popular accounts, and policy recommendations that take the patient-consumer as their fulcrum often suggest that patients pursue traditional medicine in one of two cases: out of desperation or because they are a token of a social type, the sort of person who rejects established medical treatments in favor of untested alternatives. In the first instance, these analyses suggest that, in extremis, when the self is in mortal peril, one is liable to become medically omnivorous. Conversely, when such medical fugues are narrated in relation to a priori social taxonomies, they tend to draw on an optic of resistance or rejection. For example, scholars writing about New Age bodily practices in the West, including CAM therapies, frequently point to a syncretic consumerism of culturally "other" epistemologies and aesthetic forms. Even when these are framed, on the surface at least, as a rejection of dominant discourses, such consumption is assumed to be funneled into enhancing quintessentially modern selves, informed by an economic subjecthood (Thrift 2005; Chrysanthou 2002; Fries 2008; Fadlon 2004).

Other scholars have tracked the lines of flight that reach toward the alarming peripheries of medical noncompliance. As with the rejection of pediatric vaccines, therapeutic paths that shirk conventional care are sometimes interpreted as willful, but misguided insubordination to public health recommendations and to conventionally accepted best practices. Public commentators critiquing such medical decisions are quick to point out the class dynamics that inform them: the distrust of experts and expertise attributed to a particular kind of middle-class consumer subject often described as "neoliberal," animated by an orthodoxy of individualistic self-interest and market choice gone wrong (Greenhalgh and Wessely 2004; Sobo 2015). The lure of the therapeutic margin within such centrifugal models is automatically suspect: at best, a desperate groping for a last resort option and, at worst, a site of fatal erring, textured by the lure of healers' personal charisma and persuasion, of commercial hype and publicity, of inauthenticity and ideological deception.

Centrifugal depictions of patients' movement from "centers" into "margins" are not simply a practical problem of the distribution of access to care in medical systems where biomedicine is taken to be the default. They are also a conceptual spatialization for generating specific types of arguments. Medical anthropology offers a rich scholarship that theorizes the final stops, dead ends, and limbos of patients' trajectories. Ethnographies of such spaces show that the end of the line is often a zone of social, political, and medical abandonment or entrapment, where habitual ethical orders are suspended or where they reveal their darker side, ceding way to contradictory entanglements of care and violence, of intensified intervention and neglect (Biehl 2005; Jain 2010; Garcia 2010). In this, they intersect with other biopolitical architectures of exclusion, where the logics of "making live" and "letting die," which Michel Foucault famously attributed to the modern state, begin to collapse into each other or to operate in tandem (Stevenson 2012, 2014).

While this book is attentive to the insights generated by the literature on the failures of care in order to think about the ways in which Russia's medical landscapes were being reimagined in the first decade of the 2000s, my goal is to complicate the often-implicit centrifugal models that describe the relationship between "official" and "unofficial" medicines. To be sure, traditional medicine and other forms of nonbiomedical healing offer terrains from which my interlocutors in Russia articulated critiques of the healthcare system, in no small part because it enabled patients and medical workers alike to vent their grievances and to reframe conventional healthcare as an index of the state's failures in its commitment to the population's health. However, an approach that equates the tail end of exhausted medical options with forms of care variably described as traditional and often associated with specific ethnic, religious, or cultural identities, as well as remote geographies, nestles the centrifugal model of patient circulation and medical decision-making within other kinds of enactments of centers and margins. Center-periphery logics work as normative claims across a variety of political and social domains in Russia, and they are frequently deployed in expert and everyday discourses alike to account for the country's internal layout and position on the world stage. For its part, the Soviet Union itself wrestled, both ideologically and infrastructurally, with a center-periphery model, one that was not simply geographic and infrastructural but also epistemological.[4] Marxist historical materialism and social evolutionism in its Soviet inflection inspired the frequently violent eradication of so-called cultural survivals—including religiously marked forms of healing among non-Russian populations incorporated into the Soviet project of accelerated modernization. In practice, this meant the political repression of practitioners and the destruction of therapeutic infrastructures that departed from the modern aspirations of "rational," state-endorsed medicine. The implied hierarchies of knowledge and expertise left over by these historical legacies texture debates over the role of nonbiomedical care in the present.

My point is that a framework that paints Russia's therapeutic field in terms of inevitable centrifugal flows—from official state-supported but infrastructurally failing biomedicine toward nonbiomedical margins—overshadows other potential conceptualizations. Such explanations often assume discrete steps, stops, phases. They posit in advance what occupies the end of the line—and overdetermine patients' trajectories through their terminality. Even when presented as resistance to often violently dominant paradigms, this kind of analytical cartography still recenters them. The implicit center presupposes a gravitational force—its margins are those spaces where the dissolution of its pull makes other ways of managing bodies possible, but only as a product of weakened bonds. It leaves little room for thinking about the paths it maps "positively"—for viewing them as more than flight from failure or as discontent, but, rather, as a movement *toward* something else. Centrifugal trajectories do not do well with mixtures, epistemological toggles, strategic shifts, wavering commitments, uncertainties, skepticisms, and reimaginings. They offer no lexis for theorizing passions and attachments that do not dictate a priori identities, whether defined through the framework of suffering, of neoliberal choice, or that of preexisting ethnic, religious, or cultural self-identification. They miss open-ended destinations. Other scholars have discussed the ways in which medical legitimacy and authority are precisely what is often at stake in the clinical spaces of post-Soviet medicine (Rivkin-Fish 2005b; Raikhel 2016). In this book, I ask what happens when therapeutic practices embrace epistemological and ontological ambivalence.

But is it *real* medicine?

The goal of this book is to displace the matter of traditional medicine (and medicinal matter) away from a politics of ontological certainty by asking what sorts of objects and actions are centered through different modes of therapeutic attention. In this, I want to sidestep two familiar frames that have often made traditional medicine legible, particularly in times of great social, cultural, and political transformation. The first frame reads medicine through the lens of suffering, broadly defined: in this case, nonbiomedical practices are often made meaningful in their capacity or failure to alleviate physical and emotional woes, individual or collective. Even when we take suffering to be experienced and described in culturally specific ways, a sense of needfulness—of having nowhere else to go—can foreclose the conversation much in the same way as my early inquiries about the place of traditional medicine in Russia. For many of my interlocutors engaged in the work of Tibetan medicine, the prerogative of care was often experienced through the optics of Buddhist ethics. The only correct answer an aspiring student of Tibetan medicine might give to the question of why they wished to embark upon this path, I was told, was to alleviate the suffering of living beings. However, the sorts of bodies and subjects Tibetan medicine in its many forms was asked to treat was also open to interpretation. To be sure, patients who pursued traditional therapies described their discomforts, their struggles, and the frustrations with both personal and systemic challenges to their physical well-being, to their ability to work and care for others, to their senses of self, and to their relationship with the demands of everyday life. But for many, "the end of the line" was a transfer to a different route or just one stop along meandering paths, not a terminus. In the care practices of both Tibetan medicine doctors and patients, the labor of mitigating suffering often extended far beyond the patient's ailing body. This book is thus concerned with the conditions under which the work of Tibetan medicine is done in Buryatia—the legal, practical, and ethical conundrums of making that kind of therapeutic labor possible in present-day Russia. Pulling the focus away from the question of how nonbiomedical healing—in this case, Tibetan medicine and other treatment modalities in conversation with it—works *as* medicine allows me to focus on the many types of labor that make its working possible. The question that seemed to preoccupy many of my interlocutors—*but is it real*—went beyond concerns with efficacy. Instead, it opened up efficacy to other kinds of questions. On whose terms does it work? For whom is it real?

Second, this book asks what sort of analytical purchase does "biopolitics" have in places where "biomedicine" is especially unstable and open to questioning, linked to a sense of contingency in the political and cultural regimes that appear to favor it, and thus becomes less an easily recognizable object than a polemical configuration, while still experienced as a therapeutic necessity? The deployment of traditional medicine in Russia paradoxically hinges on both a utopian optimization of extraordinary vitality—a horizon of health beyond health as we know it—and on an effort to remedy an "extra-ordinary," in the sense of "super ordinary" (Perrow 2011), state of unhealth that is itself attributed to the failures of the state's medical (and, more broadly, biopolitical) management of the population. During my research, practitioners of traditional medicine and patients did not much resist or interrogate the state's unequally distributed efforts to "make live," but rather focused on the degree to which these efforts appeared haphazard, perfunctory, and rarely successful, always on the verge of unpredictably turning into their opposite of "letting die." Instead of a politics of "bare life," the horizons of integrative medicine in Russia seemed more attuned to the problem of barely living. To paraphrase a popular joke I frequently heard during my fieldwork—often a favorite with patients—"our people will live badly, but not for long."

By paying attention to how traditional medical practices in Russia throw into relief officially accepted therapeutic configurations, I take my cue from scholars who question the limits of biopolitics, focusing on interstitial spaces where biomedicine encounters other medical practices and where the stakes of care are not overdetermined by the promissory value and emergent ethics of cutting-edge biotechnologies (Fassin 2009; Marsland and Prince 2012). This book explores the relationship between efforts on the part of states and other entities to manage "life" and individual pursuits of health that make the body proper into a site of self-intervention and manipulation. At the same time, my primary focus is not so much on tracing the implications of unequal access to biomedical treatment or to expose the structural violence of normative biopolitical discourses. My research began with the suspicion that the rising popularity of nonbiomedical practices in Russia might reveal something about the dissolution of the welfare state, about the ways in which medicine was being welded to market logics, and about how experiments with managing individual and collective vitalities might shed light on the epistemological and cosmological grounds on which the governance of bodies and subjects might operate. I follow other researchers who have suggested that health-related strategies and livelihoods provide a productive lens for examining post-socialist transformations (Petryna 2002; Rivkin-Fish 2013; Farquhar 1996; Jašarević 2017). However, attention to the contentious category of "traditional medicine" quickly revealed some of the limits of the analytical frameworks that inform anthropological discussions of therapeutic plurality in Russia and elsewhere. Translational frictions that pointed to deep epistemological uncertainties were there from the very start—my interlocutors and I grappled with linguistic confusions and shifting nomenclatures as we sought to establish the relevant contrast sets. What is typically rendered as "biomedicine" in English-language scholarship had a number of shifting designations in the landscape of post-socialist therapeutic proliferation: official medicine, academic medicine, scientific medicine, and, paradoxically, flipping the relationship entirely, "traditional medicine"—as opposed to "nontraditional" medicine. The "center," if it existed, was always a tenuous proposition. The ironies of these lexical instabilities were not lost on anyone, especially as designations for nonbiomedical healing multiplied in everyday conversations and in legal and professional ones. It seemed impossible to talk about what constitutes "traditional medicine" without also talking about *whose* traditions counted, what counted as tradition, what sorts of subjects ought to practice or use which medicine, and for whose benefit (and on whose behalf) should such therapies be deployed. Projects of integrative medicine promoted by various state actors brought to the fore distinctly political questions—what might medical integration mean in a place like Buryatia, with its histories of the Russian state's expansion into and management of Siberian regions, with collective memories of Soviet ideological control over everyday life, and in relation to present-day debates over regional sovereignty and connections to the metropole? If medical traditions were to be integrated, on whose terms would such integration take place?

It also invited other kinds of questions about both individual and collective bodies. In Russia, medical "integration" does not so much refer to privileging the doctor-patient encounter or reestablishing a socially and ecologically emplaced view of the body elided by contemporary biomedical pursuits and aimed at optimizing what Nicolas Rose has called a biologically defined "life itself" (Rose 2001). The rediscovery of the environmental situatedness of medical subjects and the return to a focus on the ecological and social permeability of life within biomedical science documented by researchers working in Western contexts (see Landecker 2011; Lock et al. 2015; Olson 2010) are not new for post-Soviet medicine. A focus on a body's milieu, broadly defined, is quite prevalent in such medical domains as restorative medicine, which owes much of its intellectual genealogy to Soviet medicine's concerns with "functional health." Encompassing a wide variety of specializations from gerontology to sports to space medicine, restorative medicine in Russia pushes toward incorporating "traditional" therapies, valued for their potential to account for the body's permeability to multiple environmental exposures. In many ways, Soviet modernity (and Soviet medicine and science) focused on the ways in which the living subject, whether human, animal, or botanical, is always overwhelmingly produced through environmental and social forces. The legacies of these preoccupations with bodies in situ within Soviet (and post-socialist) ideologies of health shape the terrains on which the presumed needs of Russia's body politic are tethered to the therapeutic possibilities of nonbiomedical practices in the present. For many of the patients and practitioners I spoke with, post-socialism operated like a preexisting historical condition with no solid treatment plan—it was a visceral affair, one where personal biological time and collective historical processes were not so easily disarticulated because they were always already materialized in enfleshed biographies. As such, the body became a productive site for reflecting on historical and social transformations and one's place in them—on how collective histories worked in and through the body, ailing or recovering. These conversations also troubled center-periphery models that depicted patients' and practitioners' journeys through the familiar optics of centrifugal flight.

As I argue throughout this book, the coherence or incoherence of medical paradigms and therapeutic approaches, as well as their geographic ties and cultural specificity, their translatability or untranslatability, their distances and similarities, their specific ways of understanding the vitalities of bodies (human or otherwise), and their anticipated trajectories, emerged as the result of a great deal of work by a variety of actors—these apprehensions were produced, maintained, and contested in dialogue across professional, disciplinary, and ontological borders. I take the practices and discourses that surround "traditional medicine" in Russia to be always already co-constitutive of what counts as "modern" medicine (or biomedicine) in the first place. In the context of the dramatic post-socialist transformations that overhauled Russia's social and political life, conceptualizing "modernity" and "progress" was often open to interrogation on intimate bodily grounds. In Buryatia in particular, where "Eastern medicine" is not simply an abstract market label but a complicated and deeply situated political claim for making sense of the region's cultural and religious histories, the work of tracing and blurring the internal boundaries of the therapeutic landscape frequently served to express competing politics of encounter between different social and symbolic worlds. By making Tibetan medicine inalienably Buryat, yet key to restoring the health of Russia's body politic, local actors articulated their region's place in space and history and renegotiated the social meaning of how bodies, medicine, and lived worlds are assembled, entangled, and held in place.

PERIPHERAL ATTENTION AS METHOD

Anthropological discussions of medical pluralism have complicated popular descriptions of different medical traditions as self-contained and isolated systems, even though such distinctions are frequently quite important to both local and international institutions engaged in arbitrating a multiple therapeutic field. Anthropologists and historians of medicine have pointed to the ways in which text-based medical epistemologies are constituted historically and socially through practices of borrowing, cross-fertilization, synthesis, and transformation. These critical accounts reject contrast sets that might pin "traditional" medicine against "modern" biomedicine, where the former acquires an aura of timeless immutability, with its implied lack of progress, against the presumed future-oriented dynamism of the latter. They also challenge the supposition that there is something inherently coherent to the therapeutic practices identified as part of a single tradition, suggesting instead that an apprehension of epistemological coherence might just as easily be an epiphenomenon of our own theoretical predilections (see Leslie 1980; Scheid and MacPherson 2011; Scheid 2002; Cohen 1995; Langwick 2008).

For its part, critical medical anthropology reminds us that medicine—and especially Western biomedicine—travels. Biomedicine is as much to be found in the spaces of patient-doctor interaction as it is in the global circulation and local uptake of clinical regimes, disease categories, pharmaceutical products, scientific protocols, and public health initiatives. Scholars have also focused on the ways in which so-called traditional medicines are put into circulation—nationalized as part of a state's official healthcare apparatus and then exported as a national product, aligned with specific political and cultural ideologies, or ushered into global markets of culturally marked therapeutic commodities (Alter 2005; Adams 2003; Farquhar 1994; Langwick 2008; Pordié 2008). Many of these critical accounts call for a greater attention toward the ways in which efforts to align and incorporate traditional therapies with biomedical and scientific regimes disrupt and challenge the rationales and forms of knowledge attributed to Western biomedicine and science (Adams, Murphy, and Clarke 2009).

Building on a body of anthropological theory that has, over the last few decades, privileged questions of circulation and flows, *Mixing Medicines* makes the case that not only does the flux of therapeutic knowledge, practices, and substances require coordinated efforts and labor, but so does making things stand still. At its core, the book tracks the politics and poetics of localization that characterize the incorporation of Tibetan medicine into Russia's therapeutic geographies, both actual and aspirational. In Russia, experiments with integrative approaches to medicine that strive to incorporate biomedicine alongside other culturally marked therapies—and to make them speak to (and past) each other—reframe all ways of being and knowing as always stubbornly rooted *somewhere*. They also invite us to think about how making something rooted in place is an arduous and uncertain process.

As in many other parts of Russia, talking about health, always potentially failing and in need of maintenance or tinkering, was never far from the surface of conversations, both superficial and intimate, professional and casual. In Ulan-Ude, such exchanges produced a collective topography.

Health, as an asymptotic, elusive, always already imperiled state of being, textured a sociality of embedded companion ailments inhabited together but visible only when one was looking for it intently. Traditional medicine in Russia is, at turns, publicly prominent and officially supported or interstitial and shadowed, a capillary permeation that extends past state-recognized institutions and weaves itself through a rich therapeutic terrain of people, places, and things in flux. It is a kind of connective tissue that saturates the mundane practices of care between family members, friends, and neighbors and sutures the sociality of strangers. It is communicable: recipes, advice, medicines, devices, plants, jugs of "medicinal" water, strange minerals of unknown origin, books, newspaper clippings, advertisements, personal stories, names, addresses, and telephone numbers of practitioners incessantly change hands—they are given, copied, saved, transferred to the next person in solicited and unsolicited exchanges, in a staggering circulation of all things medicinal. It is literally and figuratively rhyzomatic: seedlings and tubers of medicinal plants are carefully nurtured, multiplied, and passed along, probiotic cultures with evocative names like "Tibetan mushroom" spread across kitchens, populating pantry spaces with jars of murky liquid. It is a collective pursuit—both a practice of collectivity and of collecting—as people assemble care across therapeutic sites and assemble friends, acquaintances, family members, and strangers as therapeutic co-conspirators.

To engage with traditional medicine in this part of the world requires one to notice the unobtrusive name plaques that identify the potential caregivers and curers; it demands one to follow up on the repeated glance that settles into firmer eye contact in the lead-up to a conversation shared during a long, slow-moving queue. Above all, such pursuits require one to be swept up in the flows of rumor and gossip that many of my interlocutors labeled with the metadiscursive and somewhat ironic term *sarafannoye radio*, or "the sundress radio." Although this book focuses on Tibetan medicine in Buryatia, the optics required to make the complex textures of these practices visible suggest a methodological and conceptual approach that engages peripheral forms of attention. I mean this in a dual sense: on the one hand, as literal attention to margins, peripheries, and to the interstitial spaces between recognizable focal points. On the other hand, as a methodological orientation, it seeks to accommodate the uncertain flickering of something that might vanish through other ways of looking—something that is "barely smoldering" if engaged head-on. Peripheral modes of attention help orient oneself in a therapeutic environment that cuts across and vastly exceeds patients' movements in and out of medical institutions structured by the state's healthcare system or other recognizable sites of formalization. It scrambles any sense of trajectory or the idea that such trajectories are inevitable. It follows, laterally, the therapeutic tactics that bypass or wander past mainstream medical thresholds, find ways around closed doors and the circular traps of bureaucratic inefficiencies, or pick up where one promise of care terminates and another one begins.

My own entry into this local therapeutic field began with medical institutions, and much of the ethnography for this project was done at those sites where I was told to look for Tibetan medicine: at professional conferences on traditional medicine, at the East-West Medical Center, at the Buryat Research Institute, at a university research laboratory that worked on developing computerized pulse diagnosis, at a private Tibetan medicine compound, at temples where practitioners of Tibetan medicine were receiving patients, and in the largely invisible, informal spaces of practitioners' apartments and rented offices. It extended into practices that are not visibly medicinal, like the work of attending to botanical and spiritual beings on which therapy often depends, a labor that is frequently unrecognized and has a complicated relationship with commercialization. Most of the data for this book comes from participant observation and structured and unstructured interviews with patients, medical doctors, administrators, practitioners and their assistants, scientists, and Buddhist lamas at these different sites, carried out between 2006 and 2017.

In addition to these more structured ethnographic pursuits, I was quickly swept up by the therapeutic excesses of everyday life and by the chaotic circulation of patients and practitioners across institutional boundaries I had assumed were more rigid than they were in practice. As an ethnographer, it is impossible not to become incorporated into these flows or to follow them to new therapeutic spaces. They have a life of their own, and to fail to engage with their serendipity is as ethnographically limiting as it is socially vexing. Although I have attempted to discipline these therapeutic excesses, they have shaped both this book's theoretical approaches and the way in which the narrative is structured.

STRUCTURE OF THE BOOK

Mixing Medicines moves between institutional sites where I was told to look for Tibetan medicine, but it also seeks to outline a context sutured together through a complex therapeutic flux. I found Tibetan medicine to be always engaged with its fellow travelers and with the logics that attempted to recruit it or co-opt it. Each chapter details spaces of uneasy encounter between Tibetan medicine and other therapeutic, ecological, and epistemological rationales and commitments, sometimes quickly recognizable as biomedical, but frequently refracted in unfamiliar ways. I focus on spaces where multiple logics of caring and knowing, Tibetan medicine among them, are made to coexist and cohabit, to enter into dialogue, although often in different languages.

The style and structure of the book seek to accommodate and reproduce the alternating senses of dissemination and emplacement that characterize therapeutic life in Buryatia as it is refracted through the practices of Tibetan medicine. The writing seeks to do justice to both forms of ethnographic engagement: to the slow knowledge that comes from sitting in place and to the serendipity of unexpected tangents—and the insights of each mode are dependent on the other. The chapters are structured around two sets of arguments. On the one hand, the book follows the many ways in which Tibetan medicine in Russia has been deployed for thinking about the present and future and how it becomes the site of struggles with its peripheral encompassments, with articulating alternative centers and a competing cosmopolitics that challenges the spatial orderings implicit in the state's imaginaries of incorporation and inclusion. On the other hand, the book explores how a therapeutic life mediated through the practices of traditional medicine(s) is held in place through the densely collective mingling of human and nonhuman worlds—those of doctors and patients, of course, but also of machines, botanicals, minerals, texts, nonhuman others, and intimations of different spaces and times and the ways in which human bodies and subjects are theorized and experienced through the ontological uncertainties of these interstitial encounters.

Chapter 1 situates Tibetan medicine historically in Russia, focusing on its development in Buryatia and the struggles with what was, at different moments, perceived as its "otherness." Following Tibetan medicine from prerevolutionary Russia of the late nineteenth and early twentieth centuries against the theater of the Russian state's political expansion and colonial aspirations, the chapter tracks the role Tibetan medicine has been assigned in relation to Russian and Soviet visions of medical modernization. It focuses on the production of translational gaps that made Tibetan medicine useful for articulating the relationship between knowledge, medicine, and modernity.

Chapter 2 follows up on this history by examining Soviet and present-day Russian scientists' efforts, begun in the 1980s, to rationalize the diagnostic techniques of Buryat-Tibetan medicine by producing a device that would replicate the traditional practitioner's diagnostic palpations of pulses. The chapter follows these specialists' recurrent uncertainties about the kind of data—and the forms of knowledge—the resulting machines generated.

Chapter 3 explores how scientists, medical professionals, and religious figures in Buryatia make claims about the existence of a separate branch of Tibetan medicine, grounded in the region's history, as well as in Buryatia's local scientific and scholarly pursuits. It situates these arguments in relation to efforts on the part of medical institutions, both in Buryatia and in Russia more broadly, to incorporate Tibetan medicine as part of a state-endorsed integrative medicine as well as to weave it into for-profit medical sites. On this terrain of therapeutic incorporation, claims about Buryat-Tibetan medicine interrogate the relationships that characterize the political and geographic imaginaries of the Russian state—and of medical integration itself—by recentering Buryatia as a uniquely cosmopolitan therapeutic geography in its own right.

Chapter 4 follows Tibetan medicine into the clinic. It tracks patients and practitioners' strategies of managing health in a clinical space that offers a mixture of therapeutic interventions and leaves the body radically open-ended. Here, Tibetan medicine is made to align with older rationales of Soviet-era biomedicine about health being the direct condensation of detrimental and beneficial environmental exposures, and the ailing body becomes narrated as an accumulation of collective pathogenic time, which these treatment regimes aim to redress or revert. Tracking how patients and doctors negotiate these sutured therapeutic orientations, this chapter also attends to the toggling between individualized care and apprehensions of embodied collectivity.

Chapter 5 looks at the frictions at the core of projects of medical integration. It follows the ways in which local actors involved with Tibetan medicine both inside the clinic and outside of it regionalize biomedicine as a specific cultural formation, entangled with and therefore inflected by the political and ideological interests of the state. Mobilizing claims to distinct, local biologies, these practitioners suggest that the body implicit in modern medicine is not an adequate baseline for a universal therapeutic practice. In these accounts, Tibetan medicine becomes a more cosmopolitan ground for treatment—and for the possibilities of medical integration— than the one offered by modern biomedicine.

Chapter 6 focuses on the committed entwinements between practitioners of Tibetan medicine in Siberia and the plants they work into medicines. Concerned with plant labor, it follows the cultivation of therapeutic potencies by attending to "plant matters"—both the lively materialities of the different plants necessary for medicine-making and the matter of minding the entanglements of vegetal and human communities and bodies. I suggest that Tibetan medicine, as it is practiced in Buryatia, curates plants' vitalities by cultivating embodied modes of attention to human and nonhuman copresences and histories. In so doing, it makes explicit layered relations between post-socialist deindustrialization, Buddhist cosmologies, ailing human bodies, and vegetal life.

The Conclusion returns to some of the questions the book leaves open-ended. It revisits Tibetan medicine's relationship with post-socialist embodiments, reflecting on the restructuring of bodies and selves in relation to the dramatic social changes of post-socialist reforms. It also returns to the practical contingencies of Tibetan medicine in Russia—its dubious legal status, its entanglements with both medical infrastructures and labor markets, its complicated relationship to the marketization of medical care more generally, and its pharmaceutical contingencies. Finally, it juxtaposes the popularization of esotericism and traditional medicine and its challenges to official histories of Soviet rationalist progress and territorial control with the changes that have affected practitioners and patients after the economic recession hit Russia in 2016.

1

"MAY ALL LIVING BEINGS BENEFIT"

Passions of Translation

"AT FIRST YOU DON'T UNDERSTAND ANYTHING": ENCOUNTERING THE *GYÜSHI*

> The language of Mongol medical literature in general, and that of the *Durben-undusun* (*Gyüshi*) in particular, is so peculiar in its choice of words and the compactness of its expressions, that to read it with due understanding without the guidance and explanations of Mongolian medical specialists is unthinkable not only for a European, but also to a born Mongol or Mongol-Buryat. I was frequently forced, when failing to understand specific passages of this work that contained not actual medical questions, but instructions pertaining to religious teachings and to everyday life, to consult with highly learned Mongols; but they inevitably refused me an explanation, sending me instead to specialized medical practitioners, stating outright that they themselves did not understand this Mongolian language.
>
> —PYOTR POZDNEEV, *MANUAL OF TIBETAN MEDICINE*, 1991 [1908]: II

"Have you read the *Gyüshi*?" It was one of the first questions Tsyrenma, one of the Buryat practitioners of Tibetan medicine I would eventually work with extensively, asked me when I met her in 2006. At the time, she was still employed at the East-West Medical Center—officially, as a *terapevt*, a general practitioner and, less officially, as an *emchi*. Tsyrenma's office at the East-West polyclinic was unremarkably biomedical, a pleasantly airy room, with sparse institutional furniture, located on the second floor of a nineteenth-century merchant's manor in the city center. The building had gone through multiple incarnations before the municipal administration gave it over to East-West in the early 1990s, but in a city where indexing both Buddhist and Buryat aesthetics is a conscious part of cultivating cultural distinctiveness and a strategy that shapes the circuits of capital and establishes political claims about the region, Tsyrenma's workspace seemed subdued. The strongest indication that this was a site where an *emchi* practiced was the smell—the pungent aroma of herbs saturated the room, lingering despite the breeze from the window. Tsyrenma herself wore the obligatory doctor's white coat, and the plaque outside her door described her as a general practitioner, with a small addition of "Tibetan Medicine doctor; phytotherapist" written in tasteful but discreet cursive beneath it. Tsyrenma had just published her own book on the history of Tibetan medicine in Russia, originally her Ph.D. thesis, and our initial encounter was somewhat guarded. I answered her question about the *Gyüshi* in the affirmative: I explained that I read the only copy available at the Buryat National Library in anticipation of our meeting, but this did not allay her doubts. "Which one is that? There are many of them." Tsyrenma wanted to know which of the multiple available Russian translations—the first of them completed over a century ago in 1903—I was invoking.

In practice, reading multiple versions of the same text in translation was more than intellectual thoroughness or a case of scholarly acquisitiveness for my *emchi* interlocutors, Tsyrenma among them. Memorizing the *Gyüshi* by rote in Tibetan is still regarded as one of the basic prerequisites for learning Tibetan medicine in the region for both lay and monastic practitioners, and in a context where not many prospective students start off with a working knowledge of Tibetan that would enable them to read and understand the original text, translations mattered a great deal. Tsyrenma was part of a small cohort of women doctors who had apprenticed with a well-known local Tibetan medicine practitioner in a lineage-based tradition, and his approach to their tutelage was to uphold the classical model of starting with rote memorization. When I asked how this worked, she laughed. "We sat at night and we memorized it, with a dictionary. Of course, at first, you don't understand anything at all."

Translations of the *Gyüshi*, or the Four Medical Tantras—the core treatise of Tibetan medicine thought to be compiled by the Tibetan scholar, physician, and translator Yutog Yonten Gonpo the Younger (1653–1705)—exist in multiple European languages, several of them in Russian.[1] The hard copies of these books were hard to come by and rather expensive. Barring the many digitalized versions one could download from Russian internet sites that stored pirated literature, the physical books figured for my local interlocutors as objects of what I first mistook for a collector's appetite but were, in fact, a much more practical matter: how does one implement in practice something that one encounters in written fragments, across spaces of incommensurability? That sense of uncertainty—"At first, you don't understand anything at all."—lingered. Which translation is better? Whose commentary is trustworthy? Which medicinal formulas are accurate? What sort of person was the translator, and what was his or her relationship to the text, to the practice of Tibetan medicine, and to Buddhism more broadly? How could one be confident of one's (and others') understanding? How might one tell that what one learned is truly Tibetan medicine and not something else entirely? What are the ethics of treating patients if one's knowledge exists at a distance, in the spaces between multiple interpretations and historical occlusions?

In what follows, and in much of this book, I lean heavily on Russian-language scholarship on Tibetan medicine, in part because I want to resist its discursive abstraction into a disembodied medical system and highlight instead the ways in which it is always rooted and dialogical, made to speak to and about concrete, historically situated bodies and systems of knowledge and power. The conundrums faced by many of my interlocutors in Buryatia who are involved with Tibetan medicine is that abstraction itself enacts a form of what linguistic anthropologists Susan Gal and Judith Ervine have called "erasure" (Irvine and Gal 2009)—a homogenization at greater scale that obscures plural specificities, while, in practice, reinscribing a cultural origin story that patterns into a politics of authenticity and derivativeness. In Russia, where the connection between abstraction and the localization of Tibetan medicine is built into the very name of this medical practice, specificity matters—it shapes the claims to cultural distinction, to ecological and political situatedness, to religious connections, and to power differentials writ large. For many practitioners of Tibetan medicine in Buryatia who learn their craft outside of a temple-based education, Tibetan is not their first or even second language, and access to the linguistic, textual, and material resources necessary for becoming an *emchi* is often undertaken against the grain, in the interstices of other, often more pressing commitments: official employment, the necessity to make a living, caring for dependents, and the rhythms and time constraints of everyday life. Outside of a temple-based apprenticeship to become a Buddhist lama, no clear-cut or simple pathway toward acquiring a working knowledge of Tibetan medicine is easily available—and as we will see throughout the book, the institutional spaces for learning and practice are often contested, interstitial, and precarious, always unfolding on shifting terrains. They are also unequally accessible and differentially distributed— immunity from challenges, on institutional, professional, and interpersonal grounds, is often a matter of enframement, of competing social connections and encompassments, ones that reflect and sediment older histories of epistemological inequalities between centers and peripheries.

Paying heed to the ways in which doubt structures the readerly (and writerly) engagements with Tibetan medicine in Buryatia is deliberate. Knowledge produced in this mode loses the authority of a voice from nowhere, but in doing so, it sheds light on the ways in which the history of Tibetan medicine in Buryatia takes root in the present. While this chapter offers a historiography of Tibetan medicine in Russia, it is written from that same space of uncertainty. It emulates and refracts the textual attachments I found among my interlocutors, attachments that reverberate back through time—the carefully gathered written traces of Tibetan medicine were themselves traces of previous passions: those of translators, compilers, researchers, travelers, doctors, and biographers who often wrote as much with official as with personal archives, suffused with the intimacies of kinship.[2]

Moreover, circulated texts and the lives of their authors textured local social worlds. Their dissemination hinged as much on cultivating personal relations as it necessitated gaining access to state resources and research libraries. The readerly and writerly practices that Tibetan medicine inspired, and on which it depended—the collection of documents and books often difficult to find, the circulation of out-of-print editions and newspaper clippings in a choreography of equally reluctant and hopeful exchanges, the gifts of unpublished, typewritten manuscripts and self-published scholarship, and the personal and professional risks of becoming involved with a medical practice that exists at the nebulous fringes between the officially sanctioned and the expressly criminalized materialized trust, care, and an intellectual regard for a type of expertise that seemed, to its practitioners, potentially always incomplete—a vast world glimpsed through a keyhole.

In the field of Tibetan medicine in Buryatia, attention to translational and readerly practice is also attention to relations of power: between competing enactments of expertise, between disparate epistemologies that do not allow for facile equivalences, between those whose voices are enshrined through textual circulation and those that left no written or archival record. These histories do not exist separately from the practices of care writ large: practitioners read scholarly commentaries and original sources, comment on them, and constantly speak back to what remains of that history. The sense of loss, of translational distance, of an archive riddled with occlusions, is palpable.

Translational encounters between Tibetan medicine and Russia's official medical establishment enacted incommensurability and articulated a politics of relation that spoke back to the Russian state's projects of participating in European "modernity," of scientific and medical advancement, population management, and governance. This process was not unilateral: prominent Buryat scholars and practitioners of Tibetan medicine spoke back to Russia's official medical and academic establishments, to state officials, to local and metropolitan publics, and often proposed different visions of best practices and articulated their own version of what should count as science and medicine. Boundaries between different ways of knowing and caring for individual and collective bodies are not predetermined a priori, and that this chapter does not offer a story of metropolitan scientists and doctors encountering indigenous healers only to clash in a choreography of cultural incommensurability and colonial domination, though the long horizon of the Russian Empire's slow, settler-colonial expansion and governance in Siberia, and of the Soviet Union's rapid revolutionary restructuring and violence, is very much in the background of the politics of translation this chapter outlines. By attending to moments of mutual interpretation, friction, and debate between what counted as scientific medicine at any given period and those practices that such delineations came to exclude, it is possible to see the ways in which Russian, and subsequently Soviet, scientific knowledge was produced through what it came to factor out. In so doing, it too was transformed.

ELEMENTAL BODIES

This section highlights the central translational conundrums that both present-day practitioners and past scholars of Tibetan medicine in Russia have faced and negotiated. From the practical standpoint of local *emchi*, the phenomenology of Tibetan medicine does not equate easily with what present-day patients, habituated to biomedical diagnoses, expect from a medical encounter. Scholars and practitioners of Tibetan medicine in Russia usually narrate the body as a system of three "constitutions"—*rlung*, *mkhris*, and *badgan* in transliterated Tibetan (translated as wind, bile, and phlegm). During my research, I heard the Tibetan terms used interchangeably or in combination with their Mongolian equivalents—*chi* (or *khi* in the Buryat pronunciation), *shara*, and *badgan*, were, in turn, frequently rendered in Russian as *veter*, *zhelch'*, and *sliz'* in a practice of contextual double translation.[3] In what follows, I use the Russian and Buryat-language referents interchangeably, depending on the context.

"*Khi*" (or *rLung*), occasionally translated into Russian as gases (Pozdneev 1908), but more commonly as wind, refers broadly to breath, the activity of the nervous system, cognitive and emotional activity, and more generally, to movement in the body, both in terms of internal circulation and external locomotion.

Shara (or *mkhris*), typically rendered as bile, refers to the activity of the digestive and biliary systems responsible for the functioning of the liver, the production of heat in the body, and for the acuity of eyesight, which is closely linked to liver functioning.

Badgan (translated as *sliz'*, which in Russian can mean phlegm, mucous, or slime) is, most immediately, responsible for mucous membranes. More abstractly, it is responsible for the internal integrity, stability, and cohesion of bodily structures and materials, as well as the self-perpetuation of tissues. In terms of the senses, it is primarily linked to the functioning of the kidneys, which, in turn, is linked to the acuity of hearing.

These three constitutions, alternatively translated into Russian as "*nachala*" (beginnings, origins) or "*vinovniki*" (culprits) of physical embodiment, are the resulting expressions of the five primary elements: air (or wind), water, fire, earth, and space. The five primary elements are each responsible for a particular aspect of physiological manifestations. Thus, earth is responsible for stability and solidity; fire is responsible for bodily heat, digestion, and maturation; water is responsible for bodily liquids as well as a more general quality of binding and cohesion; air is responsible for movement; and space is responsible for the internal spaces and cavities of the bodies (Pupyshev 1989, 1992). Subsequently, each primary element, often rendered in the Russian literature with the Sanskrit term *mahabhuta*, is responsible for certain bodily structures and organs, as well as for the senses. Earth is linked to the sense of smell, fire is linked to sight, air is linked to touch, water is responsible for taste, and space is responsible for hearing. According to some sources, space is responsible for a sixth sense— the ability to orient oneself spatially (see P. A. Badmaev 1901). Other sources suggest that the mind is the sixth sense, responsible for recognizing abstract objects (Pupyshev 1992). The three culprits are thus also linked to the five primary elements, in that wind is the manifestation of air, bile is the manifestation of fire, and phlegm the manifestation of a combination between earth and water.

In Russian-language literature concerned with the translation and interpretation of Tibetan and Buryat canonical medical treaties, this bodily phenomenology has to do with the process of digestion, broadly speaking, where food and medicines that pass through the digestive tract undergo complex processes of triage between an "essence" and a "remainder." At each subsequent stage, the essence moves to a different location in the body, where it is once again sorted into "essence" and "remainder" and so on. Disruptions of these processes result in improper separation and therefore the pollution of the essence with the remainder, which then disrupts the subsequent stage and results in illness (Kosoburov 2011). Digestion in this sense is not limited to the activity of the gastrointestinal tract, but, rather, ties together bodily tissues in a constant becoming of mutual derivation and transformation.

A second phenomenological dimension that is important both in the scholarship on Tibetan medicine and, even more so, to clinical practice is the contrast between heat (*zhar* in Russian) and cold (*kholod* in Russian)— and, less explicitly, warmth and coolness. The qualities of the three culprits are, in fact, expressions of these two dimensions in that *shara* (bile) is inherently hot and *badgan* (phlegm) is inherently cold—qualities that directly result from the primary elements these constitutions manifest. Wind tends to be described as "cool," although under certain conditions it might acquire a hot quality. Each of the culprits has five manifestations, each responsible for a particular process of becoming in the body, and in the case of wind, it also has a directionality (in the sense that there might be a wind directed downward or upward). An increase in wind might act upon the two other culprits and thus exacerbate them, increasing either *shara* or *badgan*, and thus bringing them out of balance, which, in turn, causes their pathological expression in the form of illness. In this sense, although illnesses might have an external cause, such as *karma* or interference from nefarious spirits, all pathological bodily processes can still be classified as hot or cold in nature. In the therapeutic practices of *emchi* in Buryatia, a common way of describing these pathological processes is to locate heat or cold in a specific organ—for example, as "cold in the kidneys" or "heat in the lungs." These expressions also tend to be understandable, on the level of a daily bodily phenomenology by patients in Russia, in that a sense of "coldness" easily connects to a vernacular understanding of certain pathological processes linked to excessive cooling (Rus. *pereokhlazhdenie*), in the same way that heat can be easily identified as an inflammatory process. I do not mean to suggest here that the vernacular use of "heat" and "cold" in the etiology of banal, everyday illnesses is motivated by the same logic as heat and cold in Tibetan medicine, but, rather, to summarize how practitioners of Tibetan medicine in Buryatia translate what they do to patients (and the occasional ethnographer), what they choose to emphasize, and what they choose to omit. The emphasis on these two dimensions of heat and cold in the therapeutic practices of Tibetan medicine in Russia makes it familiar for patients. This familiarity is partially mediated by a genre of popular self-help literature in Russia, which has incorporated Tibetan medicine into a practice of DIY self-healing and wellness, one that reinterprets processual bodily concepts as a rigid physiological and psychological typology. Because this literature dispenses practical self-diagnostic and lifestyle advice on how to manage a "windy" constitution or an excessively "phlegmy" nature, it tends to be quite popular with patients (cf. Choyzhinimaeva 2010a, 2010b; Sidorov 2008; Vostkokov 1998).

Buddhist philosophical concepts underpinning the practice of Tibetan medicine were not always verbalized during therapeutic encounters. To be sure, considerations for the interconnectedness and phenomenological scaling of cosmic phenomena, embodiment one among them, matter for practitioners who need to know the principles of assembling medicines, devising long-term treatment plans, and adjusting medication depending on the patient's reaction. However, the majority of practitioners I had contact with tended to translate their diagnosis back to the patient into a familiar biomedical terminology, and unless the patient showed a keen interest in Tibetan medicine, they left it at that. While this practice of reverse translation has implications for the institutional deployment of Tibetan medicine, making it only partially and unevenly visible in medical practice, this is not necessarily a reflection of how much practitioners rely on Tibetan medicine logics for therapeutic work. To return to Tsyrenma, who flawlessly code-switched between biomedical and Buddhist idioms depending on her patient, linguistic usage is not always a reflection of epistemological commitments. When I asked her how much she still relied on biomedicine to establish a diagnosis and devise a treatment plan, she laughed with a dismissive wave of her hand. "I forgot most of it [biomedicine] by now."

As we will see, the history of Tibetan medicine in Russia is marked by efforts to make it "make sense" to European audiences and is centered on translational practices that would make it converse with Western medical knowledge—at different moments, with anatomy, physiology, endocrinology, pharmacology, epidemiology, and microbiology, depending on what was at the forefront of the authoritative medical mainstream of the time. At other moments, like in the Soviet 1980s and early 1990s, concepts taken from physics and cybernetics were mobilized to decipher the epistemology of Tibetan medicine. The legacy of these engagements, where Tibetan medicine captured the cryptographic ambitions of Soviet and Russian scientists, is still relevant to its contemporary practice in Buryatia, and many of the projects of studying it are expressed in the language of "deciphering" and code breaking as a particular kind of translational orientation.

While a focus on the materiality and the social biographies of textual artifacts runs through the different historical periods this chapter outlines, the periodization itself focuses on the public visibility of Tibetan medicine in Russia with an eye to how its incorporations and exclusions have been mediated. In this sense, the history of Tibetan medicine in the region is one of uneven and interrupted projects of translational institutionalization, both within the medical sphere and outside it. After a brief history of Buddhist expansion into the Transbaikal region, I begin with prerevolutionary Russia at the end of the nineteenth and beginning of the twentieth centuries, examining efforts made by practitioners and scholars to introduce Tibetan medicine to a European audience and the epistemological and social tensions that emerged at the sutures of these encounters. At the turn of the twentieth century, Buryatia became an important geopolitical player in the Russian Empire's efforts to extend its influence into Asia—specifically, into Tibet and India—and to carve out a place in the theater of Europe's colonial expansions. Tibetan medicine was an integral part of this process as it encountered the Russian state's efforts to simultaneously formulate policies toward the empire's indigenous subjects while modernizing the medical delivery system in territories considered peripheral. I then examine the debates about Tibetan medicine under state socialism, from early attempts in the 1920s to make it commensurable with the pharmacological interests of the Soviet state, to its relative disappearance from public view from the late 1930s to the late 1960s, to its reemergence as an object of scholarly interest and often secret professional passion in the 1970s and 1980s. Finally, by the 1990s, Tibetan medicine became the object of political conflict in Buryatia, bringing to light struggles over religious and cultural patrimony, custodianship, and regional distinction.

MEDICINE AND EMPIRE

The Transbaikal territories, which include the administrative region presently known as Republic Buryatia, were incorporated into the Russian Empire following a series of treaties beginning in the second half of the seventeenth century. Scholars typically consider the formation of the Buryat people as a distinct ethnic community of Northern Mongol clans to have taken place in the context of the Russian state's delineation of the border with the Great Qing, though local scholars debate whether ethnic identity among the Buryat should be viewed through the optics of migration or autochthony (Dagbaev 2010). Buddhism is thought to have arrived in Siberia at around the same period: radiating from the religious and cultural centers of the Manchu Empire, the Gelugpa school of Tibetan Buddhism is thought to have been propagated by itinerant lamas who ventured north, moving along well-established pilgrimage routes across what only subsequently became rigorously policed polities. Throughout the eighteenth century, increasing tensions between the Russian and Manchu governments led to stricter control over the Russo-Mongolian border. By the

1740s, the Russian state's previous laissez-faire attitude toward Buryat religious life was replaced by efforts to regulate and institutionalize the Buddhist church within the confines of the imperial administration, sequestering it from foreign influences. The imperial decree thought to mark this separation was reportedly issued in 1741 by Empress Elizaveta Petrovna, officially recognizing the "Lamaist faith" (Alov and Vladimirov 1996), which exempted lamas from taxes and ensured freedom of confession for the Buryat population—or, at least, freedom from coerced conversion to Russian Orthodoxy. Buryat scholar Nikolai Tsyrempilov also notes that it set quotas on the number of Buddhist lamas and forbade contact with foreign clergy under the penalty of death (Tsyrempilov 2012, 247), though Buryatia's ties with the rest of the Buddhist world were never fully severed (Bernstein 2013). Buryat historians of medicine have suggested that the Buddhist lamas who introduced Buddhism to the Transbaikal region also provided medical care to the local population who had little access to other forms of healthcare (see Abaeva 1998; Ayusheeva 2007). However, tightening border control had a practical impact on the processes of institutionalization of Tibetan medicine, disrupting the access Buryat scholars and religious aspirants might have had to the medical schools in the Buddhist monasteries of Tibet and Mongolia (Aseeva 2008, 33).

Prior to the nineteenth century, no unifying official state policy regulated the relationship between ethnically Russian settlers and indigenous Siberians. The first official state decree concerning Russia's indigenous populations was the "Act of Governing Minority Populations," drafted and introduced in 1822 by Mikhail Speranskii, a prominent lawmaker and political figure in the administrations of Tsar Alexander I and, subsequently, Tsar Nikolai I. The Speranskii Treaty was part of a broader effort to reform the management of Russia's Siberian regions. It prescribed free trade and the freedom of confession for indigenous Siberians and subdivided all indigenous populations into three subtypes based on a lifestyle typology that categorized different groups into "sedentary," "nomadic," and "roaming" populations, mapping them against the preexisting system of estates (Rus. *soslovie*), which underpinned Russia's social organization.[4] Under this framework, Buryats were considered nomadic and were incorporated into the imperial administration of Russia's eastern territories via a system of nested self-governing units aggregated into Steppe Dumas.

The image of Siberia in the imagination of western Russia was itself subject to change—from the optics of a colonial frontier styled after Western European colonial expansions to more ambiguous and critical symbolic geographies of national self-fashioning emerging in the nineteenth century.[5] Throughout the eighteenth and nineteenth centuries, medicine, and in particular the management of epidemiological threats, was an integral concern to the broader project of state building and governance in the Russian Empire's eastern settler-colonial frontier, especially after the abolition of serfdom in 1861 brought in an influx of peasants from western regions into southeastern Siberia, leading to conflicts over land tenure and increased contact between settlers and local Siberian groups. Steppe Dumas, the main governing bodies of the Buryat people, were informed of infectious disease outbreaks, some of which were endemic to the region, and some of which had traveled along trade routes with China, India, and the Middle East. Records of plague, smallpox, syphilis, and dysentery among both ethnically Russian and indigenous Siberian populations date back to the 1700s (Bashkuev 2016). However, while occasional compulsory vaccination campaigns among autochthonous Siberians, in particular vaccinations against smallpox, were sporadically mandated by tsarist decree, by the time of the Speranskii Treaty, the policy of noninterventionism regarding indigenous Siberians living close to the border with Mongolia also meant that Buryats largely fell out of the state system of healthcare provisioning, mostly by omission. Buryat scholars note that the limitation on Russian administrators' travel into Buryat settlements, posited by the Speranskii Act of 1822, meant that Buryats did not have recourse to the emergent medical infrastructure available in ethnically Russian settlements (Bashkuev 2016, 136), turning instead to shamans and Buddhist lamas practicing Tibetan medicine. According to local scholars, *emchi*-lamas did not solely provide medical help to their Buryat coreligionists, but they were also receiving patients from among the Old Believer communities, who had fled to Siberia following Patriarch Nikon's religious reforms, which precipitated the schism of the Russian Orthodox Church in 1653. According to records from the late eighteenth century, Old Believers refused medical care from physicians trained in European medicine (Gordeeva 2013, 325), though they did not object to seeking care from Buryat and Mongol *emchi*, largely because plant-based medicine was considered religiously acceptable.

European travelers in the eighteenth century took notice of Tibetan medicine. German explorer, chemist, and botanist Johann Friedrich Gmelin is often credited with introducing the Tibetan medicine of Transbaikalia to a European scholarly public. He wrote in his diaries about his encounters with Tibetan medicine during his travels in southeastern Siberia (1733–43), when he took part in the Second Kamchatka Expedition, a massive state-sponsored undertaking headed by Jonassen Bering and aimed at exploring the potential connection between Asia and the Americas (Sokoloff et al. 2002). In addition to compiling a herbarium for the St. Petersburg Academy of Sciences botanical gardens, Gmelin published a monograph on Siberian flora, later used by Linnaeus in his work on plant classification. In his travelogue, Gmelin recounted an encounter with a Buddhist lama who impressed him with his ability to treat eye diseases and with the ways in which he processed metals for medicine-making (Gordeeva 2013). But a more focused concern with Tibetan medicine on the part of Russia's political apparatus emerged by the late nineteenth century, when Buryatia became an important geopolitical player in the Russian Empire's ambitions to expand its influence in Asia.

By the second half of the nineteenth century, the number of lamas and *datsan* (Buddhist temples) in Buryatia had grown rapidly. The creation of specialized *manbo-datsan* (medical schools) within larger temple complexes also enabled the further training of *emchi* lamas. Medical knowledge was not only transmitted in the institutional context of temples; it often took the form of discipleships, in which secret instructions and commentaries were passed on from a prominent practitioner exclusively to one particularly worthy student (Ayusheeva 2007). The development and institutionalization of Tibetan medicine in the Buddhist temples of the Transbaikal region are thought to have begun in earnest in the second half of the nineteenth century. Much of the work undertaken in Buddhist *datsan* was archival in nature, focused on translating Tibetan and Mongol canonical texts and their commentaries, explanations, and illustrations into Buryat, as well as compiling formularies that developed local substitutions of the original medical formulas in order to deploy local flora instead of the often tropical or subtropical *materia medica* only available through trade with India, China, and Tibet. Some sources suggest that by the end of the nineteenth century, a total of 700 lamas practiced Tibetan medicine, a number that would grow into the thousands by the beginning of the First World War (Zhamsuev and Banchinova 2008, 185).

In the Transbaikal region, the problem of what to do with Tibetan medicine became an important political question for the imperial administration. By the mid-nineteenth century, efforts to institutionalize Tibetan medicine as an integral part of *datsan* education had begun in the area's largest temples. Local monasteries were engaged in active translational work of the canon of Tibetan medicine, adapting Tibetan religious treatises into Mongolian. According to D. B. Dashiev, himself a later translator of the *Gyüshi* into Russian, the Aginsk Buddhist Monastery produced a Mongolian version of the treatise under the supervision of the lama G. J. Dylgyrov in the 1860s (Dashiev 2009). In 1869, Galsan-Zhumba Tuguldurov (?–1873), himself a practitioner of Tibetan medicine, invited Choy Maramba, an accomplished *emchi* teacher originally from Mongolia, to help found a school of Tibetan medicine at the Tsugol' Buddhist *datsan* (Aseeva 2008). Prior to this, Tuguldurov headed the Aginsky *datsan* for ten years and authored a Tibeto-Mongol medical dictionary.[6]

In 1905, after the administration of Emperor Nikolai II passed a decree granting the freedom of confession among Russia's various non-Christian subjects, the question of what should be done about Tibetan medicine in traditionally Buddhist regions percolated up the institutional ladder following Buryat and Kalmyk representatives' request to institute this medical practice officially as part of local monastic schooling. Russia's Medical Council, the highest professional organization dealing with legislation of medical activity at the time, had to decide whether Tibetan medicine should be legalized among those indigenous populations who already used it. The council decided against legalization, but also against outlawing it, suggesting instead that official state policy should promote the modernization of medical provisioning among the empire's ethnic and religious minorities (Grekova 1998).

Interest in Buddhism was also rising among Russia's metropolitan academic elites throughout the nineteenth century, hand in hand with scholarship on the Russian Empire's "Asian" territories. Buddhist studies as an academic discipline emerged in Russia at the beginning of the nineteenth century, first in Kazan University and subsequently relocating to St. Petersburg as part of the Oriental Studies Institute. Russia's "Orientologists" (Rus. *vostokovedy*) were a network of often socially prominent scholar-activists and political figures. Since studying the "Orient" was inseparable from political interest in it, these scholar-activists saw themselves as contributing to and setting up an ideological platform for Russia's organic spiritual expansion into Asia, which they contrasted with the forceful military invasions attributed to British strategists in the context of the "Great Game" (Snelling 1993). Prominent Buryat religious and political figures, such as Agvan Dorzhiev, who had served as the Thirteenth Dalai Lama's personal adviser, were invited to St. Petersburg. There, under the patronage of the Orientologist lobby, Dorzhiev promoted the construction of the first Buddhist temple in Russia's "Northern capital."[7]

THE POLITICS OF TRANSLATION

In what follows, I consider debates around the nature of Tibetan medicine through a focus on the two most popular translations of the *Gyüshi*—Pyotr Badmaev's interpretive effort to create a dialogical foundation that could unite Tibetan medicine and European medicine (1903), and Aleksei Pozdneev's philological study and translation of the same original text (1908). I discuss these two texts because, on the one hand, they are fundamental to the history of Tibetan medicine in Russia and, on the other, because they remain to this day essential to the reading practices of many practitioners in Buryatia. It should be noted that the two translators—Badmaev and Pozdneev—had very different professional agendas.[8]

By the turn of the twentieth century, and along with Buddhism itself, Tibetan medicine caught the attention of Russia's political elite. Sultim Badma (later baptized Aleksandr Badmaev), a Buryat from the Chita region, practitioner of Tibetan medicine, and the senior lama of the Aginsk Steppe Duma, was invited to St. Petersburg and opened a Tibetan medicine pharmacy and clinic after successfully stopping an epidemic of typhoid fever raging through the Transbaikal region. According to one of his biographers, it was precisely Badmaev's ability to address those matters of medical concern for the state administration—namely, the spread of epidemics—that attracted the attention of the governor of Siberia, N. N. Muravyev-Amurski, who supported Badmaev in obtaining a medical license (Arkhangelsky 1998). In St. Petersburg, Badmaev undertook a three-month internship at a military hospital and passed his medical exams in order to bring his medical activities in line with official regulation of medical practice, receiving the diploma of a military medical assistant. Subsequently, in 1871, he encouraged his younger brother, Zhamsaran, who later converted to Russian Orthodoxy and was baptized Pyotr Aleksandrovich Badmaev, to join him in St. Petersburg and help him with running his clinical practice and pharmacy. Pyotr Badmaev married into a Russian aristocratic family and became a prominent, if controversial figure among St. Petersburg's political and social elite. He treated a number of well-connected patients, securing patronage and support (Saxer 2004), while becoming imbricated with the Russian court and, later, vilified over accusations of his association with Rasputin. He also served as a political adviser to the monarch on matters of the Russian Empire's relations with China and Mongolia and undertook scholarly work, completing a translation of the *Gyüshi* into Russian that is still in circulation among practicing *emchi* in Buryatia.

Writing about the process of translational "othering," Walter Benjamin argues that the translator's task is to retain the "echo" of the intent of the original language within the structures of the target language (Benjamin 1997, 159), thus producing a text that frustrates the linguistic expectations of the translation's audience. At first glance, Badmaev's translation of the *Gyüshi* begins with an opposite effort—to make the (admittedly) unfamiliar conceptual language of Tibetan medicine recognizable to a European audience by substituting the Tibetan or Mongolian referents for its principal concepts not simply with Russian linguistic equivalents, but with an explanation of how they might fit into a European understanding of the body. However, Badmaev's text is simultaneously doing something else: in its meticulous usage of the medical terms of what Badmaev understands to be conceptually compatible with European medicine, sometimes to the point of absurdity, his version of the *Gyüshi* works to defamiliarize the particular epistemic commitments of nineteenth-century medicine in Russia. The impression of conceptual unwieldiness of Badmaev's lexical choices reflects a careful avoidance of an anatomical, static view of the body.

Insofar as the circulation of discourses and ideas is always mediated through the possibilities of both linguistic and conceptual recontextualization (Gal 2003; Hrycak 2006; Venuti 2000), it is possible to understand Badmaev's Russian-language version of the *Gyüshi* as an effort to make the concepts of Tibetan medicine simultaneously familiar to, yet on some fundamental level incommensurable with, those of European biomedical discourse. Roger Hart's discussion of the collapse of linguistic and cultural difference in the case of seventeenth-century translations of Chinese texts and concepts by European missionaries might be helpful in this respect (Hart 1999). Addressing the question of incommensurability, Hart notes that the extent of "othering" or distancing present in the act of translation is enmeshed in ideological frameworks, which themselves are interlinked with and inflected by concrete social relations of power. The distancing produced through translational projects creates a sense of conceptual incommensurability, projecting it onto the language itself, while simultaneously deriving confirmation from the evidence thereby found for the seeming incompatibility of cultural forms. Badmaev worked to conserve some of the epistemological moves that distinguish Tibetan medicine from European medical epistemology precisely because his goal was to change the premises of European medicine from within. In combination with his penchant for a trenchantly sarcastic writing style, this orientation likely worked to antagonize some of his colleagues.

Much of Badmaev's efforts to advocate for Tibetan medicine center on critiquing his contemporaries' focus on germ theory and infectious diseases. On this topic, Badmaev offers a mordantly ironic description of European medicine's epidemiological focus:

> One should not imagine that, according to the teachings of the Tibetan science of healing, medicines constitute some kind of special substance, that, no sooner is it introduced into the organism, can immediately cure a deregulation of nourishment in the organism, i.e., illness. Representatives of European medicine are still in search of some kind of specific [element], capable of immediately changing a pathological process in the organism. According to enlightened European medical authorities, all pathological phenomena can be reduced to the appearance of disease-inducing microorganisms within the organism. [Some] of these microorganisms are already discovered and studied, and some of these specially processed microorganisms can be introduced into a healthy body to prevent its future illnesses. According to this theory, if we ever find all the microorganisms for every single kind of pathological bodily phenomenon, and introduce them all at once into the body, then our goal will be achieved, i.e., the organism will have reached a state of

complete imperviousness to illnesses for which these microorganisms are responsible. (Badmaev, Gusev, and Grekova 1991, 37)

What follows is an explanation of the ways in which Tibetan medicine encourages a contextual and processual view of pathogenic etiology, suggesting that the proper functioning and flow of the three constitutions make the body less susceptible to "colonization" by foreign microorganisms. Badmaev deploys a militarized immunity metaphor to explain why, according to Tibetan medicine, disease-causing agents do not provide a sufficient explanation for the phenomenology and causality of illness:

> The living organism is a colony of microorganisms of different nationalities, all connected through independent purposeful activity directed toward self-preservation. If one suddenly introduces into this colony an unknown and entirely different colony of microorganisms, it might strike a significant blow against the microorganisms of the organism. As a result of this sudden event, the microorganisms of the organism will be unable to sustain their fight against these invaders and might die, which results in the death of the organism. (Badmaev, Gusev, and Grekova 1991, 38)

Badmaev rejects the link between specific biomedical manifestations of illness and particular medicinal substances. Food and medicine, he conjectures, are not qualitatively different, and both act upon the functioning of the three constitutions central to how Tibetan medicine views the materiality of human bodies. As a result, to search for the medicinal essence of plant and food substances is to misunderstand the complex flows of absorption and transformation that allow the body to maintain itself. To consider medicinal substances as belonging to a fundamentally separate category of efficacies from lifestyle, food, and the daily embodied habits of thought and emotions is thus to misunderstand the body's phenomenology (Badmaev, Gusev, and Grekova 1991, 38). A search for what he calls the "specificities" (*spetzifikum*) of medicines to match them to particular disease categories is, according to Badmaev, a profoundly unscientific exercise (Badmaev, Gusev, and Grekova 1991, 39).

As we have already seen, the fears of epidemics coming from the "foreign" East were central to Russia's administrative and public health efforts at the peripheries of the empire, and arguments about the danger of foreign invaders to individual and collective bodies relied on collapsing bacterio-logical and xenophobic tropes (Saxer 2004, 41). In this sense, Badmaev's descriptions of a harmoniously functioning collectivity of "multinational" microorganisms can be read as an argument about the (political) health of the nation, at the same time that it strives to amend a European approach to an ailing body. According to Badmaev's grandson and writer Boris Gusev, attacks against Pyotr Badmaev and his translation were mostly perpetrated by surgeons, who accused him of offering treatment to patients with cancer who subsequently missed the crucial window for a timely operation, and on the part of pharmacists, who faulted him for stealing their clients and for using "poisons" in his practice (Badmaev, Gusev, and Grekova 1991, iv). Badmaev's detractors critiqued him for both his activi-ties as a physician and for his assembling and prescribing of herbal-based formulas of his own making. On both accounts, the popular press and important public figures in the medical profession emphasized that thera-peutic and pharmaceutical activity could not be undertaken by an unli-censed practitioner who might be using harmful or toxic ingredients or composing his pharmacopeia on principles that, as Grekova cites, are "patently absurd, of which it is repulsive to even talk" (Grekova 1998). Repulsive or not, the mediation of Badmaev's therapeutic efforts in the press was itself a source of alarm: some of the authors worried that, whether vilified or vehemently defended in printed discourse, Badamev's already considerable popularity was benefiting from free advertisement.

In a brochure published in 1911, called "Response to the Unconvincing Attacks by the Members of the Medical Council against the Medical Sci-ence of Tibet" (Badmaev [1911], cited in Badmaev, Gusev, and Grekova 1991), Badmaev attempted to rebut some of his critics and convince the medical community to seriously consider both the theory and the practice of Tibetan medicine on the basis of his own therapeutic success in St. Petersburg. The brochure is a condensed explanation of the diagnostic and treatment principles, the distinctions in disease etiology in "European" and "Tibetan" medicines, and a series of case studies that illustrate the successful treatment of patients when "European" medicine has failed to either correctly diagnose patients or to alleviate their suffering. Despite its conversational tone, Badmaev's answer is careful to address those matters important to European medicine. Thus, the case studies that he recruits as evidence focus on what Badmaev identified as a series of incorrect diagnoses followed by the dismissal of the patient, resulting in his or her needless suffering. He begins by listing a series of fallacious tuberculosis diagnoses on the part of European practitioners, where symptoms like fever, loss of appetite, coughing, blood in the phlegm, and "hysteria" are in fact signs of a number of interrelated conditions that appear isomorphic to tuberculosis at the moment of the doctor-patient encounter, but do not, in fact, stem from the infection. As we will see in Chapter 2, this concern with the isomorphism of diagnostic categories in European medicine still reverberates through present-day discourses on how Tibetan medicine is ascribed value.

After listing a number of misdiagnosed cases that he successfully treated, Badmaev moves on to improperly diagnosed syphilis, improperly diagnosed cancer, and cases of paralysis that European practitioners had written off as hopeless. In fact, this is the overarching theme of Badmaev's rebuttal: in all the cases he lists, it is not so much "European medicine" that fails, but European doctors who give up on the suffering patient, too intent on the likely correctness of their (predictable) diagnostic categories (like tuberculosis and syphilis) and too preoccupied with their epistemological commitments to the latest scientific fad to act through an ethics that privileges healing over professional posturing—to look deeper. By explaining how he was successfully able to identify and address cases where European physicians were blindsided by the epistemic practices of European clinical medicine, Badmaev is constructing an account of himself as a talented and attentive clinician, one who uses deductive methods in conjunction with his knowledge of Tibetan medicine to correctly diagnose and treat his patients. In other words, for Badmaev the epistemology of Tibetan medicine—its take on the body, its disease categories, and its pharmaceutical arsenal—enable him to recuperate patients that have fallen through the cracks of European practitioners' "business as usual."

I understand this move as an effort on Badmaev's part to challenge an assumed relationship between scientific and clinical practice, countering his critics' insistence that before—and whether—Tibetan medicine can be deployed clinically, its efficacy must be thoroughly investigated through experimental methods outside the clinic. In Badmaev's account, his clinical success provides sufficient evidence for the necessity of incorporating Tibetan medicine into European medical science. But more importantly, Badmaev is also insisting on ethical praxis as the core of any medicine, a space capable of supplying its own metrics of efficacy outside of the laboratory.

Badmaev concludes the pamphlet on an ironic note, which in fact highlights the isomorphism between the hegemony of European science and of European colonial ambitions:

> I fully acknowledge that this [Tibetan] medical science will become the whole world's asset only when talented European specialists will begin to study it. In addition to knowing languages in which it is presented, it is necessary to explore everything oneself, to be a dedicated physician and to know well both the European and the Tibetan medical systems. Unfortunately, European learned physicians are too busy each one in his specialty to really devote time to studying the Tibetan science of healing. Besides, it is hard to study an unknown subject, to seek a truth elaborated and put to words somewhere over there, in far-flung Asia, in languages few understand (Badmaev [1903] 1991, 34).

Pyotr Badmaev's commercial success and wide popularity with patients, his proximity to the court, his political activities in Buryatia, and, notably, his sustained written petitions to the emperor to uphold the treaties that secured Buryats's land rights, his criticism of the local administration in the Far East for corruption, and his efforts to secure the building of a railroad through the Transbaikal region made him the target of ire on the part of Transbaikalia's gubernatorial administration. Between 1986 and 1899, the governor of the Transbaikal region Sergei Dukhovsky wrote a volley of complaint letters to the minister of Internal Affairs Ivan Goremykin, accusing Badmaev of rudeness, profligate expenditure, and of fomenting interethnic conflict. At the heart of the complaints was a struggle over land tenure. Duhkovsky worried that a local newspaper, printed in both Russian and Mongolian script and distributed through Pyotr Badmaev's trading house in the Transbaikalia, would, in Dukhovksy's words, lead "the dark masses of the *inorodtsy*[9] . . . to develop unfounded ideas about their rights, and to an expectation of their prompt realization that, in the event that the land question will be resolved not in accordance with their expectations, might lead to unrest among the Buryat" (Dukhovsky 1896). Goremykin, for his part, attempted to defuse the matter, suggesting that Badmaev's activities in the region were crucial to the interests of the crown, and urged the local governor to refrain from interfering (Goremykin 1897).

Tensions between the "scientific" potential of Tibetan medicine and its "religious" content provided fodder for critiques on the part of the professional medical community in St. Petersburg and motivated efforts to dismiss Tibetan medical knowledge—and Badmaev's clinical practice—as little more than an elaborate profit-driven scheme to fool the population. Similarly, the cultural and ethnic markedness of Tibetan medicine made it vulnerable to a colonial discourse on the "backwardness" of the non-European subjects of the Russian Empire. During the last decade of the 1800s, Badmaev's medical activities became a focus of newspaper polemics. Anthropologist Martin Saxer has argued that in the scholarly atmosphere of nineteenth-century Russia, biomedicine had not yet acquired the kind of hegemonic power that would eventually result in a self-evident rejection of Tibetan medicine as unscientific (Saxer 2004, 17). Pyotr Badmaev undertook efforts to promote Tibetan medicine as a scientific form of knowledge of interest to European scholarly audiences and to make its canon available for those unable to read the original texts in Tibetan, which caused a backlash on the part of St. Petersburg's professional medical community. The polemics that erupted around Badmaev and his practice were a struggle over epistemic legitimacy and over what should count as acceptable scientific evidence. Many of these debates had a tautological quality, and a different set of standards was applied to Badmaev and to the practices of his European medicine colleagues. Badmaev's contemporaries questioned the medicinal qualities and content of the formulas he prescribed as well as the integrity of Badmaev himself. A number of St. Petersburg journalists visited Badmaev's practice undercover, masquerading as patients, and wrote derogatory exposés regarding the long queues, the unorthodox examination methods, and the mysterious substances he dispensed. Many of these attacks betrayed profound political anxieties over the Russian Empire's "Europeanness," and with it, its status on the world stage. While some commentaries centered on what should count as proper "science," others used racialized language to dismiss Tibetan medicine outright: "It is entirely possible that the 'Tibetan plant powders' work very well for thick-skinned Mongols and others who believe in the Dalai Lama, but for us, who consider ourselves a cultured nation, it is embarrassing to use the medicine of Asian savages," one such account scoffed (Grekova 1998, 73). Lawsuits against Badmaev, who practiced privately and thus did not have the institutional backing of a medical organization, were publicized in newspapers. Badmaev himself used the press to refute these accusations, unleashing scathing critiques against Russia's medical establishment and medicine-as-usual, citing his successes in curing patients deemed hopeless by the conventional medical mainstream of the time. In response, medical professionals objected that clinical therapeutic success could not serve as a reliable indicator of a medical system's efficacy (Grekova 1998, 71), while individual failures to cure were taken as evidence of Tibetan medicine's ineffectiveness in general, and of Badmaev's questionable ethics in particular.

While Badmaev's *Gyüshi* precipitated a volley of popular and professional debates about the value of Tibetan medicine to Russia's medical publics, Aleksei Pozdneev's version had an entirely different social trajectory and ultimately outlined a space in which Tibetan medicine's encounters with Russia's scientific establishment did not cause the same kinds of controversies.[10] Unlike Badmaev, a physician with a thriving practice who advocated for the official recognition and scientific study of Tibetan medicine, Pozdneev was an ethnographer and orientologist with scholarly interests in Mongolia, and his discussions centered on culture, philology, and the technical aspects of the text and certainly not on the popularization or defense of Tibetan medicine itself. In many ways, their goals and their anticipated audiences were orthogonal: while Badmaev was actively seeking often provocative dialogue with physicians trained in what he called "European medicine," Pozdneev's goal of putting the *Gyüshi* into circulation was self-avowedly scholarly, and he actively distanced himself from being seen as an advocate of Tibetan medicine.

Pozdneev never aimed his translation at the general readerly public, nor at medical professionals, and not even at a narrow circle of his academic colleagues. In his introduction to the translated text, he explained that the manuscript languished in a drawer because the original project was meant to satisfy Pozdneev's own scholarly curiosity, and he did not expect it to circulate or find much of an audience outside of narrow specialists. Pozdneev's work on the treatise began in 1876 in preparation for a professorial position at the faculty of Mongolian languages in St. Petersburg. As Pozdneev writes, the original project was purely linguistic: by studying the "medical literature of the Mongols," he hoped to expand his discipline's knowledge of medical terms and expressions (Pozdneev 1991). However, the Mongol-language version of the *Gyüshi* he had encountered turned out to be incomprehensible to him and to some of his informants. This peculiar phenomenon, Pozdneev explained, was because of the practice of translating Tibetan medical texts undertaken by Mongol Buddhist monks themselves. Instead of doing what he calls "a translation proper," Mongol scholars of the *Güyshi* performed a literal translation that refused to modify the original Tibetan grammar, simply substituting Mongolian words to preserve the Tibetan sentence structure (Pozdneev 1991, 2). The resulting text was largely unreadable without consulting the Tibetan originals, which is what Pozdneev did, according to his own account under the tutelage of the Buddhist monk Lobsan-Galsan, then living at the Ogiy-nuur monastery in north-central Mongolia. Lobsan-Galsan, Pozdneev notes, had also undertaken a corrected translation of the *Gyüshi*, supplementing it with an extensive commentary, which was incorporated into Pozdneev's Russian-language text.

Pozdneev's decision to publish his translation, entitled *The Essence of Healing: The Foundations of the Eight-Part Secret Teachings* and abbreviated in print to *Manual of Tibetan Medicine* is, in fact, directly linked to Pyotr Badmaev's activities, both as a practitioner and a translator himself. According to Pozdneev's account, in 1898, the wealthy Russian merchant A. V. Kokorev, who was interested in Badmaev's efforts to popularize Tibetan medicine, expressed his support for Pozdneev's translational project. Kokorev had read Badmaev's version and asked Pozdneev to publish his own. Pozdneev describes his initial response to this request as follows: "I answered him that, in composing my translation, I was motivated by a single goal—to personally become acquainted with the language of Tibeto-Mongol medical texts, and absolutely did not intend to popularize the concepts of Tibetan medicine, or to report detailed information on it" (Pozdneev 1991, iv). For Pozdneev, the only utility of making the *Gyüshi* widely available was in the pharmaceutical information it might contain. Still, he stated that the translation would need extensive editing before it could appear in print, notably because, in order to be useful, the *materia medica* listed in the canon, and presumably unknown to a European audience, had to be identified. Kokorev shouldered the expenses for the editorial process, offering financial support that enabled Pozdneev to conduct supplementary fieldwork in Buryatia and, subsequently, Mongolia to correct and complete the manuscript. At both ethnographic sites, Pozdneev worked directly with practitioners of Tibetan medicine and proceeded to acquire samples of medicinal plants described in the *Gyüshi* in order to help scholars at the Imperial Academy of Sciences identify the ingredients listed in the text. In Buryatia, he collaborated with Choyzon Dorzhi Iroltuev (1842–1918), the Pandido Khambo Lama from 1895 to 1911, and the founder of the Atzagat Buddhist school of medicine. Iroltuev himself was a scholar and practitioner of Tibetan medicine and authored his own *chzhor*—a compendium of medicinal formulas—printed in Tibetan and classical Mongolian.

Despite Pozdneev's original optimism that the botanical identification of the medicines he presented to the Imperial Academy of Sciences would not take long, the process turned out to be arduous. By 1906, a considerable work of identification had been completed by the Imperial Botanical Garden, as well as the Geological Museum of the Imperial Academy of Sciences—with seemingly little trouble over the status of Tibetan medicine itself, now that it was divorced from its cultural, political, and religious contexts. Pozdneev notes that identifying the botanical components was significantly facilitated by the fact that much of the *materia medica* appeared to be imported from China and India, and the St. Petersburg Botanical Garden had substantial collections and information on the medicinal fauna of these regions (Pozdneev 1991, viii).

"OVERCOMING THE PAST":
TIBETAN MEDICINE AND SOVIET PHARMACOLOGY

The dual trajectories of quiet and largely uncontroversial pharmacological research into Tibetan medicine and the public tensions over its place in the clinic shaped by the two translations of the *Gyüshi* eventually collided after the Russian Revolution. While the newly minted Bolshevik government had distinct ideas about the bourgeois obsoleteness of national identities, the impetus to combat imperialism and its ideologies meant that the task of governing the sprawling territory of the former Russian Empire required an apparatus of knowledge production about its multiethnic constituency. Soviet ideology styled itself quite explicitly against the racialized and racializing logic of European imperial colonialism. Marx and Engels defined the national state as an inevitable but temporary stage of bourgeois political and economic accretion along the teleological axis of capitalism's historical evolution toward an eventually cosmopolitan class antagonism. By contrast, in their interpretation of scientific Marxism, Lenin, together with Stalin's definitive 1929 intervention on the "national question," articulated a materialist vision of the nation as a "historically constituted, stable community of people" that shared language, territory, economy, and psychological mindset (Stalin 1929) and that would naturally gravitate together into coherent units along the affective bonds of "popular sympathy." The newly established Soviet socialist state enshrined a quasi-Herderian materialist reworking of national fragmentation into the concept of nationality (*natsionalnost'*), defined through territory, language, biologized ethnicity, and economic organization roughly hinged together in the world's first example of what historian Yuri Slezkine felicitously called "institutionalize[d] ethnoterritorial federalism" (Slezkine 1994, 415).

Cosmopolitan proletarian identity was meant to eventually override all other forms of identity rooted in bourgeois logics, including racial, national, and gendered divisions. Against detractors who rejected nationalism as a form of bourgeois false-consciousness, both Lenin and Stalin eventually formulated a nationalities policy that was, in theory, designed to encourage ethnic sovereignty and self-determination for all the nations of the Soviet Union, albeit with the hopes that attachments to national self-identification would eventually wither away in favor of class solidarity and a global socialist ethics and self-awareness.[11] Yet, not all nations—or nationalities—were seen as equal. Different social groups were mapped to different points in the linear imaginary of a dialectical unfolding of history. Nor were all forms of nationalist affect legitimate, since "oppressor nations," whether in their domestic or colonial inflections, were solely interested in expansion and the furthering of their bourgeois interests, whereas "oppressed nations" were clamoring for sovereignty and the right to self-determination. Lenin saw the granting of political autonomy to "oppressed nations" as key to furthering the goals of the revolution, since the "natural" nationalism of such groups was seen to be devoid of content (or "culture"—since culture was thought to shift along with the economic base). Soviet nationality policy was thus an exercise in aspirational cultural standardization cast as historical acceleration that, in practice, enabled ever more minute fragmentation into geographically defined identities—where each national group had to have a language, literature, theater, educational system, and national dress and be firmly locatable on the map.

While smaller ethnic minority groups of the Soviet Union were not able to claim a titular territory, Buryats were numerous enough that, by 1923, the Buryat Autonomous Soviet Socialist Republic was created in the Trans-baikal region. However, while certain cultural expressions were officially promoted under the aegis of Soviet nationality policies, traditional medical practices were not part of them—the logic of developing national conscious-ness was rooted in what Francine Hirsch has described as "state-sponsored evolutionism" (Hirsch 2005, 103). Bringing biomedicine to remote areas of the Soviet Union became an opportunity for both demonstrating the supe-riority of modern scientific medicine and a strategy in accelerating the cultural enlightenment and social progress of the USSR's various peoples. As Paula Michaels summed up in a pithy parallel, "Pilots took peasants on airplane rides to prove that there was no God in heaven, while doctors used modern pharmaceuticals to demonstrate that germs, not evil spirits, caused disease" (Michaels 2000). Soviet biomedical propaganda strove to narrate local disease etiologies as harmful superstitions and nonbiomedi-cal practitioners as cynical charlatans and exploiters of the gullible masses.

Soviet medical doctors and their *mission civilisatrice* did not appear in the remote territories of the USSR in a vacuum, since the new communist government inherited Russia's long history of interacting bidirectionally with its ethnic "others," as well as part of the Russian Empire's scholarly apparatus and those ethnographic experts eager to collaborate with the new government and its utopian visions. For their part, medical reformers in Siberia found themselves in a complex local environment, with its own deeply entrenched medical practitioners, cosmologies, and social institu-tions. Although some current Russian scholars express the view that the Soviet "medical model" was characterized by its total intolerance of any "rival" practices (Mikhel 2004), medical and scientific publications in fact manifested a constant intellectual and ideological engagement with these apparently unwanted competitors. In the 1920s, a discourse on Soviet health care as radical experimentation emerged.[12] This spirit of experimentation, rife with utopian visions of embodied collectivities, was not altogether hostile to traditional medicine. Similarly to the constitution of Qigong in China (Palmer 2007), Soviet discourses on "traditional medicine" imag-ined a historical past (often existing contemporaneously with the "pres-ent") from which the keys to future medical and human progress could be extracted. Tibetan medicine was in a somewhat privileged position in comparison to other "ethnomedicines." Until the 1930s, it still had influen-tial supporters in St. Petersburg who advocated for its utility to the new

Soviet state, and throughout the 1920s and 1930s, the battle over its legitimacy was waged over whether it should be considered a cultural survival or a similarly contemporaneous medical epistemology developed by fellow toilers, with equal claims to "modernity" as its European equivalent.

From the perspective of its supporters, the greatest liability of Tibetan medicine was its association with Buddhism.[13] By the 1930s, there were about forty-five Buddhist monasteries operating in Buryatia, and practicing *emchi* were recorded in thirty of these (although the list appears incomplete) (Ochirova 2001). According to this data, 357 lamas were recorded as practicing Tibetan medicine in temples alone (Ochirova 2001, 120), though this number would not include those practitioners who were not officially affiliated with a large temple complex.[14] The practice of Tibetan medicine in Buryatia was neither standardized nor centralized across the region, varying from one Buddhist complex to the next.

One of the most famous and ultimately most controversial sites for the practice of Tibetan medicine in Buryatia was the Atzagat Buddhist monastery, about thirty miles to the east of Ulan-Ude (then Verkhneudinsk). Founded in 1825, the monastery was located near an *arshan* (a sacred and medicinal spring in Buryat) that became an integral part of the medicinal practices at the site. The Atzagat medical school was founded by Choyzon Dorzhi Iroltuev (1842–1918) after his service as the Fifth Pandido Khambo Lama (1895–1911) had ended. Like many of the prominent Buryat lamas at the time, Iroltuev authored his own *chzhor* of medical formulas and did other translational work. He was also noticed by Emperor Nikolai II when the latter was touring the Far East with his family in 1891. After treating the members of the emperor's family, Iroltuev was awarded two St. Stanislav medals in recognition for his services.

In 1921, Agvan Dorzhiev, an important political and religious figure in the "reformist" school of Buryat Buddhism and one of the cofounders of the Atzagat medical school, made efforts to reorganize the school of Tibetan medicine to correspond with the political demands of Soviet antireligious agitation (Ayusheeva 2007; Aseeva 2008). The aims of these transformations were to separate the learning of Tibetan medicine from the *datsan* complex and to integrate it more firmly into secular Soviet society both practically and epistemologically by introducing it alongside the principles of European biomedicine in schools.

By 1924, after Iroltuev's death, Dondub Yendonov (1870–1973), a *gabzhi* (or *geshe*) and teacher of Tibetan medicine, joined the Atzagat school. In 1925, the Atzagat complex numbered about twenty practitioners of Tibetan medicine (Semichov 1932, cited in Mitypova 2006). Yendonov was asked by the temple administration to gather eight lamas from different Buddhist complexes throughout Buryatia and develop a single unifying program for teaching Tibetan medicine throughout the Buryat-Mongol Republic (Zhamsuev and Banchinova 2008, 202). In addition, Yendonov had a keen interest in European medicine and spent some time at an otolaryngology hospital in Saratov in 1929. As a result of this work, he authored a medical atlas for the Atzagat medical curriculum that tried to bring together the principles of European anatomy and the concepts of Tibetan medicine.

Although Atzagat quickly became both a clinical site for treating patients and a research base for St. Petersburg scholars working on Buddhism, it was also undergoing a process of hybridization that would make it more recognizable to the Soviet authorities. For his part, Dorzhiev helped organize a medical facility at the site of the Atzagat monastery, and the clinic combined the dispensation of Tibetan medicine with European

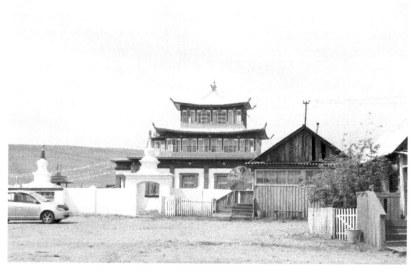

Figure 1. Atzagat Temple, reconstructed (Photo by the author, July 2017)

balneological therapies. The medical facilities at the site included a stationary clinic, a pharmacy, several warehouses for storing ingredients, a school, a bathhouse for using the *arshan* water, and a water-powered mill for grinding the *materia medica*.

Atzagat might not have looked entirely unfamiliar or undesirable from the point of view of the Soviet state. In 1919, the People's Committee for Health Protection (Narkomzdrav) passed a decree entitled "About health resorts and therapeutic regions of national importance" that nationalized all preexisting health resort facilities. In the early 1920s, the Soviet government was reforming and expanding the tsarist-era infrastructure of sanatoriums, converting them from spaces of leisure for a wealthy aristocratic elite to sites where ordinary workers could enjoy "useful"—often strictly regimented and medicalized—relaxation. The emerging disciplines of balneology and resort medicine divided the territory of the USSR according to the different regions' therapeutic effects. In Siberia, the management of therapeutically relevant ecological features was under the administrative responsibility of "Sibkursan," an institution in charge of documenting the therapeutic landscape and discovering new sites beneficial for the toilers' health. Active identification of therapeutic locations began in the early 1920s, and "natural" phenomena, such as sunlight, elevation, mineral waters and muds, climate, scenery, and certain local food products were classified as therapeutically efficacious and were mobilized to bolster the population's flagging health (Semashko 1934). The institutionalization of sanatoriums in the Baikal region continued full-force in the after-war years, when many of the local health resorts were reorganized into hospitals for war evacuees. At the same time, Soviet balneology was developing scientific protocols and metrics for classifying the efficacy and use of "natural" factors in the treatment of patients, as well as developing a treatment methodology for different illnesses, matching the properties of specific ecological features, like the mineral content of water, to disease categories.

By 1931, the Atzagat clinic had treated over seven thousand patients (Ayusheeva 2007, 96). Although the Soviet regional government in Buryatia actively worked to diminish the influence of Buddhism in the region—for example, by heavily taxing monasteries—Tibetan medicine was in an ambiguous position. On the one hand, it was popular with the local population, and frequently still the only source of accessible health care, and local Soviet officials were therefore reluctant to outlaw it. On the other hand, it was suspected of reinforcing the authority of local lamas and Buddhist faith more generally.

In 1934, the All-Union Institute of Experimental Medicine (AIEM), located in Leningrad, opened the Bureau for the Study of Oriental Medicine after continuous lobbying by Nikolai Badmaev, Pyotr Badmaev's nephew and disciple, in defense of the scientific study of Tibetan pharmaceuticals and medical practice (Grekova and Lange 1994). Botanicals were precisely what was at stake for the state and for the medical community: interest in Tibetan medicine and especially in its *materia medica* coincided with a very immediate economic concern. Since the 1920s and throughout the 1930s, the Soviet Union was plagued by severe shortages of basic pharmaceuticals. Meanwhile, the Soviet state hoped to supplement its income by aggressively exporting medicinal botanicals to Europe (Conroy 2006).

Nikolai Badmaev himself had enthusiastic supporters among the Soviet elite. Much like his uncle, he treated prominent political and cultural figures, among them Maksim Gorky, a writer with strong backing from the Communist Party who became a patron to Badmaev's activities and an advocate for scientific research into Tibetan medicine (Grekova 2002, 80). The bureau planned expeditions to Buryatia—specifically, to Atzagat—to gather plants and conduct archival and ethnographic research. In fact, the AIEM had been engaged in the study of the pharmacology of Tibetan medicine for several years prior to that, as had the Botanical Institute of the Soviet Academy of Sciences, which sent an expedition to Atzagat in 1931.

The result of this 1931 expedition, headed by botanist Adele Gammerman and her assistant, orientologist Boris Semichov, had negative consequences for the Atzagat clinic and for Tibetan medicine in Buryatia more generally. A controversy broke out after Semichov published a scathing article in the 1932 issue of *Soviet Ethnography* on the results of their study. The article, entitled "Tibetan Medicine in the BMASSR," set out to assess the utility of the clinic and medical school in particular and the utility and value of Tibetan medicine more generally. Directly addressed to Buryatia's Narmokzdrav, the article begins with a description of the institution and concludes with policy recommendations. Citing what he describes as the unsanitary conditions of the medical facility, the "ignorance" of the principles of bacteriology and hygiene on the part of the lamas, the suspicious ways in which the pharmacy seemed to operate on a model of private entrepreneurship, the apparent lack of standardized schooling and the ways in which the students appeared to loiter aimlessly around the temple complex, and, finally, the "irrational" and "religiously dogmatic" premises of Tibetan medicine and its view of the body, the article concluded that, in the words of Semichov himself, "Tibetan medicine isn't a science, and thus does not have a right to exist" (Semichov 1932, 225). Semichov urged the local Commissariat of Health to create conditions for facilitating the "natural death" of the Atzagat temple, which, in his opinion, occupied a useful therapeutic site that would be suitable for a state-run sanatorium (Semichov 1932, 227). The only recoverable element, for Semichov, was the *materia medica* deployed in Tibetan medicine. The plants and minerals used locally might require careful laboratory analysis, he stated. Beyond this pragmatic goal, the study of the compendium of Tibetan medicine texts would belong to the domain of abstract historical scholarship—a pursuit that the state, according to the author, could not presently afford (Semichov 1932, 225).

A year later, an odd scandal brought Tibetan medicine to the attention of a general Soviet public. In 1933, *Izvestia*, the official daily periodical of the Soviet government since 1917, reported on the public trial of a group of power-plant managers and engineers, some domestic and others British, accused of conspiracy to sabotage a number of power plants throughout Russia, with the intent of creating a political diversion (Vitvitsky 1933). The show trial caused serious tensions between the Soviet Union and the United Kingdom, and the threats to interrupt all diplomatic and trade relations between the two states were voiced in the British press. Reporting on the reactions in the foreign media, *Izvestia* stated that the "reactionary British press" was putting forth a set of outlandish accusations about the interrogation methods of the Soviet State Police (OGPU). They had claimed, *Izvestia* reported, that the agents of OGPU used the formulas of Tibetan medicine "to weaken the will" of the accused British subjects and thus were able to produce a confession. Although tangential to the expert debates that surrounded Tibetan medicine at the time, the article signals a shift in the attitudes toward the topic: Tibetan medicine was progressively being reframed as superstition, and, in the logic of performing modern, scientifically backed thinking, the article accused the British press of profoundly irrational obscurantism.

In the mid-1930s, Tibetan medicine still had enthusiasts and defenders in professional scientific and medical circles, but the controversies over its status as a legitimate form of knowledge further destabilized its position.

In 1935, after a public lecture by Nikolai Badmaev, the "Initiative Group for the Study of Eastern Medicine and Physical Education" was created, bringing together a variety of experts: psychologists, neurologists, and physiologists, as well as an economist and the director of a laboratory for the study of radioactive substances (Grekova 2002, 119). The group sought official recognition from the Narkomzdrav and advocated for the scientific study of Tibetan medicine as a valuable resource. Although the bureaucratic process proceeded haltingly, eventually the Committee for Health Protection called a general meeting of a special medical council to discuss the status of Tibetan medicine and to evaluate the initiative's proposal to further develop scientific research into the practice, with the long-term goal of incorporating it into the state's pharmaceutical arsenal. The meeting took place in March of 1935, and the members of the initiative presented their reports in defense of recognizing Tibetan medicine as a separate branch of the sciences, one that merited closer scrutiny and eventual integration with European medicine.

The resulting argument over Tibetan medicine between representatives of the National Commissariat of Health and the Initiative Group was not a matter of straightforward opposition between European medicine and indigenous modes of healing. Rather, it expressed itself as a series of epistemic contextualization and recontextualizations concerned with establishing what might be counted as legitimate forms of *scientific* knowledge—and what sorts of people were capable of it. In March 1936, the Initiative Group, comprised of Nikolai Badmaev and his supporters in the St. Petersburg medical and scholarly community, filed a report in anticipation of the meeting with Narkomzdrav's Scientific Medical Council. The report was compiled by Vasilij Pavlovich Kashkadamov, a Russian hygienist and physiologist whose research on plague in India in 1899–1900 brought him into contact with Ayurvedic medicine and its pharmacology. Kashkadamov's argument that Tibetan medicine presents an interest to European science, not only as a source of potential pharmacological innovation but as a medical knowledge system in its own right, anticipated and sought to counteract potential claims about its "backwardness": "Any European educated doctor," he wrote in the report, "becomes persuaded that Tibetan medicine has reached astounding levels of development, and therefore making doctors familiar with it is a matter of utmost importance." His own interest in Tibetan medicine, he confesses, was informed by the comparison of two hospitals in Bombay, one based on a European model mostly serving Western expatriates and another based on what he calls "local medical traditions." Kashkadamov notes that both approaches were, in his evaluation, effective in managing bacteriological threats and patients' convalescence. In an interesting harnessing of the *Gyüshi*'s injunction that the Buddha's teaching of Tibetan medicine was given to "benefit all living beings," Kashkadamov aligned Buddhist ethics with Marxist rhetoric, proposing a synthesis that harnessed the political language of Soviet progressivist optimism and geopolitical competition:

> In our country, courageous routine-breaking thought forges new paths in all domains of scientific, social, and economic life, it seeks to use all possibilities for the benefit of the toilers—possibilities that were met with indifference in prerevolutionary Russia. With the same courage and breadth we must break through medicine's conservatism, we must approach the study of Indo-Tibetan medicine with energy and dedication, based on the broad foundations available to our country, at the speed of our country, before we are superseded by the West, which is already turning its attention to this problem. It is necessary to create a synthesis of knowledge compiled by both West and East, and on the basis of this synthesis we must build a single medical science for the benefit of the toilers of all the world. (Kashkadamov 1936)

Even more forcefully, Nikolai Badmaev's own writings in the same report insisted on the legitimate scientific status of Tibetan medicine as a form of medical knowledge with its own historical trajectory distinct from, but no less valid than, that of European medicine. Much like modern European medicine, Badmaev argued, Tibetan medicine traces one part of its lineage to ancient contacts with Hellenic medicine. However, unlike European medicine, it was never interrupted in its development by medieval Christianity, and therefore unfolded on its own terms. Badmaev details Tibetan medicine's arrival into Russia, focusing on the long history of its willful importation from the country's peripheral regions toward its metropolitan center. His account of the logic of this movement articulates a medical geopolitics: while the ability of notable local practitioners of Tibetan medicine to contain bacteriological threats at the peripheries of empire earned them initial notice and eventual support among state officials, he argues, it was their skill in treating recalcitrant chronic conditions among metropolitan populations that ensured their lasting professional and medical success. Between the lines, and much like his uncle, Badmaev offers a sly critique, one that ventriloquizes socialist logics of class antagonism and anti-imperialist rhetoric to bring into the view the grounds of legitimacy: what counts as a scientific approach in medicine is never exempt from the centripetal forces of the metropole. The reason Tibetan medicine took root in the metropolitan center, even in the absence of full state endorsement, is that it could treat the social elites. Badmaev systematically uses the term "the medical science of Tibet" to refer to Tibetan medicine, though the choice of terms appears to be a carefully calibrated bid for an optics of recognition in anticipation of his audience's potential reaction.

Much like his uncle, Nikolai Badmaev was concerned with the dismissal of the therapeutic principles of Tibetan medicine and with its reduction to nothing more than a source of ethnobotanical knowledge that might expand the pharmacopeia of European medicine without lending legitimacy to the reasoning behind *why* it works clinically. In 1935, his article in defense of Tibetan medicine was published in *Izvestia*. The article attempted to convince the public that Tibetan medicine had at its disposal a long history of successful research into the body, including insights into the development of the fetus that preceded European embryology. Badmaev also pointed out a history of using surgical procedures and effectively mobilizing medical substances to reinforce the body's self-healing capacities to restore the functions of specific organs in recalcitrant cases like diabetes, where European insulin therapy would in fact result in the permanent deregulation of the pancreas. Most importantly, Badmaev argued, Tibetan medicine used botanical substances in ways that did not lend themselves to analysis with the scientific methodology of contemporary European pharmacology. Plants are combined with each other, and the entire plant is used, instead of its "active essences." He critiqued the laboratory as an inadequate space for determining the therapeutic efficacy of Tibetan medicine formulas, suggesting instead that the clinic was better suited for it:

> There are no reasons to believe that the "active essence" of a medicinal plant, obtained through chemical means, can perfectly replace the plant itself, which includes many other substances, not to mention that it is doubtful that the medicinal properties of plants are left unchanged

under the influence of reactive substances through which the extraction of these "active essences" is produced. We cannot consider the experimental laboratory method exhaustive. A healthy animal, artificially infected with some kind of illness, cannot provide a picture of the complex process that progressively develops under the normal conditions of life in a human organism, where the processes of disturbance and destruction happen at the same time as the process of self-preservation of tissues. (N. Badmaev 1935)

Based on the methodology for the study and clinical deployment of Tibetan medicine that the report of the Initiative Group articulated, its members were not optimistic about the sort of response they expected to receive. Both Kashkadamov and Badmaev insisted on the creation of an entirely independent clinic, one where diagnosis would be established solely on the basis of Tibetan medicine. For its part, the Scientific Medical Council issued invitations to a number of independent scholars and experts to present their own assessments alongside the members of the Initiative Group. Many of these external participants were either lukewarm or downright hostile to the proposal. The lengthy report filed by Genokh Kogan, a professor at the Vitebsk Medical University, specially invited to weigh in on the matter by the assistant commissioner of the Medical Council Rakhovsky, begins with a rambling racialized critique of Traditional Chinese Medicine—as well as Chinese culture more broadly. Kogan generalizes Tibetan medicine alongside all other "Far Eastern Medicines" as products of "feudalist backwardness," mostly suitable as topics of interest for historians of medicine, but not for the medical community.[15] Despite his dismissal of the pharmacology of Asian medicines, Kogan concludes that "we cannot wash our hands of Chinese-Tibetan Medicine, while we are still persuaded that we might find, in its huge pharmaceutical arsenal, something that might enrich our own reserves. This familiarization should not present any great difficulty, since Chinese-Tibetan Medicine has never held and doesn't presently hold any 'secrets,' those secrets allegedly kept by its current practitioners can just as easily be read in books" (Kogan 1936).

As with its predecessor in 1905, the Scientific Medical Council rejected the Initiative Group's proposal of synthesis, leaning heavily on Kogan's report to decide how the study of Tibetan medicine ought to proceed in the future. It categorically rejected the proposal that Tibetan medicine could be considered scientific or that its theories of the body and efficacy have any value beyond those of an ethnographic curiosity. It nonetheless called for pharmaceutical investigation—no longer at the hands of the original members of the Initiative Group, but in those of the commentators the Scientific Medical Council had invited to weigh in on the original proposal. What the council did recognize was the utility of studying the pharmacopeia and techniques of Tibetan medicine under strict laboratory conditions after "purifying them of all religious sediments," including Tibetan medicine's unscientific view of the body.[16]

The centrality of Tibetan medicine in the scientific work of the bureau at the AIEM was eventually eclipsed. Following some internal political maneuvering, the bureau expanded its focus from Oriental medicine to traditional medicine more broadly, a change that implicitly demoted Tibetan medicine from the status of a methodical text-based tradition to that of idiosyncratic "empirical" skill. Nikolai Badmaev's role became more peripheral, as he was demoted to the status of consultant. Nevertheless, in 1937, with the support of G. N. Kaminsky, then the head of the People's Commissariat of Health, a clinic for Tibetan medicine was opened in Leningrad. It was short-lived—it existed for only two months. In March of 1938, following an avalanche of arrests of the Bolshevik Party's own members, including many of Badmaev's influential patients, and the arrest and replacement of Kaminsky himself, the clinic was disbanded. Reports on the inefficiency and reactionary nature of Tibetan medicine appeared in the press (B. Reyn, *Krasnaya Gazeta*, cited in Grekova 2002). On April 20, 1938, Nikolai Badmaev was arrested by the state police. He was subsequently accused of counterrevolutionary conspiracy and Japanese espionage, which was a fairly typical charge at the time, and executed on February 26, 1939.

During the war and post-war period, Tibetan medicine disappeared from the limelight of public, political, and scholarly attention. One domain where its study continued during the Soviet 1940s and 1950s was in the activity of botanists and pharmacologists documenting the uses of medicinal plants among the different people of the USSR (Gammerman 1966; Gammerman and Semichov 1963; Gammerman and Shupinskaya 1937). Adele Gammerman, the botanist in charge of the Atzagat expedition in 1931, and her team continued pharmacological research into identifying the plants used in the pharmacopeia of Tibetan medicine.

In Buryatia, public invisibility did not necessarily mean complete obscurity. Based on conversations with my local consultants and interlocutors, many remembered having either a relative or an older acquaintance who would receive patients unofficially and prescribe medicines. Accounts of other nonbiomedical healers, such as shamans, suggested that practitioners continued to treat patients under the radar of the Soviet state—I was frequently told that in rural and remote areas especially, the state had neither the capacity nor the willingness to scrutinize these "folk" activities too closely. My interlocutors often mentioned that, while the risk of getting caught and accruing a fine was present, actual persecution was rare, primarily because everyone in the area, the party officials included, consulted these practitioners themselves and had no interest in self-sabotage. These narratives of remembered healers are important in another way—they figured prominently in explanations for why someone had decided to pursue training in Tibetan medicine in the present. Sometimes mobilized into logics of rebirth and lineage, these ancestral bodies became anchoring sites for recovering and articulating a continuity of practice and knowledge that withstood the politically hostile climate of the post–World War II Soviet years.[17]

A theoretical turn toward the usefulness of studying traditional medicine, and especially the "literary" medical traditions of Asia, reemerged in the late 1950s. In 1957, a group of Soviet neurologists from the Soviet Union's metropolitan centers traveled to China during a professional exchange, where they were tasked with learning about Chinese acupuncture, and with importing its methods back to the Soviet Union (Osipova 2003). While the relationship between China and the USSR soured by 1958 and professional exchanges in medicine were significantly reduced (Ratmanov 2010), these collaborations enabled the foundation of what later became known as the Soviet school of reflexotherapy, institutionalized by the Soviet Ministry of Health in the Moscow-based Central Scientific-Research Institute of Reflexotherapy in 1977. By that point, reflexotherapy was taught as part of the medical university curriculum in a number of university departments around the country. Reframed in terms of a Pavlovian framework of neurological reflexes, the acceptability of Chinese acupuncture created a precedent for the clinical study of Tibetan medicine, especially in those regions, like Buryatia, where a substantial archive of Buddhist medical texts was available. Official approval from the state came once again via a renewed interest in the pharmacology of Tibetan medicine. In 1968, P. B. Baldanzhapov founded the institute of social sciences at the Institute of Mongol Studies, Buddhology and Tibetology in Ulan-Ude. The research center focused on the study of the primary sources of Tibetan medicine, among other Buddhist canonical texts. Using his personal connections in what local scholars employed at the research center often described as an incredibly daring political gambit, the new director located and recruited former lamas, recently released from the Soviet state's carceral apparatus, and employed in entirely different walks of life, to act as consultants for the researchers at the institute. Among the specialists in Tibetan medicine recruited as "junior scientific collaborators" were D. D. Badmaev, L. Ya. Yampilov, Zh. Tz. Tzybenov, Z. H. Zhapov, M. D. Dashiev, and G. B. Gombozhapov. These practitioners, in turn, gained followers among the scientific intelligentsia of the research center, taking on some of them as apprentices and disciples.

In 1974, the national periodical *Pravda* described the activity of the research institute, outlining the rediscovery of the "ancient heritage" of Tibetan medicine in Buryatia. No longer narrated as ancient superstitions, Tibetan medicine texts were now described as a "cipher," a secret knowledge purposefully encoded by the authors of the canonical treaties to keep it from the public in an effort to preserve their class interests (Sokolov 1974). In 1975, the Buryat Science Center (BSC) founded an institute for the study of biologically active substances of Tibetan medicine that conducted both translational work and biochemical research (Makarova 2001). By the late 1980s, scholars in Russia were developing research methodologies and scientific protocols in order to integrate "Eastern" medical principles into biomedicine and to "decipher" its encoded knowledge in the hopes of incorporating some of its elements into practical healthcare. The Buryat Science Center was actively publishing research literature on Tibetan medicine in philology, botany, pharmacology, physics, and translations of primary texts.

While in Buryatia Tibetan medicine was the object of rigorous scientific investigation for several decades, as well as a modality of discreet medical practice, often undertaken under the radar of the state, by the late 1980s and early 1990s it had, once again, captured the public imagination in a way that seemed radically different from the kinds of questions the Soviet scientists were asking of it, and its place in relation to a distinctly *Buryat* cultural and religious heritage became a contested question. The final section of this chapter details these transformations—if Tibetan medicine could be partially preserved and carefully explored in the safely "apolitical" space of historical and philological research (as long as no claims were made about its right to a contemporaneous existence alongside the hallmarks of Soviet modernity and social progress), after the fall of the Soviet Union, these distinctions became rapidly repoliticized.

THE ATLAS OF DISCORD:
TIBETAN MEDICINE AS CULTURAL HERITAGE IN THE 1990s

On the night of May 4, 1998, a group of young Buddhist monks and their lay supporters picketed the courtyard of the Odigitrievsky Cathedral—a majestic eighteenth-century Russian Orthodox temple perched on the bank of the Uda River in the historical heart of Ulan-Ude, Buryatia's capital. Preceding by about two months the devastating economic collapse that would sweep Russia in August of the same year into a tidal wave of currency devaluation, unpaid salaries, hikes in the prices of consumer goods, and a stark dip in life expectancy registered post factum on demographers' charts (Brainerd and Cutler 2005), and a year before the Second Chechen War would bring ethnonational separatism into the center of political conversations, the picket had a somewhat surprising focus. At the time of the protests, the basement of Odigitrievsky was used to stockpile various religious and cultural artifacts that had not made it into Buryatia's National History Museum's narrative of the region's past. The picketers were concerned with the fate of one such artifact: the Atlas of Tibetan Medicine, a set of seventy-six Buddhist companion illustrations to the seventeenth-century canonical Tibetan medicine text *The Blue Beryl* (Tib. *vaidurya sngon po*), itself a commentary on the *Gyüshi*.

The Buryat Atlas, as it is often referred to locally, is a late nineteenth-century copy of an original set of illustrations (Tib. *thangka*) produced in Tibet by Desi Sangye Gyatso (1603–1705), regent to the Fifth Dalai Lama and author of the Blue Beryl commentary. The original was believed to have been destroyed by Chinese communists during the Cultural Revolution but was allegedly rediscovered later in Lhasa. The Buryat copy, likely commissioned in Tibet by Tsaniid-Khambo Lharamba Agvan Dorzhiev, a prominent political and religious figure of Buryat Buddhism and adviser to the Thirteenth Dalai Lama Thubpten Gyatso, was transported from Tibet to Buryatia at the turn of the twentieth century and presented to the medical school of the Tsugol Buddhist Temple, where it was kept until 1926 (Zhambalova 1997, 5). In 1926, the Atlas was transferred to the Atzagat Buddhist Temple, where it remained until the temple's destruction in 1936. The set, minus one lost page, survived Stalin's antireligious purges and the destruction of most of Buryatia's Buddhist monasteries in the 1930s and 1940s and currently stands as one of the most complete sets of the Desi's illustrations. Presently, the Atlas is recognized as one of the greatest treasures of Buryat Buddhism. However, for much of the twentieth century, it languished in the basement of the Odigitrievsky Cathedral. Odigitrievsky had not fared much better during Stalinist antireligious purges than its Buddhist counterparts. In 1930, after its property and icons had been confiscated and its prior executed, the cathedral's basement was turned, with a great deal of historical irony, into storage for the Anti-Religious Museum housed on the first floor (Zhambalova 1997, 23).

In the late 2000s, Buryatia's local administration liked to emphasize the region's social stability and cordial ethnic relations—a part of what constituted "Buryatia's brand" (*brend Buryatii*). As such, the picket, a decade old by that point, had a long afterlife, and was often recast as an episode of unusual political upheaval for the region. But it was also one of the most vivid events in the history of tangled translations, appropriations, movements, and controversies over the fate and history of Tibetan medicine in Buryatia, for which the Atlas came to stand as a synecdoche. The picket erupted in response to the scheduled departure of the Atlas on a yearlong tour of U.S. museums. In a final desperate effort, the protestors created a human chain around the cathedral, hoping to physically impede the Atlas's prospective departure from the republic.

By the time the protestors had occupied the cathedral's courtyard, debates about the legitimacy of the Atlas's international exhibition had raged in the local press for months. What made the May 4 picket qualitatively different, consolidating the events into a political incident with a long and fraught memory, was the violent response from the local government. In an effort to put an end to the protest, the administration of Leonid Potapov, Buryatia's president at the time, sent a Special Rapid Response Unit (SOBR) to retrieve the crates containing the Atlas from the museum's repository in the basement of the cathedral. The special ops beat and dispersed the picketers, most of whom were Buddhist monks and teenage disciples (Bur. *khuvarak*), loaded the crates onto a KamAz truck, and sped off toward the airport.

State violence directed against religiously marked bodies, captured on grainy nighttime photographs and as shaky, blurry footage and fed back to local kitchens and living rooms through Russia's central TV channel NTV, stunned Buryatia's public, fomenting a polemic in the regional and national press in the weeks and months that followed. Regional newspapers framed the conflict over the Atlas as one that pitted the Buddhist Sangha of Russia, headed by Khambo Lama Damba Ayusheev, against Buryatia's adminis-tration. The region's government, with the support of the local scholarly community and museum workers, signed an agreement with Pro-Culture, an international NGO that served as a broker for planning international exhibits. Early in May, Buryatia's administration reneged on the agreement after concerns were raised about the legitimacy of Pro-Culture and the legality of the entire operation. The national magazine *Kommersant'*, which covered the events, listed the penalty for defaulting on the contract with Pro-Culture at U.S. $3 million. Russia's federal government intervened with a reminder to local officials in Buryatia that the Atlas was in fact an artifact of *national*—and not just regional—significance.[18] As a result, Potapov's administration backtracked and reinstated the agreement. The contract was finalized in secret, entirely bypassing the Sangha and its potential objections (Zhukovskaya 1998), and thus precipitating the alter-cation on May 4 and the subsequent scandal.

Because the "Atlas Affair," as the local newspapers quickly dubbed it, took place a month and a half before scheduled regional elections, politics occupied the foreground of its media coverage. The regional press became a platform for multiple, often antagonistic voices. Newspapers printed opinion and testimony pieces sent in by representatives of the different factions involved: regional administrators, museum workers, academics, and religious figures. The regional administration issued vague statements chastising "certain candidates" for "playing the nationality card" and propagating "disinformation" to score political points.[19] The head of Bury-atia's Ministry of Internal Affairs (MVD) explained to reporters that the use of force was justified, since the pickets were "well organized," and Khambo Lama Ayusheev himself had escalated the situation by appear-ing on a local radio program with a call to the general public to join the protests.[20] As the rhetoric reached its boiling point over the weeks that followed, the local government shifted to a narrative of geopolitical securitization, invoking the specter of ethnic nationalism fed by unspecified nefarious agents, and wrote of the mobilization of "religious fanatics" in an effort to play out "a scenario of destabilization" accompanied by an "information war."

A different interpretation centered on whether the Atlas should be considered a religious or a cultural artifact (Batomunkuev 2004). The Buddhist Sangha of Russia and its representatives argued that the Atlas was a sacred Buddhist relic, commissioned in the nineteenth century with funds gathered by Buryat Buddhist congregations. Therefore, they argued that the Sangha—and not the National Museum of Republic Buryatia—should be the Atlas's sole legitimate custodian and the arbiter of its circulation and availability for viewing. In a stark reversal of previous trends, leaders from the local academic community wrote to local newspapers to argue that the Atlas was a rare and unique *scientific* document, and not religious at all: a testimony to the important place of Eastern scientific thought in a cosmopolitan history of science and of Buryatia's contribution to the global pursuit of knowledge. The scholars called for the Atlas's careful study and wide circulation, not religious veneration and control.[21] To muddle matters further, His Holiness the Fourteenth Dalai Lama, Tenzin Gyatso, had penned a letter, subsequently reprinted in a local newspapers, in which he aligned with this latter, cosmopolitan take on the Atlas, commending the Buryat government for its decision to share this unique example of Tibetan medical culture with the global scholarly community, thus raising awareness of both Buryatia and of the Tibetan art of healing.

Other critics situated the Atlas protests in relation to the zeitgeist of the "roaring 90s"—the sense that "shock therapy" neoliberal reforms, for which the first decade of post-socialism in Russia is often remembered, had made everything potentially available to the logics of commoditization, cultural patrimony included. Marianna Vladimirovna, one of the curators of the permanent exhibit of the Atlas at the National Museum, explained to me that the heightened emotions surrounding the protests had little to do with the Atlas in particular or with Tibetan medicine more generally, and everything to do with local and national political ambitions harnessing the social anxieties brought on in the aftermath of the Soviet Union's collapse. "It was the 'bedeviled 90s,' [Rus. *likhie devyanostyye*], you understand. This was when all sorts of historical rarities were being expropriated [*vyvozilis'*] abroad." She was certainly not alone in offering this interpretation—in fact, the political economy of international art circuits had been at the heart of the original debates about the fate of the Atlas. Some local cultural heritage specialists asked who stood to profit from the Atlas's American exhibit. A member of the local chapter of the All-Russian Society for the Protection of Historical and Cultural Monuments (in Russian abbreviated as VOOPIIK) speculated in an opinion piece published in *Pravda Buryatii*, one of the oldest and most established local newspapers, that the Atlas's departure would be the latest heist in a string of thefts of valuable artifacts from the region's museums that had gutted local collections since the early 1990s. Minimally, those opposed to the Atlas going on international tour on secular, rather than religious, grounds focused on the legal and financial underpinnings of the transaction, arguing that neither Buryatia nor the National Museum stood to gain anything from the artifact's travels. Buryatia's print media framed it as yet another instance of exploitation of an indigenous minority population in a long history of colonial expropriations and trickery the world over: an exchange of priceless cultural patrimony for "glass beads."[22] A focus on financial gain was also the frame favored by Moscow newspapers.

Like other important Buddhist treasures (Bernstein 2013), the Atlas has, at various points, served as the ground for articulating Buryatia's contributions to the Buddhist world. In more recent years, since a discourse on formulating a distinct regional brand for Buryatia began to shape some aspects of Buryat Buddhism, the Atlas came to occupy a central role in guiding the flows of tourists and capital into the region. However, my interlocutors in the practicing *emchi* community often noted that, its turbulent biography notwithstanding, most of the *tanghkas* were largely inaccessible for public view—its current status was that of a historical artifact firmly kept under glass in a museum, and only some of the *tanghkas* were available on display. Much like Tibetan medicine in Buryatia, over the roughly 100 years of the Buryat Atlas's existence, most of the controversies that surrounded it have centered on the problem of its duplication, reproduction, and mobility—and who should be its rightful custodian.

In telling its history in Russia, I wanted to be mindful of Tibetan medicine's own capacity for recruiting allies, advocates, and converts. By focusing on the politics of legibility of nonbiomedical therapies, I have argued in this chapter that Tibetan medicine in Russia has been continuously made and unmade *as* medicine. As a set of therapeutic, ecological, bodily, and religious practices, as well as a corpus of written texts, it has been directly and indirectly co-opted into a number of regional and national institutional experiments with frequently incompatible agendas. Its translations, adaptations, and recruitments parse these therapeutic practices into movable and immovable parts—into "historical heritage," "medical technology," "religion," or "pharmacology." Struggles over its definition redefine it across epistemic borders—they shape what counts as "medicine" in the first place, and what sort of medicines are seen to "count."

Much like its Atlas, Tibetan medicine in Buryatia straddles multiple social and symbolic worlds. Struggles over its definition and proper deployment reveal how local therapeutic knowledge is continuously produced, contested, and redefined—which is to say, its particularities are both constantly negotiated and renaturalized—in relation to institutional projects that strive to incorporate it while retaining (or constantly reproducing) their claims to universal applicability. In Chapter 2 I focus on efforts to develop the Automated Pulse Diagnosis Complex—a project where competing ideas about making Tibetan medicine "portable" (both figuratively and literally), while uprooting it from the particularities of its embodied practices, created an uneasy dialogue between Soviet and post-socialist researchers and practicing *emchi*.

2

"TO SEARCH FOR THE SOLELY RATIONAL"

Engineering Tibetan Pulse Diagnosis

SEEING THE PULSE

The pulse diagnosis lab was housed in a surprisingly sunny spacious room, hidden behind a massive aluminum door at the end of one of the dimly lit concrete hallways in a seemingly abandoned section of the austere Soviet-era research institute. As I sat with the current director of the lab, chatting about the institutional history of the Automated Pulse Diagnostic Complex, which his laboratory has been developing since the early 1980s, Vitaly Vasylievich pointed to a poster hanging on the wall, a black-and-white photograph of a hand holding another, index, middle, and ring fingers resting on the inside of a wrist. It is hard to read the image without immediately recognizing its citational quality: it is the standard representation of traditional pulse diagnosis used in Tibetan medicine. Above the photograph, where the two hands faded into a dark background, ornate letters spelled out "Tibetan Medicine." In the director's narrative, the poster served as an anchor, a memento of one of the moments of professional triumph for him and his lab. It was printed specifically for the visit of Tenzin Choedrak in 1990, who, at the time, was the Dalai Lama's personal physician. Dr. Choedrak visited the lab's clinical base at the Hospital of War Veterans in Ulan-Ude to observe the research into Tibetan medicine that Buryatia could offer. Once Dr. Choedrak was on site, the physicists did not want to squander the opportunity to obtain a consultation from a renowned practitioner. To this end, Dr. Choedrak read patients' pulses alongside the Automated Pulse Diagnostic Complex (APDC). In the early 1990s, the device was a set of cuffs outfitted with sensors, connected to an enormous unwieldy wall-sized computer installation, "big as a wardrobe," as Vitaly Vasylievich joked. The lab director recounted Tenzin Choedrak's reaction as follows:

> He became fascinated with the graph—the read-out of the pulse wave, and as it turned out, he had never seen the "pulsogram" curve before. He listened very carefully to our descriptions and explanations, and when we explained what the [APDC] diagnosis suggested, he became really delighted, since it was just as his own. He then turned to the (Buryat) lamas accompanying him [both were *emchi*], and told them "You have to help these guys." We took it as a sort of blessing.

Whether Tenzin Choedrak's excitement was indeed because of seeing the pulsogram for the first time or the result of the convergence between his own interpretation and that of the researchers is difficult to say. However, that the incident was a condensed moment of professional and scholarly success for Vitaly Vasylyevich and his team is significant. For the group of radiophysicists, engineers, and doctors working on "objectivizing" Tibetan medicine, the ability to make the pulse visible in ways that reflected the principles of pulse diagnosis was a source of professional and intellectual pride.

In this chapter, I examine the tensions and slippages that spring from attempting to encode diagnostic palpation into an imaging device. The frictions, misalignments, and resistances that arise from these projects of *objektivizatziia*,[1] or "objectivization," are not simply a matter of epistemological distance between different practices of generating authoritative knowledge or between divergent takes on the human body and its constitutive processes characteristic of different medical traditions (Kuriyama 1999). Scholars have long noted that the task of incorporating traditional medical modalities into a biomedical mainstream is a process that mobilizes practices of authorization such as double-blind control trials, which more often than not function as gatekeepers for what counts as valid forms of evidence and efficacy.[2]

What interests me instead is what the APDC is "asked" to do by its creators and users, and what these questions might tell us about the paradoxes inherent not only between, but also within specific practices of knowledge-making. In order to understand the hopes and desires invested into the design and deployment of the APDC by its developers, it is insufficient to view the device as simply a site where "modern" medical knowledge co-opts or colonizes "traditional" practice, seamlessly absorbing and transforming it without leaving an epistemological remainder. As we will see throughout this chapter, the logics of Tibetan medicine were never fully factored out—nor was a seamless translation necessarily desired by those participating in the project of automating and computerizing this style of pulse diagnosis. As such, it is useful to locate the APDC in relation to a history of Soviet scientific imaginaries, ones that often explicitly and consciously sought to articulate a developmental trajectory distinct from that of "Western" science (Krementsov 2006, 2011). Second, the APDC can be understood as the materialization of the convergent—and sometimes divergent—"epistemic cultures" (Cetina 1999) of radiophysicists, engineers, clinicians, and *emchi* practitioners, and of the resulting claims about what the pulse is (or should be) in the first place.

Designing the APDC was concerned with making Tibetan medicine *real*, in a uniquely Soviet rationalist inflection: a project of epistemic validation that was premised on reimagining it away from the optics of religious "superstition" and toward a logic of code breaking and uncovering the "truth" beneath its religious symbolism. It was also concerned with making Tibetan medicine portable: for taking it away from the particularities of any given practitioner's embodied palpation skill and with bringing it, ideally, into any standardized clinical space. However, as we will see, projects of dissemination also produce rootedness in unexpected ways and in unlikely places. Although the pulsometer is presented and deployed as an imaging technology that claims to standardize pulse diagnosis, its design and recruitment into various research projects center around its prosthetic function. In turn, these prosthetic qualities complicate the possibilities of "factoring out" the embodied skills of the *emchi*, on which the pulsometer is modeled, or the equally embodied expertise of its users. As I explore later, the pulsometer is a kind of symbiotic prosthesis that demands of those who use it as a diagnostic tool a new embodied engagement of Tibetan medicine and its multiple practitioners, exceeding the boundaries of the laboratory and forging surprising alliances across epistemic borders. The device also does other work, such as authorizing the traditional knowledge of Tibetan medicine, paradoxically not simply by demonstrating that there is more to the pulse than biomedicine typically notices, but because to access this excess of meaning, and to be able to adequately interpret it, one needs to have—or slowly approximate, by mediation of the pulsometer—the embodied and largely inalienable expertise of the *emchi*.

Both Western and certain Russian-language accounts of Soviet scientific projects have tended to focus on the peculiarities of Soviet and postsocialist science, either by pointing to its tight entanglements with the state's military interests and to the difficulties of transitioning to an R&D model or by cataloguing the irrationally scandalous "dead ends" of scientific efforts too heavily marked by the state's ideological demands.[3] By contrast, I am intrigued by the possibilities of excavating, at the heart of Soviet aspirations to a rationalist, scientific modernity, with its claims to bearing (and perfecting) the ideals of European Enlightenment (without all the capitalist and colonial baggage), a different set of epistemic practices—ones that neither affirm a universalist narrative of scientific progress nor relegate "non-Western" (or non-capitalist) science to "non-science." By paying close attention to the internal workings of the pulsometer, both literally and figuratively, I am interested in complicating narratives that frame endeavors of scientific and technological incorporation of "traditional" knowledge as always and necessarily exercises in epistemic colonization. My point is that the pulsometer is an "other" to both the traditional practices of Tibetan medicine in Buryatia and to Euro-American biomedical imaginaries, but that its creation and implementation shed light on the ways in which Soviet and present-day physicists, engineers, and clinicians attempted, certainly from their own situated perspectives, to seriously engage with epistemological alterity.

THE PULSOMETER AS UNRELIABLE WITNESS

Within Ulan-Ude's varied therapeutic geography, which comprises a diverse range of practitioners, from lamas and shamans to biomedically trained doctors, as well as a number of "traditional healers" who straddle these more standard categories and thus resist easy classification, the ability to use the pulse for the purposes of diagnosis is often taken to be the marker of an *emchi*'s professional identity. While patients sometimes listed specialists in Traditional Chinese Medicine as another kind of pulse expert, the ability to diagnose "by the pulse," often without relying on other means, tended to stand in metonymically for the whole of what it meant to be practicing Tibetan medicine.

While pulse diagnosis is widespread in TCM, the practitioners of Tibetan medicine I interviewed in Buryatia frequently reminded me that the Tibetan style of pulse-taking was unique, methodologically and conceptually distinct from pulse diagnosis deployed in other medical traditions. By contrast, both practitioners of Tibetan medicine and researchers whose careers are tethered to its study argued that "modern" (Western) medicine conceptualizes the pulse in a narrow, specialized way, as solely indicative of the state of the cardiovascular system. This distinction was not always framed as a sign of epistemological incommensurability. Instead, both practicing *emchi* and scientists tended to attribute it to the peculiar historical amnesia characteristic of "modern" medicine: in its pursuit of ever more cutting-edge pharmaceutical technologies and surgical interventions, biomedicine had forgotten its Galenic roots.

Yet, these differences frequently became a source of deep puzzlement, especially for those practitioners who came to Tibetan medicine from a scientific or biomedical background. *Emchi* and researchers alike seemed to draw a kind of troubled pleasure from the apparent incommensurability between the different kinds of diagnostic palpations. "You don't take the pulse in the same points in TCM," Tsyrenma told me during an afternoon discussion over beer. "But even in those points that overlap, they don't correspond to the same organs. And yet, both diagnose correctly—how is that possible?" Tsyrenma's comment echoed frequently through my conversations with different practitioners, as well as those researchers interested in "deciphering" and standardizing Tibetan medicine for clinical use. Invoking divergent correspondences between the "points" on the wrist where the practitioner's fingers press into the skin to detect the texture of pulsations and distinct therapeutic cosmologies that recognize the expressions of primary elements—or, in the case of "modern" medicine, none at all—my interlocutors frequently mused that "Tibetan," "Chinese," and "Western" medicine all managed to arrive to the same conclusion, even when their respective practices of pulse taking indexed incompatible methodologies and epistemological assumptions about the origins of illness, the nature of bodies, or the determinants of health.

In part, this sense of puzzlement is predicated on a linguistic peculiarity—that pulse diagnosticians in different traditions are largely doing the same thing, which is to say, "listening" to the pulse (*slushayut pul's* in Russian). By contrast, most patients and practitioners I interviewed in Buryatia used a different phrase—*smotret' po pul'su*, or "to look on the basis of the pulse." While pulse-taking is by no means the only way in which Tibetan medicine practitioners determine from which ailments their patients suffer, in Buryatia it has become iconic of the *emchi*'s practice. Scientists and medical doctors, as well as some practitioners who tend to critique the ways in which biomedicine generates knowledge about patients' bodies, see the merits of pulse diagnosis in its noninvasiveness and relative simplicity. In part, these very qualities make Tibetan medical knowledge about the pulse appear esoteric. For practicing *emchi*, listening to the patient's pulse is as important and time-consuming as listening to her words. For patients, an inability to read the pulse exclusively, which is to say, to be unable to derive an accurate and convincing diagnosis without relying on information gathered outside of the immediate, tactile, and usually silent encounter of pulse-taking, is often construed as a sign of therapeutic incompetence. Although the majority of patients who visit an *emchi* tend to have some form of biomedical diagnosis at their disposal, it is not uncommon to withhold it in order to check if the *emchi* might figure it out on his or her own. In a therapeutic context where the "realness" of Tibetan medicine is constantly questioned, checking the pulse goes both ways.[4]

Canonical Buddhist texts on Tibetan medicine, such as the *Gyüshi*, *Vandurya-Onbo*, and *Lhantab*, discuss pulse diagnosis as a source of information that may speak of many other aspects of life, taken broadly, and not exclusively about illness. Each organ has its own pulse, and the pulses of different *nyes pa* (culprits) have their own distinct characteristics. Each person has her own unique "innate" pulse, which may be male, female, or neutral, and it is this background that will give relevance to any subsequent interpretation. Pulse-taking as it is described in the Tibetan medical canon blends the line between diagnosis and divination (Connor and Samuel 2001), and the pulse can be read for many different insights—for example, to distinguish different types of bodily and psychological constitutions, to predict a couple's likelihood of conceiving a boy or a girl, to divine the length of one's life and the time of death, to anticipate the outcome of treatment, or to detect the presence of nonhuman agencies causing the disease.

It is as oriented toward the future as it is toward the present. A similar logic applies to urine diagnosis, another method often associated with Tibetan medicine, but practiced much less frequently in Ulan-Ude, partly because of its "inconvenience"—the practice of "*sdavat' mochu*" (Rus.), "turning in urine" for testing—is so strongly associated with a biomedical setting that most Tibetan medicine practitioners in the city are reluctant to request it from their patients and will do so only in extreme cases, or when an accurate diagnosis eludes them. While both urine and the pulse may speak of much more than specific biomedical diagnoses or immediate bodily processes, in the day-to-day experiences of Ulan-Ude practitioners and patients of Tibetan medicine, "hearing the pulse" to detect illness and determine treatment is the main diagnostic modality.

The experience of pulse-reading stands in stark contrast to the ways in which the body is made legible in biomedical practice. Pulse-reading skirts the materialities of bodily tissues and fluids and focuses on elusive flows. It is both fundamentally local and momentary, yet it is often made to speak of the recurrent tendencies of particular bodies and geographically localized populations—Russians, Buryats, Tibetans, "Westerners." Both patients and researchers often mentioned to me that a skilled practitioner requires no complex medical technology or equipment, no physiologically and psychologically traumatic interventions into the body, no expensive and time-consuming tests, and no team of additional experts to generate a fairly accurate interpretation of her patient's ailments and medical history. Pulse-taking cuts across the bureaucracies of medical infrastructures, the separation of lab work and clinic, and the uphill battle of obtaining a referral. Ironically, the desire to mechanize pulse diagnosis would introduce exactly those elements of additional mediation that both researchers and patients articulate as undesirable characteristics of the medical encounter.

Most research projects organized around Tibetan medicine in Russia take for their main goal the "objectivization" and "deciphering" of *emchi* knowledge and practice. Local scientists and scholars working with Tibetan medicine conceptualize their activities as having two components— making Tibetan medicine speak in the language of "Western" biomedicine and "cracking" its "code" through the methods of modern science. For contemporary researchers involved in this field, the problem is thus not whether Tibetan medicine "works" or whether it might contain something "valuable"—and, arguably, this question was not at the forefront for those earlier debates over Tibetan medicine I detailed in Chapter 1. Most contemporary scholarly accounts published in Russia, and in Buryatia especially, argue that the question is moot—the fact that Tibetan medicine had been successfully used in the region for far longer than Western medicine and, some scholars argue, has contributed to the spread of Buddhism serves as proof of its utility (see Nikolaev 1998). The stakes, in many ways, have remained the same then and now—the question is whether it works for the right reasons.

Popular literature and film on Tibetan medicine in Russia tend to emphasize a sense of secrecy, as the title of "Secrets of Tibetan Medicine" characterizes a number of different works that promise to unravel its hidden message. In other words, Tibetan medicine as a set of textual artifacts salvaged and archived in the aftermath of Stalinist antireligious repressions, but also as a local form of lived knowledge and practices, captured what Chadha (2010) referred to as the "cryptographic imagination" of researchers and scientists. In discussing the influence of military deciphering technologies on the ways in which archaeologists conceptualized the nature of ancient scripts, Chadha argues that in the aftermath of World War II, translating ancient scripts became viewed as a type of code breaking, best served, much like the military projects of deciphering, by a scientific, mathematical approach to linguistic signs and the deployment of computers.

Translating Tibetan medicine in Buryatia, whether defined as a practice of commensuration or of code breaking, is as dependent on a preexisting history of conceptual assemblages and entanglements between Soviet medicine and certain branches of science, notably radiophysics and magnetic fields research, as it is on current projects of clinically deploying "Eastern" medicine in state healthcare institutions. As I have argued in Chapter 1, efforts to translate the therapeutic practices associated with Tibetan medicine to a variety of different media, languages, and therapeutic contexts have a long history in Russia, and especially in Buryatia. Developing the pulsometer is one such project. It has been one of the major directions of scientific research into Tibetan medicine in Buryatia for almost three decades. By the time of my fieldwork in Ulan-Ude, several generations of the automated pulse diagnosis complex had replaced their predecessors, and different versions were deployed both for therapeutic and for research purposes in at least four major institutions in the city: the East-West Medical Center; the Buryat Science Center; the State University; and the Hospital of War Veterans.

For the last thirty-some years of its multiple incarnations, the pulsometer has remained curiously always on the brink of emergence, neither fully authorized in clinical practice in Russia nor relegated to dusty oblivion as yet another useless dead end. While it is deployed in clinical settings, the APDC locally bears the veneer of a technology of the future, one whose potential applications are yet to be mined to their fullest. Nor is the APDC an entirely "local technology," on the model of the "local biologies" or culture-bound syndromes catalogued in the medical anthropology literature (see Kleinman 1980; Scheper-Hughes 1992; Lock and Nguyen 2018). One of its versions is registered in Russia's patent system, and its deployment in research settings successfully recruits federal financing. There is also a history of developing a pulsometer in Chinese medicine, although its popularity in clinical practice seems to have dwindled (Farquhar 2014). For scientists working on the APDC, the goal was to harness the cultural heritage of Buryatia's involvement with Tibetan medicine by designing a unique pulsometer, one that would be distinct from the Chinese counterparts based on the pulse-taking practices of TCM.

Conceptually, this chapter straddles the pulsometer's multiple entanglements in the Tibetan medicine community of Ulan-Ude, following the histories of its creation and testing in order to illuminate some of the ways in which "pulsometry" in present-day Buryatia is mobilized to address and comment on how Tibetan medicine might come to bear on the vitality of bodies and populations. I explore the questions and claims that scientists working with the pulsometer ask of the device in order to turn it into what Isabelle Stengers has called a "reliable witness" (Stengers 2003), a technical assemblage that the experimenter can mobilize to affirm the factuality of the phenomena that are put into question and to distinguish facts from artifacts. With the pulsometer, these two elements of the device's "witnessing" map onto different domains of application that are not separate in practice. To put it more concretely, as a *measuring* device at the research and design stage, the pulsometer would need to "objectivize" the pulse by confirming that the pulse of Tibetan medicine may speak to more than blood flow in the ulnar vein and artery as exclusively a correlate of the body's cardiovascular status. In other words, it must generate an image of the pulse—the pulsogram—such that it can be analyzed to index multiple processes within the body, not just the work of the heart and vascular system. Conversely, as a *diagnostic* tool in a clinical setting, the pulsometer must generate information about recurrent and systematic bodily states rather than ephemeral circumstantial changes: "data" must be easily sortable from "white noise," fact from artifact. Throughout the local histories of its design and use, the pulsometer systematically merged the lab and the clinic, failing to disaggregate its usefulness as a "witness" to the Tibetan pulse, from its ability to extrapolate from the pulse to the body. As I will argue, it is precisely this apparent failure that makes it a surprising site for forming new kinds of alliances and bridges between communities of experts, connecting the otherwise separate worlds of praxis of scientists and *emchi*.

As a diagnostic modality, pulse-taking in Tibetan medicine does not lend itself easily to conversion into a medical object, alienable from the concrete moment of the encounter between the practitioner and the patient. There is nothing about the pulse as it is apprehended by Tibetan medicine practitioners in Buryatia that an expert can present to the patient or to other experts without the mediation of another moment of pulse-taking by another observer, on a body that, at this new moment in time, has already subtly changed. For the physicists working on the APDC, showing the pulsogram became an opportunity to measure a phenomenon seen as imprecise and subjective with existing scientific tools. Meanwhile, the "pulsogram"—the graphic representation of the oscillations in the skin surface above the "pulse points"—became a snapshot of a moment, one that would mediate the event of pulse-taking such that it could theoretically be converted into an autonomous medical object, much like an X-Ray or an MRI image: one that could be archived and revisited. The possibility of "seeing" the pulse—rather than hearing or feeling it—became at once a way in which its diagnostic potentials are validated for researchers interested in "objectivizing" Tibetan pulse-reading and a way to circulate it as a record of a clinical event.

Like many other medical images, the pulsogram requires interpretation and translation.[5] Unlike its "static" counterparts, the pulsogram is an image of *time*, rather than *space*—a number of temporally aggregated pulsations in the form of an oscillatory function. The temporal nature of this image has two sets of implications. First, the pulsogram requires an interpreter who will link the changes in the oscillatory function's profile to broader conclusions about the body. For the purposes of clinical practices, the pulsogram requires another image to represent it, a two-step translation that converts the recording of the pulse into a schematic image of the body's internal processes and states. Second, unlike those images that represent *spaces* inside the body, whether static structures (like the X-ray) or frozen images of metabolic flow (like the MRI), the pulsogram reveals no self-evident truth about the body. It requires a series of frequently experimental or hypothetical mathematical manipulations that might shed light on what the pulsogram says back to the canonical literature on the properties of the pulse, to the patient's physiological and emotional experiences, and to the *emchi*'s embodied skill of taking and interpreting the pulse. As a result, the image of the pulse is neither self-explanatory nor an easily mobilizable rhetorical text. "Objectivizing" the pulse—that is, making it "objective" by detethering it from the subjective apprehension of a specific practitioner at a particular moment of encounter—does not yet equate to "objectifying" it by turning it into an autonomous medical object able to speak "for itself." It is thus not the image of the pulse wave, but the imaging technology (the device that generates the pulsogram) that figures at the center of the hopes and hype of deploying a "scientific" version of Tibetan medicine in Buryatia.

By pointing to the ambiguities inherent in the pulsometer, I do not mean to suggest that the device was the result of "bad science" or improperly conducted research and design. Instead, I argue that what makes the pulsometer efficacious for a number of different projects in the community is precisely that it is an *unreliable* witness, one that had to constantly recruit other experts to bear witness to itself. In other words, the trouble with the APDC, as well as the reason for its productiveness, is not just that the images it generates require authoritative interpretation—in this sense, it would be no different than any other imaging technology. It is that it constantly defers the possibility of final and definitive interpretation—whether of the pulse or of the body—and therefore mobilizes a number of other allies in a gridlock of mutual authorization.

FROM "WITCHOLOGY" TO RADIOBIOLOGY: EASTERN MEDICINE AND SOVIET IMAGING PROJECTS

The effort to mechanize Tibetan pulse-taking was started in Ulan-Ude in 1983 by a professor of physical and mathematical sciences, Dr. Chimit Tsyrenovich Tsydypov (1925–91), and his team of researchers. Originally focused primarily on radiophysics, Tsydypov's interests progressively expanded to include biophysics, and the last project of his long research career became the "objectivization of the diagnostic methods of Tibetan medicine"—in practice, the development of the "Automated Pulse Diagnostic Complex." The original project of creating the APDC owes much to a particular legacy of Soviet medical imaging technologies. Tsydypov's research was articulated against the background of an emergent scientific field, one that brought together radiophysics and biophysics. Formulated by Professor Yuri Vasylyevich Guljaev, the director of the Radio-Engineering and Electronics Institute (REI) of the Soviet Academy of Sciences, and Eduard Godik, the head of the Radioelectronic Diagnostic Methods Laboratory in Moscow, the new field was labeled "biomedical radiophysics," and its main goal was the scientific investigation of paranormal phenomena and, in particular, of ESP. The specific project of studying ESP was given the title "the physical fields and radiation of the human body."

According to Eduard Godik's memoir, in 1981 the REI began a new research project, prompted by a directive coming "from above": to figure out the scientific basis for "extrasensory perception" (Godik 2010). Godik, the leading scientist who had been assigned to this task by his hierarchical superior Y. V. Guljaev, explained the sudden interest in these distinctly "nonmaterialist" phenomena on the part of the party elite with reference to the stagnation of Soviet society, and specifically of its ruling class. Much as prerevolutionary Russia had been fascinated with spiritism and the occult, Godik argued, so were the aging party cadres of the 1970s and 1980s and the Soviet population more broadly captured by the seemingly miraculous capacities of the *extrasensy*.

Godik was a graduate of the prestigious physics department of the Moscow State University; he specialized in the properties of semiconductors and had little interest in what he jokingly referred to as *ved'mologiia*, or "*witchology*"—despite the constant media hype around "unexplainable" phenomena like remote healing and telekinesis that peppered the Soviet media. In hindsight, Godik suggests that the Soviet governmental elite's panics around Brezhnev's aging body brought this popular interest to scientific visibility and secured support—if not full-fledged financing—for research into discovering the nature of the human "biofield" and the various kinds of "information" it might contain.

This concern with "information" as a property of living organisms is closely entangled with the discourses of Soviet cybernetics, as well as to a broader interest in "extrasensory" experiences (and laboratory experiments), investigated by both Soviet and American defense intellectuals in the 1960s and 1970s (see Lemon 2018; Velminski 2017). While cybernetics as a discipline was reviled under Stalinism, by the late 1950s the attitude toward it had progressively reversed, and cybernetics became envisioned as a potential meta-discipline capable of uniting disparate scientific fields, like mathematics, physics, biology, and linguistics. Gerovitch (2004) documents the establishment of "cyberspeak"—what he terms a pidgin language in the scientific "trading zone" that Soviet proponents of cybernetics hoped would eventually permeate all scientific domains. Envisioned as an organizing meta-level theory, Soviet cybernetics made room for and recruited forms of knowledge previously rejected by Soviet ideology, such as genetics, and recast such problematic scientific pursuits in the "coded" language of "cyberspeak" (Gerovitch 2004, 213). Conversely, "radio-physics" and "radio-biology" often stood in for genetics and molecular biology.

The REI was chosen to host the project of ESP investigation and had several well-known *extrasensy*, notably Juna Davitashvili, one of the most famous mediums in the USSR, and subsequently Russia, affiliated with it for research purposes. For Godik and his initially small team of young recruits selected from the top physics departments of the state, the goal was to show the "objective" reality underlying certain phenomena that had the general public and many of his academic peers convinced that there were forces at work that contemporary science had no way of explaining.

The new research project took off rather successfully, although, according to Godik, his team struggled to procure financing, a laboratory space, and equipment in the context of the late Soviet bureaucracy. The project recruited a number of *extrasensy* as collaborators in the experiments and applied and perfected techniques of remote sensing taken from military and cosmic science to assess the changes happening in the bodies of *extrasensy* and their clients. At the core of their scientific query was the question of the "biofield," a shorthand term that had been in circulation in the popular media and among the lay population to designate a hypothetical force field surrounding all living organisms, and whose interaction with other biofields might account for the efficacy of *extrasensy* healing. For Godik, however, the task was not to look for an unknown force, but to focus on the known properties of a living organism—namely, its bioelectric activity, and with the ensuing electromagnetic thermal radiation. Because assessing the bioelectric activity of bodily organs on the surface of the body is complicated by the variable conductivity of bodily tissues (so, for example, muscles do not conduct electricity as well as fat), obtaining a picture of what goes on "inside" the body by measuring its surface currents is a challenge. Instead, Godik and his team focused on measuring the electromagnetic fields of the body, since magnetic radiation passes through tissues more or less unimpeded (Godik 2010, 21). This research required the team to come up with methodological innovations. In order to increase the sensitivity of their measurements, the team used an infrared thermal imaging device that recorded changes in surface temperature but had to increase its precision by improving the frequency to twelve frames per second to create a "dynamic" representation of minute fluctuations in body temperature.

It is outside the scope of this chapter to detail the different experiments that Godik's team conducted: not all of them targeted ESP, and some, such as the development of thermal mammography, eventually found a secure place in biomedical practice. Instead, I will focus on one specific aspect of their research, most indicative of the ways in which their findings prompted the team to reconsider the nature of bodies, health, and medical knowledge and to ultimately turn to "Eastern" medicine as the next horizon of research. Dynamic thermal imaging was important in analyzing the processes that took place when an *extrasens* treated a patient without touching the skin. The team measured the changes in temperature for patients suffering from obliterating endarteritis of the feet caused by smoking. Seeing the gradual improvement in skin surface temperature that followed the *extrasens*'s hand movement over the patient's legs, a change made visible with the help of their "tweaked" thermal imaging equipment, Godik formulated several working hypotheses by way of a possible explanation. First, the improvement could be simply because palms also emit infrared radiation and act as a kind of "shield" against thermal loss from the skin surface, thus increasing the temperature of the area they are moving over. This explanation appeared viable while the team worked with healthy patients—there was no statistically significant difference between the heating effects of the skin surface induced by the *extrasens*'s hand and from that of a "regular" researcher not endowed with the elusive "gift" of ESP. However, the hypothesis became more problematic when a seriously ill patient responded only (and dramatically) to the *extrasens*'s manipulations. At this point, Godik proposed a psychological explanation, akin to the placebo effect. It is possible, he concluded, that the *extrasens* subtly cues the patient's subconscious to self-regulate through a variety of nonverbal gestures that accompany the "healing" hand movements. However, in a later experiment, once again with a patient suffering from smoker's foot, the team had received a request from the Chinese embassy to test a qigong master visiting the Soviet Union. Working with his hypothesis that it was the immediacy of the interaction between patient and healer that enabled the healer to psychologically "mobilize" the body's self-regulatory capacities, Godik proposed for the qigong practitioner to position himself near the patient. To Godik's surprise and confusion, the practitioner declined, and sat out of view. The recording equipment, once again trained on the patient's feet, recorded the changes in surface temperature as Godik silently cued the qigong master to begin or terminate his "influence" on the patient. The equipment recorded changes that corresponded to the intended periods of "influence," which forced Godik to reconsider and expand his working model.

From these different experiments, Godik and his team drew several conclusions. First, that the human body was a complex self-regulatory system, and its capacity to "perceive" information was not limited to those signals it could consciously apprehend. From this perspective, he writes, the term "extrasensory" no longer irritated him as much as it had at the beginning of his and his team's research efforts. It is quite possible, he decided, that an informational exchange was happening between the patient and the qigong master at a level that had nothing to do with visual cues—this was not a problem for physicists, then, but for psychologists and physiologists. Second, contemporary medicine and science were becoming increasingly specialized, and therefore finding experts capable of a "systemic" approach to the body, as opposed to burrowing deeper into the body's micro-structures, was becoming a serious challenge for conducting the kind of interdisciplinary "systems" research that the team had set out to do. Third, different senses were mutually imbricated, and the totality of sensory perception could be organized in different ways, not to mention trained, as the qigong master's skill seemed to suggest. As proof of this interrelatedness of the senses, Godik lists pulse diagnosis in "Eastern medicine":

> The core of diagnostics in Eastern medicine, which is to say pulse diagnosis, differentiates between about a hundred different sound images: from "hollow" pulse to different kinds of fillings, like "bubbling" and so forth. At the same time, the pulse is not perceived with the ear, but through the tactile receptors at the end of the fingers. . . . But the result is "colored" and distinguished in the auditory spectrum. The interaction between different analyzers, not just of the tactile and the aural, but of the visual as well (the simplest example is the reading of music) increases the potential for pattern recognition by combining the strengths of different sensory modalities. (Godik 2010, 106)

That other medical traditions offered radically different sensory assemblages—a conclusion Godik eventually used to explain his lab's findings—promised that their study could shed light on the phenomena that his team had been able to document, but not explain. It is precisely in Eastern medicine that Godik sought to find a "systemic" view he felt lacking in contemporary Western medicine and science—one that trained the kind of "spontaneous" and random manifestation of healing skills he had documented among the *extrasensy* he worked with and elevated it to the level of art. He saw his laboratory as ideally suited for further research into Eastern medicine—both as a response to a perceived urgency linked to Eastern medicine's projected disappearance under the onslaught of globalization and Western science and because the equipment and methodology they had developed could show the way forward in integrating traditional and modern medicine, thereby transforming the former from an "art form" into a "technology."

Tsydypov had met Godik in Moscow and had several discussions with him on the phone regarding the possibility of "automatizing" Tibetan medicine pulse diagnosis—Godik was both supportive of and excited about this proposal (Godik, personal correspondence, 2011). After several trips and meetings in Moscow, Tsydypov managed to secure approval for his new project in Buryatia, in spite of the skepticism among his colleagues in the other departments of the Buryat Science Center. In its first stages, the lab consisted of four researchers, one office doubling as lab space, and two research themes: the "objectification of Tibetan pulse diagnostic methods" and "the influence of magnetic fields on the human body." In relation to the latter project, it should be noted that research into the effects of electromagnetic radiation was also carried out at REI, under the administrative supervision of Nikolaj Dmitrievich Deviatkov (1907–2001), who was later credited with developing the first electromagnetic therapeutic device "Istok." Eventually, electromagnetic therapy was officially recognized by the Soviet Ministry of Health and then by Russia's Ministry of Health as a valid form of complementary treatment for various pre- and post-surgery health concerns.

Since its inception, the APDC has been a surprisingly cosmopolitan machine, considering the selectively permeable borders of the Soviet state and its impeded internal flows. Following Tenzin Choedrak's visit, a contract for collaboration and "expertise exchange" with Men Tsee Khang in India was drafted but was forgotten in the tumult of the collapse of the Soviet Union in 1991. Around the same time, in 1989, and then in the early 1990s, a large delegation of specialists from the Medical University of Huhhot (Inner Mongolia, China) came to observe the research and assess its effectiveness. Several of the visitors were recruited to lend their expertise, and the head of the delegation spent time testing his palpation skills against the APDC. As in the case of Tenzin Choedrak, consensus was found—the APDC came to the same conclusions as the pulse diagnostic specialist.

The device survived the turbulent early nineties and continued to develop. In 1993, the laboratory submitted an application to Russia's Federal Bureau of Intellectual Property, Patents, and Commercial Orders and received a patent in 1997. The APDC was submitted under the heading of "Pulse Measuring Device" and was classified with other medical technologies designed to record the heartbeat: no reference to Tibetan medicine or explanations as to why the pulse was recorded in six separate places were mentioned. In 2005, the Russian minister of economic development and trade Herrmann Graf, while on an assessment tour of the Russian Far East for investment potential, came to visit the research facility and underwent diagnosis. After this visit, Graf's team issued a favorable assessment of Buryatia's potential for developing tourism and "health tourism" related to Tibetan medicine in particular.

Over the years of its development, the APDC took many forms and recruited a number of technologies, devices, and specialists. Its shiny white plastic body is made in Novosibirsk. The role of the thick plastic is to insulate the sensitive electronics from external interference and mechanical damage. In one of its earliest incarnations, the APDC's body was a metal instant-coffee can—a visibly marked "Western" commodity, gained in a rare feat of procurement in the Soviet economy of shortage and scarcity of foreign products. The APDC's sensors—the black piezo-ceramic semi-spheres on the cuffs, aimed to mimic the fingertips of the expert *emchi*—were made by a laboratory in L'viv in Ukraine. Most of the microchips that constitute its inside were imported from China and Taiwan. The software that handles the data was written locally, but originally required several large superconductor-based computers—the "huge wardrobe-sized monsters" that Vitaly Vasylievich recalled with amused fondness—to process it. With time, the computers got smaller and more efficient, the cuffs transformed from a pneumatic "sleeve" to adhesive Velcro, and the coffee can remained only in the memory of the original researchers.

As the pulse diagnostic machine materialized these disparate transnational networks and flows, and despite its anticipated horizons of standardization-enabled circulation, it remained stubbornly and productively localized and localizing. The next section outlines some of the difficulties and anxieties generated around the production of knowledge enabled by the APDC. It uses ethnographic description to trace the establishment of a research project that attempts to use Tibetan pulse diagnosis, among other diagnostic modalities, to evaluate the state of health of the student population at a local university. Tibetan medicine practitioners working in more traditional settings question its validity, insisting that even though it might measure *something*, that something is probably not what is meant by Tibetan pulse diagnosis. Presently, the APDC still generates critiques and skepticism that resonate closely with those that emerged around its inception in the early 1980s.

By the time the APDC project was conceived in the 1980s, research into Tibetan medicine had already been underway in Buryatia, especially in the field of Tibetan pharmacology, and predated Tsydypov's proposed project by almost fifteen years. As such, Tsydypov's efforts entered a preexisting field of active and well-established scholarship at the Buryat Science Center, especially in the humanities, social sciences, and botany, and it initially generated skepticism and resistance. The skeptics came from different fields of expertise—historians of Tibetan medicine, physicists, and biomedical doctors—and shared a surprising consensus. Doubt was articulated on epistemological grounds. Viktor Pupyshev, a recognized local scholar and translator of Tibetan medical literature and later Tibetan medicine practitioner, cautioned against the imposition of "our" scientific categories onto the ways in which the body was articulated through Tibetan medical knowledge:

> We have developed our own forms of description and understanding, and the assertion that only through these forms everything can be described and understood would seem rather strange. Yet, we often stubbornly attempt to pour the phenomenon of Tibetan medicine into the molds of our habitual systems, ignoring, as we do so, the tenet about the identity of form and content that we all [claim to] accept. . . . Here, to search for the solely "rational" in Tibetan medicine, along with the expected limitations we postulate in advance, may turn out to be a quest for the familiar and a denial of all that might not fit within the frames of our habitual system, and potentially challenge them. (Pupyshev 1989)

For the physicists developing the APDC, the problem lay precisely in sorting the rational from the irrational, the "real" from everything else. In a sense, the task of "objectivizing" knowledge was not a new concept for Soviet science and was not solely applied to thinking about "traditional" or "nonscientific" forms of expertise. A similar orientation toward "Western" (which is to say, non-socialist) science was in circulation in the scientific community at the beginning of the Cold War. This was a creative strategy espoused by some researchers in response to party invectives promising to "surpass and overtake" Western science, while developing a distinctly Soviet and politically appropriate philosophy of knowledge (Gerovitch 2004).

Vitaly Vasylyevich, Tsydypov's student, explained to me that the conceptual problem for the research, from its inception, was the feeling that "pulse-taking" is a type of art. Echoing Godik's own formulation on the subject but coming to a less optimistic conclusion, Vitaly Vasilyevich initially suspected that because pulse diagnostics was an art, or embodied skill, a scientific approach would have a hard time explaining it, let alone reproducing it. As research progressed, however, the scientists became increasingly sure that hard science—and especially physics—could contribute significantly to getting to the heart of the pulse.

In some senses, scholars in the social sciences and humanities who cautioned their physicist colleagues against rash assumptions about what the pulse is were preaching to the choir. From the beginning, the scientists and researchers working on the pulsometer approached the device in a relatively open-ended fashion. First, they accepted the idea that there was something about the pulse that could be read beyond its expression of the state of the cardiovascular system and that the answers to what that something might be were already available in the Tibetan medicine canon, provided one could "decipher" it. In other words, despite the researchers' claims to "objectivize" the pulse, the APDC team never put in question whether the pulse had diagnostic properties. The task, then, was one of drawing correspondences between the qualities of the pulse described in the Tibetan medicine literature and accounted for by practitioners and the characteristics of whatever data the pulsometer would generate. Second, rather than assume ahead of time what, specifically, the pulsometer would measure, researchers working on the APDC approached the device as a "mimetic" project—their goal was a maximally precise emulation of the *emchi*'s skill. The question that the pulsometer asks, then, is not whether the pulse is diagnostically relevant, but whether the sensors of the APDC can imitate the *emchi*'s sensitive fingers and whether its software can match the *emchi*'s mind. In practice, reverse-engineering the *emchi*'s touch and thoughts meant that the researchers would try to envision what sorts of materials, electronic circuits, and physical concepts and phenomena might best stand in for what the *emchi* was doing. In 1988, Tsydypov wrote that the trouble with trying to "extract information" from the pulse through technological methods is that the pulse diagnostician:

> works in a sort of dialogical relationship: by varying the pressure, and the area of contact between the fingertips and the skin . . . , he alternately "interrogates" the 12 internal organs; he then laminates the results of this "survey" in his mind with the person's "congenital pulse" and, taking into account the season and daily biorhythms, comes to a conclusion about the state of the patient's body in its totality. (Tsydypov 1988)

Thus, before the problem of how one might be able to make the machine truly interactive could be solved, the task was to emulate the *emchi*'s fingers on the patient's wrist and to determine what the sensors that stood for the diagnostician's fingertips would, in fact, "sense." What kind of *data* would provide information for the diagnostician? While the scholars at the Buryat Science Center who worked on translating and interpreting Tibetan and Buryat texts intimated that the pulse in Tibetan diagnostics was not necessarily linked to blood flow but suggested a different system of channels that did not quite map onto a Western biomedical anatomy, the physicists at the lab were operating within a familiar phenomenology—that of radiophysics. Tsydyov himself remained cautious about jumping to conclusions, however: "We can't yet state with confidence *what* is in fact the carrier of information about bodily states—is it only the mechanical movement of the arterial wall?" (Tsydypov 1988, 17). Without a fuller project of "deciphering" canonical texts and interpreting the "theoretical premises" of Tibetan medicine, what Tibetan medicine meant by the pulse remained uncertain.

These conceptual difficulties did not prevent the project from moving forward, and the way in which the researchers solved this impasse is important for understanding what the APDC in fact is. At first approach, the design of the original pulsometer might look like an effort at biomimicry, not so much in that it is an imitation of "natural" (albeit ecologically situated and adapted) life processes, but rather a mimetic replication of the *emchi*'s bodily skill. To imitate, one needs a model—not necessarily in the sense of an "original" from which a copy is made, although this aspect figured prominently in the design of the APDC, but also as an organizing conceptual description of what is to be imitated. In this sense, the physicists working on the pulsometer already had a model of the *emchi*'s body: reduced to its relevant elements, the Tibetan medicine practitioner was a set of precise sensors outfitted with an information-processing unit. For Tsydypov, the difficulty in objectifying Tibetan medicine lay in the technical challenge of mechanically replicating what he called the "hypersensitive biological sensors"—the *emchi*'s fingertips. In other words, at its inception, the APDC was a "technomimetic" device: a machine imitating a body that was already a machine.

From this perspective, canonical texts could be used not as theory to be decoded, but as an instruction manual to the *emchi*-machine: instead of interpreting what pulsation in Tibetan medicine actually is, one could follow these texts as guides to technologically replicate the *emchi*'s touch and pragmatic interpretation. By reproducing the exact steps prescribed in the canon and recreating an electronic surrogate for the *emchi*'s expert fingers as precisely as possible, one would presumably be able to record data without needing to know what, specifically, is in fact being measured. The work of interpretation would then be done later by mapping it against the results from already available methods of biomedical imaging and by recruiting expert pulse diagnosticians to create a database of corresponding pulsograms and physical conditions. To create the surrogate for the *emchi*'s internal database, the physicists needed the clinic. By the late 1980s, the project had a clinical base at the Republican Clinical Hospital for War Veterans, a steady flow of test subjects, and the collaboration of a few biomedical doctors.

In practice, there is of course no way of building a device that is data-neutral, one that simply "perceives" without differentiation and does not already always interpret the information it receives. In order to "see" the pulse, one requires a series of conversions, or what linguistic anthropologist Webb Keane has called "translational ideologies" (see Keane 2007). For researchers attempting to produce the image of the pulse, these conversions necessarily occur between distinct and discrete modes of sensing: from touch to hearing to seeing. This is not necessarily the result of researchers conceptualizing these different senses as belonging to entirely separate realms of experience, but to the fact that in order to engineer a sensing device and an interpretative frame to process the data the sensor will generate, one must come to a decision about what the sensor will be measuring.

At the basis of the APDC was the hypothesis that the *emchi* was in fact reading a "pulse wave" as arterial blood was pushed from the heart through the radial artery toward the periphery and back again. Physicists and engineers working on the pulsometer conceptualized it from the start as a kind of prosthetic device that would reinterpret and replace the *emchi*'s embodied skill—the pulsometer as a virtual enhancing extension, to elaborate on Elizabeth Grosz's discussion of prosthesis (Grosz 2005), of a situated (Soviet, modern) body's inability or unwillingness to learn the sensory skill of the practitioner of Tibetan medicine. As a device enabling prosthetic sensing, the APDC had to replicate touch and convert it into sight via sound in order to make the pulse legible.

Because a variety of factors may, in fact, influence the characteristics of a pulse wave, including arterial blood pressure, the speed and intensity of cardiac contractions, the elasticity and tone of arterial walls, the textures of the pulse would presumably be varied enough to reflect the state of the body. But taking a wave to be the "ground" of analysis additionally complicated interpretation: as it travels along the blood vessel, the pulse wave would be reflected from the walls and interfere with itself, thus creating harmonics whose presence had to be accounted for, in some way or another, analytically and electronically, and subsequently tied to a diagnostic scenario (Boronoev, Dashinimaev, and Trubacheez 1988).

Physicists working on the project understood the *emchi*'s specific training to involve a type of "listening" to the pulse wave through palpation and proposed to analyze its characteristics, subsequently matching them to biomedical diagnoses. The very possibility of translating between one sense and another, between "hearing," "feeling," and "seeing," was crucial to the scientists' imagination of what the *emchi* was in fact doing and how science could replicate it and improve on it. In a sense, the interchangeability of different modes of "sensing" the pulse is reflected in the Russian expressions used to describe the process: the common term for qualifying what the *emchi* does is "*slushat' po pul'su*" (listening on the basis of the pulse) or "*smotret' po pul'su*" (to look based on the pulse). Thus, the *emchi*'s fingertips were equated to "biological sensors," while the *emchi* was construed to translate the feelings in the fingertips to sound: "The Eastern doctor listens to the artery as if it were a string resonating with the various physiological processes of the organism" (Logvinov 1988).

More recent accounts of the history of the pulsometer reveal the extent to which decoding and encoding the skill of the *emchi* already depended on viewing the practitioner as a kind of cyborg. In invoking the figure of the cybernetic organism, I draw on the one hand on Donna Haraway's reflections (1994) that the hybridity of the cyborg is one that rejects (or subverts) the utopia of primordial holism in favor of connections and the making of messy boundaries. On the other hand, I want to pay close attention to the imaginaries that informed the design of the pulsometer. It is precisely because the *emchi* was already understood in the idiom of cybernetics that the APDC functions as it does. In accounting for its history, a recent description of the APDC describes the device as follows:

> The end-goal of the research is the creation of a cognitive informational-calculative Tibetan medicine complex, represented in the synthesis of the automated pulse diagnostic complex (APDC) and an expert diagnostic system (EDS). The main purpose of the [diagnostic] complex is the imitation of the actions and thinking of the Tibetan doctor during the entire cycle of the therapeutic process: diagnosis, nosology, treatment. (Boronoev 2010)

Although, as we can see from the previous description, the model of the APDC assumes a certain Cartesian dualism in the sense of a stark division between mind and body, the final device aims at supplanting the entirety of the *emchi*'s embodied skill—from palpation to interpretation. In this sense, neither were scientists developing the device seduced by a promise of "holism"—they accepted the idea that their model was one of multiple interconnected functions whose relationship had to be theorized and engineered—nor did they hope to extract certain aspects of *emchi* embodied knowledge, but not others. Their project was one of total replication, or imitation—to create a functional prosthetic Tibetan medicine diagnostician.

THE CLOCKWORK *EMCHI*

In its present incarnation, the pulsometer is a white plastic box with a set of simple controls in the back: a fan, an on-off switch, a computer connection port, and two cables that extend to about a foot and a half away from the metal panel. At the end of each wire is a set of white Velcro cuffs, vaguely reminiscent of running shoes. Where the cuff wraps around the outside of the wrist, the cloth material sections off into three strips that can be individually tightened. On the inside of the wrist, a solid block of plastic is held inside the cuff to help keep it securely fastened to the skin. On the inside of the plastic block, pressed against the skin, are black rubber half-spheres of about two centimeters in diameter, three for each cuff. The pressure of these sensors against the skin can be adjusted by tightening or releasing the screws that run through each segment of the plastic block. For the duration of the diagnosis, the patient sits in a relaxed position, cuffs circling her wrists, her palms facing upward. One must maintain a relaxed position while simultaneously keeping the back relatively straight and the breath relatively even to optimize the accuracy of the device.

The six sensors, designed to imitate as closely as possible the fingertips, record the oscillation of the arterial wall. The "pulse wave" is then analyzed by a computer program that isolates its main characteristics—amplitude, frequency, contour—and compares them against a preexisting database of "normal" and "pathological" pulses. The final read-out is a series of colored pie charts that provide information about the state of different organs. Classically, Tibetan medicine recognizes five solid and six hollow organs, their pulse accessible at six different points, three on each wrist. Each point provides information on two organs simultaneously: the practitioner's fingertip is symbolically divided in half, such that the right side of the fingertip diagnoses one organ and the left one diagnoses another. In total, there are thus twelve pulses that relate to the functioning of each specific organ, except for the kidneys, where the pulse for the left and right kidneys are read separately (hence, twelve pulses). The final pie charts are meant to be self-explanatory, readable by doctors or technicians without a close knowledge of Tibetan medicine. The segments of the pie chart represent each organ with which Tibetan medicine is concerned and display whether it is functioning at optimal level or not. Excesses and deficiencies are displayed as asymmetries in the pie-chart segments: an optimally functioning body forms a circle, and all pathologies break its geometry, making it appear "shapeless" and irregular.

The series of experiments, entitled "Development of a monitoring system of student health using traditional medicine methods," were funded by a grant from the Russian federal government under the aegis of the

"Health Priority Project," an initiative started by Vladimir Putin in 2007 in response to the dire results of population and demographic studies. The HPP was especially concerned with the health of Russian youth, even if it largely formulated these concerns in the behavioral terms of "social ills" and "risk groups"—the state saw the future health of its population put at serious risk by what was being reported as rampant drug use, smoking, and high rates of alcohol consumption among students. In response to calls for programs that would help solve these problems, the scientists at the Institute for Innovative Technologies, an offshoot of the mathematics and computer science department at a local university in Ulan-Ude, proposed a project that would use a noninvasive procedure—Tibetan pulse diagnosis— to monitor students' health and aid in gathering statistical data about different student populations and their proneness to certain conditions. The advantages of this method, according to the IIT research team, would be twofold. On the one hand, unlike standard biomedical imaging technologies, such as the X-ray, ultrasound, ECG, blood analysis, and the more technologically intensive and expensive procedures like the CT scan, Tibetan pulse diagnosis, and a few other diagnostic methods that IIT mobilized, would be noninvasive. For Ayur, the diminutive, nervous, fast-talking mathematician and head of both the research project and the Institute, this "noninvasiveness" acquired a rich meaning, quite beyond its typical medical referentiality of a procedure that stays on the surfaces, without penetrating underneath the skin. Ayur was Buryat, but he spent most of his youth in Novosibirsk, where he was trained as a physicist and mathematician. Nonetheless, his interest in Tibetan medicine—and his dedication to finding scientific ways to engage with it and make it more widely available in Buryatia—were closely tied to his ethnic identity.

Students, Ayur felt, are a particular population, characterized by specific health patterns because they have neither the time nor the desire to take care of their health. "Running from one doctor to the next," a behavior locally described as a sort of pastime for the elderly and the idle, is not something that students are willing to do. Ayur commented that this has to do with the sense that doctors are frequently rude or judgmental, especially so when confronted with a younger demographic, and the procedures somehow humiliating—they are invasive in every way, encroaching on the young person's privacy. Tibetan medicine techniques, Ayur suggests, are ideally suited to this population for two reasons:

First, pulse diagnosis demands no invasive procedures, such as stripping down. Second, it can locate illness before it manifests itself clinically, and therefore prevent it.

In other words, Ayur conceptualized students as a particular type of "patients in waiting" (Sunder Rajan 2006), whose illnesses were not yet manifest because of their youth, and because of their unwillingness to go looking for them. For this reason, and because pulse diagnosis offered a way to anticipate disorders down the line based on evaluating physical tendencies in the present, they were, as a clinical population, not only conveniently available, but also a logical choice. In the long term, once all the procedures were in place, Ayur envisioned his research as something that would permit a mass-scale constant monitoring of the student population of SU—not so distinct from the preventative principles of "dispenserization" (*dispensarizatziia*), one of the hallmarks of Soviet medicine. It would discover what types of students might be more prone to certain types of diseases and injuries while helping prevent these problems before they could seriously impede academic and athletic performance. It would, moreover, map the student population according to the "constitutional types" that Tibetan medicine describes and thus offer them effective strategies in managing their own health and diet. Ayur often referred to himself as a "typical wind," with a great deal of irony, recruiting me into reading this constitution's signs on his physical appearance and deportment, and blamed his own afflictions on the predispositions on this *nyes pa* type, using his sense of success at managing the unruly culprits of his particular embodiment as proof of the usefulness of Sowa Rigpa. The rest of his lab engaged each other—and the interloping ethnographer—in frequent diagnostic banter, squinting and issuing bodily typifications that Tibetan medicine could help read from bodily surfaces: "You look like a wind-bile to me. Better not drink too much [alcohol], or heat will rise (*zhar podnimitsa*)." In August of 2009, when I began participant observation at the IIT lab, the research was still in the first phase of the experiment: its main goal was the calibration of all the technologies of envisioning and mapping bodies, populations, and habits that IIT had recruited.

At any given time, there were about ten students crammed into the long narrow office, which was cluttered with an assortment of miscellaneous computers, devices, tea kettles, and empty coffee cups. The students present were the first test subjects after the initial calibration tests, which the team had conducted on each other, and on whatever willing passerby would volunteer their time and wrists. Most of the students present were also semivoluntary participants. For some of these students, this was a personal favor to Pavel, one of the graduate students working on the project. As the captain of their wrestling team, he was expected by his supervisors to commandeer team members' time and physical presence. Partially, though, they were also the usual suspects—athletes are a frequently mobilized target research population at both SU and other institutions in Ulan-Ude for experiments that take Tibetan medicine as both analytical framework and object of study. For Ayur and his team, these students were also a convenient population, because the diagnostic technologies used to classify their bodies interpreted them with a predictable bias. As Pavel explained the color-coded pie chart that consistently showed red, "Athletes run a bit hot."

As Pavel recorded the readout from the computer screen on a paper, the students moved on to the next station, a desk crammed between a wall and an oversized couch in the long narrow room. There, Sergei waited with another incarnation of the pulsometer. This device is a small steel box made out of what appeared to be the body of a gutted hard drive. It sported no cuffs or piezoceramic sensors, but came with its own first-generation Asus netbook, specially dedicated to running the software necessary to interpret the pulsogram. The new device—referred to as "Computerized Pulse Diagnosis" or CPD, had a single sensor, which was, in fact, made from the earpiece from a set of headphones—literally, a technological chimera of "hearing" and "touching," since it was intended to record the pulse wave based on sound rather than pressure. Sergei, a radio-physicist who used to work for the Buryat Science Center but moved to Irkutsk and became a Tibetan medicine practitioner, developed the device, partly based on his experience with the APDC and partly from an extensive study of the Tibetan and Sanskrit classical texts on Tibetan medicine. He used the CPD in his practice to diagnose patients and provide them with medicines, advice, and recommendations about changing their lifestyle and diet.

Ayur and his team hoped to eventually replace the APDC with the CPD, not only because they felt that it was smaller and more portable, but also, and perhaps more importantly, because the ownership of APDC is a contested issue. While SU owns an APDC unit, it is officially assigned to a different department, and borrowing it for long-term research often amounts to a logistical and bureaucratic nightmare. In addition, Ayur sees the APDC as really belonging to its original developers—Tsydypov's lab at the Buryat Science Center. This claim of ownership extends far beyond the rights of use and can potentially taint any scientific research that might be carried out using the APDC, making its originality questionable and ushering in suspicions of plagiarism. The researchers at IIT frequently emphasized the specificity of their research methods in an effort to draw lines of distinctions between themselves and the research done at the Buryat Science Center. The strong link between the machine and its developer also extended to CPD, such that the IIT was actively looking to hire Sergei on a more permanent basis, and not only to purchase a prototype from him.

This strong connection between the developer of the device and the device itself is a curious feature of the pulsometer. After all, the aim of "objectifying" or standardizing a skill or practice is that a device could then replace the original, embodied expert and circulate freely between contexts and research sites, producing standard data regardless of where it is located or where it came from. Thus, for example, an electron microscope would be expected to perform similarly, with a known margin of error, independently of the research design that deploys it or who developed it, provided the technician who uses it follows the instructions. By contrast, neither the APDC nor the CPD is so easily alienable from its original creators.

Away from all the wires and screens, on the other side of the door, in the more spacious but equally crowded lobby, Tsyrenma and I sat at different ends of a desk. While I was charged with taking the students' blood pressure, after some suspicions about whether "Americans" knew how to use blood pressure monitors were cleared up, Tsyrenma sat with her hands folded, only a pen and pencil in front of her. Tsyrenma was classically trained in Tibetan medicine by one of the locally recognized Buryat keepers of the tradition. In 2009, she had left her job at East-West to practice at one of the Buddhist temples in Ulan-Ude. In addition to her practice at the temple, she was helping Ayur with his research after a mutual acquaintance recommended her as a potentially ideal consultant, since she was also a trained and licensed general physician. Tsyrenma's role was to palpate pulses as students circulated among the four different stations, each monitored by one of the members of the team: two versions of the pulse diagnostic system, one electroacupuncture reader, a thermometer, and a blood pressure monitor. The different data would then be compiled into a database, each result, including Tsyrenma's insights, checked against all the others and compared for consistency.

Ayur's research team took consistent deviation—along the lines of athletes running "hot" to be a significant research finding. On the one hand, it allowed the researchers to classify certain bodies and populations and connect their specific habits to the read-outs from the devices they used. Something about what athletes did made their bodies consistently different, a difference that "Tibetan medical technology" could identify. Much in the same way, Lydia, one of the senior mathematicians on the team, often observed that the thin young women that were occasionally recruited to participate in the tests were consistently found to have "cold in their kidneys" and an excess of "wind." She puzzled frequently at this consistency— "For some reason the girls are always nervous when they come in." While this led to some off-color jokes on Sergei's part as to why that could be the case, these findings were especially important in light of the constant sense of epistemological vertigo that using a single device for longitudinal studies created. In the initial phase of the experiments, each device was tested for how it performed over time on a single subject. The results were consistently inconsistent, fluctuating widely depending on the intensity of the pressure on the sensors and on various minute, temporary, and often intractable bodily fluctuations (digestion, levels of caffeine, breath, tiredness, psychological ease). Ayur's team thus took the consistency of output across devices (as opposed to with each single device) as something that eased the vertigo and anxiety of not knowing which measurements were significant and which were noise or an artifact of measuring. Cross-comparative studies allowed the data to appear "really there."

One of the main problems that the team saw in using the "old" pulse diagnostic device, the APDC, lay specifically in the ways in which it was designed to imitate the fingers of the *emchi*. As was described in the previous section, the idea behind APDC design is a type of reverse engineering— an imitation of what the skilled *emchi* is able to read with her fingertips. The device thus attempts to imitate the *emchi*'s hand—the three sensors on both cuffs stand for the fingertips of the practitioner; the device hardware and software are the *emchi*'s mind. Therein lies the difficulty. Unlike other technologies of diagnosing, especially the more conventional technologies of biomedical imaging, in the case of the *emchi* the moment of encounter between patient and diagnostician is two-sided and interactive. Ayur's own explanation of the difficulties of "objectivizing" pulse reading touches upon the impossibility of a perfect imitation. Upon my question about what the pulse diagnostic complex in fact records, he began with an explanation of how the process happens for a practitioner:

> Imagine when the *emchi* applies pressure to one of the points, he is sending a "wave" to the body, which gives a response. Based on the type of response he gets, he calibrates the pressure of his other fingertips to get more information. The practitioner does a systemic analysis in his head to determine what's wrong with the person and issues a diagnosis.

While a model where the *emchi* is already a kind of machine—a set of finger-sensors outfitted with a computer and a database of pulses made the project of automated pulse diagnosis conceivable in the first place—it left a technological remainder: the communicative aspect of reading the pulse. As Ayur described in somewhat mechanized terms, the *emchi* is constantly fine-tuning how deeply the fingertips are pressed into the flesh of the wrist in order to read what the pulse does in response to this pressure. Because the old APDC failed to approximate this constitutive interactivity—it wasn't as accurate a device as the *emchi*, because it was not as dialogical—Ayur was looking to find something better. In this way, the CPD was a closer approximation, because its readout was dependent on the level of pressure and reintroduced the capacity to vary it. The trade-off was that it required a significantly higher degree of embodied skill on the part of the researcher. Sergei's presence in the lab was thus as much for research as for training others to use the CPD.

The pulse itself is an elusive, yet highly tactile phenomenon. It can be absent on the surface, but surge forth furiously at a different depth. It can pulsate strongly at the lightest touch and disappear at the first pressure. It can feel hollow, full, sticky, slippery, light, heavy. Each side of the fingertip reads a different organ, such that the *emchi* should be able to catch the minute differences in sensation between the left and right sides of her index finger, if she is to differentiate between the pulse of the lungs and that of the large intestine, for example. Taking the pulse is very much a type of bodily knowledge, or what Csordas has called a different "somatic mode of attention" (Csordas 1993). As I understand it, it is a knowledge that is difficult to verbalize. Tsyrenma, whom I often asked to describe her experience of learning Tibetan medicine and especially pulse diagnosis, seemed to think that it is both easy and hard. Easy because it is not that complicated to memorize the different types of pulse there are or to remember the correspondences between the points on the wrist and the internal organs they reflect. Hard, because each pulse appears different and unique at first and behaves as its own thing—to make it speak of more than the very particular and largely illegible characteristics of a specific body at a specific moment, to see in it something as patterned as a discrete illness is a challenge. Frustrated with my pestering, Tsyrenma resorted to an example: "Back in the day, in Tibet, *emchi* would teach pulse-taking by making their disciples stand at a river crossing and take the pulse of every single person that came around." She, of course, didn't learn by standing at a river crossing, but by examining the flow of patients who came to consult her as a doctor. She would take the pulse after her teacher and check whether she was able to "feel" the movements of the culprits in the same way he did. Learning to distinguish the qualities of the pulse at each pulse point and to recognize them as particular kinds of processes in specific organs make up much of the *emchi*'s embodied skill. For example, one must be able to recognize a "wind pulse" (*pul's vetra*) or a "bile pulse" (*pul's zhelchi*) by their relative rapidity, depth, hollowness, viscosity, and other qualities that are learned through tactile approximation and calibration with a mentor. For practitioners in Buryatia, knowing the pulse is first and foremost a matter of extended practice and cannot be easily quantified or qualified. Thus, in a conversation with Tsyrenma's teacher, he reminded me that diagnosing by the pulse is also a matter of intuition, which itself might be a sign of properly Buddhist subjectivity.

The pulsometer makes no such distinctions. There are no sides to the sensors; the pressure against the skin of the wrist is fixed in all points and evenly distributed, unlike the pressure of the fingertips, where, according to the classical formulation of the *Gyüshi*, the index is "on the skin," the middle finger "is on the flesh," and the ring finger "is on the bone." It knows the rich textures of the pulse only via one method—it records the pulse as an oscillatory function. A complex algorithm analyzes the function and converts it into something that a doctor or researcher might find intelligible: a histogram or pie chart, each organ represented by its own column or section. The columns hover around a "normal" mean—those going above are represented as red, those going below are blue. Within the acceptable standard deviation (calculated based on all the previous uses of the device), they stay green. The red and blue code for heat and cold—terms used in Tibetan medicine to denote the pathological modus operandi of different organs.

Over the thirty years of its development, the researchers designing the pulsometer were concerned with making the device speak of the body as would the *emchi*, but without having to rely on the *emchi*'s techniques and forms of knowledge. In order to achieve this goal, APDC underwent something oddly reminiscent of the kind of discipleship Tsyrenma described. Most of the experiments on the Pulse Diagnostic Complex involved the recruitment of Tibetan medicine practitioners and specialists to monitor the pulse of the participants in parallel with the machine. Over repeated trials, APDC software was "taught" to recognize what the practitioners were seeing: different kinds of pulse waves were recorded and classified, their characteristics analyzed and mapped against the Tibetan medical diagnosis of the expert. Yet, while several hypotheses and even some degree of consensus exist regarding on what, specifically, the *emchi* bases his or her diagnosis, there is no "theory" to describe the relationship between the "pulse wave" and bodily states and no perfect mathematical formula that would adequately reflect the pulse wave itself. "There is no algorithm that accurately describes blood flow," Sergei would tell me when I asked him about his mathematical manipulations of the pulsogram. In practice, this makes the types of images provided by the software that treats the data from the pulsometer sufficiently self-explanatory only in terms of Tibetan medicine. They still require an interpreter—someone to not only read the graphs and relate them to the types of discourses on affliction that most patients are familiar with, but to determine whether the device is being too sensitive or too inaccurate, whether it is speaking of the body's actual processes or of irrelevant fluctuations. Is the pulse it reads a reliable witness, and what is it a witness to? This, too, is a question that practicing *emchi* are constantly asking themselves as they palpate the patient's pulse, a knowledge that comes with years of practice—of standing, day in and day out, at the river crossing.

Two ethnographic events capture the stakes of developing the APDC and its subsequent deployment. As my fieldwork was drawing to a close, I sat with one of the doctors at the East-West Medicine Center. The doctor was an old acquaintance who used the pulsometer extensively in his practice. In hushed tones, he announced that he'd let me in on a secret. Chuckling, he pointed to the plastic body of the machine: "See, the pulsometer has taught me Tibetan medicine," he confided. Of course, it was the doctor himself who had taught himself Tibetan medicine, not in the classical transmission style of apprenticing with a Buddhist *emchi*, like Tsyrenma did, but by avidly reading Tibetan medicine texts, interfacing with colleagues who had worked with Tibetan medicine practitioners, and following whatever seminars and workshops on the subject he could access. However, this incident points to the sense that it is precisely the ambiguities inherent in the APDC and the demands that it puts on its users that contribute to an epistemological space where the authority and legitimacy of Tibetan medicine in Buryatia are reproduced and consolidated.

The second event happened after an especially frustrating afternoon of inconsistent data at the IIT lab. As Tsyrenma and I were leaving, she joked, offhandedly, "Every time I'm here, I feel like they're testing *me*." The logics deployed by IIT scientists refigured Tibetan medicine as, on the one hand, able to provide a privileged vantage point to apprehend and anticipate the systemic dysfunctions of the body before they became manifested as a clinically diagnosable illness and, on the other, constantly undermined this very vision by viewing signs of pathology as always potentially technological "white noise." Paradoxically, this placed the traditionally trained Tibetan medicine expert—Tsyrenma—in a position of heightened legitimacy, as the only truly reliable source for authorizing the relevance of the collected data. In their relationship of mutual authorization, the traditional expert and the pulsometer affirmed the validity of Tibetan medicine as a privileged approach capable of remedying the pathologies of post-socialist healthcare and address present-day concerns with the health of the nation. Yet, the productive ambiguities of the pulsometer were contagious, its uncertainties potentially extending and amplifying Tsyrenma's own uncertainties.

It might be tempting to view the pulsometer as a scientific curiosity or as another example of what happens when Soviet science, excessively captured with its own ideological necessities, attempted to engage with its "others." The previous discussion aimed to complicate such an interpretation by asking what made the pulsometer so productive that it has largely transcended the situated histories of its development and still manages to recruit allies. It is not simply that experts versed in the embodied knowledge of Tibetan medicine resist efforts to extract and mechanize their expertise. In fact, they are sometimes enthusiastic, if cheerfully skeptical, collaborators in scientific projects of "objectivization." Instead, by tracking the social lives of the pulsometer, I have attempted to show that by asking certain questions about the pulse, the body, and the skills of Tibetan medicine practitioners, scientists involved with the APDC have inadvertently created a technological object that limits the very possibility of extraction and standardization it is supposed to enable. Functioning as a prosthetic extension of the clinician or researcher's body, the pulsometer still requires of its users to learn, at least partially, the kind of embodied expertise that characterizes the traditional skills of the *emchi* and to recruit practicing *emchi* for making sense of their results.

Over the last thirty years, researchers designing the pulsometer were concerned with making it speak of the body as would the *emchi*, but without having to rely on individual *emchi*'s variable techniques and forms of lived experience. By pointing to its many technological and social entanglements, I suggest that what makes the pulsometer efficacious is precisely that it is maintained as an *unreliable* witness, one that has to constantly recruit other experts—whether embodied in devices or people—to bear witness to itself. In other words, the trouble with the pulsometer, as well as the reason for its productiveness, is not just that the images it generates require authoritative interpretation—in this case, it would be no different from any other modern medical imaging technology, reliant on what Daston and Galison have called the "trained judgment" of the expert (Daston and Galison 2007). Instead, what is striking is that it constantly defers the possibility of final and definitive interpretation—whether of the pulse, or of the body—and therefore mobilizes a number of other allies in a gridlock of codependent authorization.

Although circumventing the *emchi*'s individual skill had been one of the original goals of the pulsometer project, the recurrent presence of the practitioner of Tibetan medicine in the laboratory spaces structured around it is not simply a matter of recalcitrant redundancy, but a necessary extension of the device itself. In this chapter, I have tried to show that rather than making the traditional expert superfluous through the perfect imitation and subsequent automation of her diagnostic abilities, the pulsometer has come to function as a prosthesis for the sensory conversions that scientists imputed to practitioners of Tibetan medicine. If the relationship between mimesis and automation is always threatening to reverse itself, the pulsometer performs its own ambiguous articulations, blurring the directionality of the prosthetic relationship. At the very least, it encourages us to think how such devices are themselves enhanced and extended through the actors and practices for which they are supposed to substitute.

While the pulsometer has systematically recruited practicing *emchi* for authorizing its data, the horizon of its transition from automation to autonomy as a self-sufficient imaging technology remains perpetually deferred. In 2011, when I returned to the field, Ayur and a colleague were actively discussing the possibility of designing a portable version, complete with a smartphone app, to turn the device into a household item—as commonplace as a thermometer or a blood pressure gauge. There were, it seemed, future horizons to its portability. In tracking the social lives of this device, I have attempted to show that by asking certain questions (while skirting others) about the pulse, the body, and the skills of Tibetan medicine practitioners, scientists involved with "objectivizing" Tibetan pulse diagnosis have inadvertently created a technological object that productively limits the very possibility of extraction and standardization it is supposed to enable. In turn, it is precisely its failures at the perfect standardization of pulse diagnosis that allows the pulsometer to buttress the legitimacy of Tibetan medicine as a lived practice in Buryatia, opening up both conceptual and infrastructural spaces for articulating its potential futures, ones that leave room for, in Pupyshev's words, something other than the "solely rational." It is to these articulations of Buryatia's potential futures, and Tibetan medicine's place in them, that I turn to in Chapter 3.

3

"THE MEDICINE OF THE FUTURE, NOW AVAILABLE"

Geographies of Medical Integration

THE COSMONAUT'S GAZE

The official banquet, held in celebration of the conference "Development of Traditional Medicine in Russia," organized in Ulan-Ude by the East-West Medical Center in August 2010, was punctuated by an abundance of toasts. As is typical of such events, one or another prominent official would stand up, at seemingly equal intervals, animated by a sense of social decorum and hierarchy that a relative outsider like myself learned to expect without ever being able to fully anticipate or interpret, and proceed to hold up a drink while waiting for the assembly's attention. The lengthy, complex pronouncements uttered on the occasion ranged from the thankful to the self-congratulatory: the conference, the participants reiterated, had been a success. Local officials raised their glasses in honor of their guests, who had traveled to Ulan-Ude to affirm their shared commitment to furthering the development of traditional medicine in Russia and beyond. Guests celebrated their hosts' gracious hospitality. As some of the Buryat participants discreetly sprinkled alcohol from their untouched glasses in the customary offering to local "*khoziaeva*" or place spirits—inhabitants of and active presences in the region's landscape—metropolitan guests marveled at the untouched "wild" beauty of Buryatia's nature and lauded the region's largely unexplored potential as an ecological paradise and future destination for resort travel and ecotourism. These pronouncements seamlessly blended

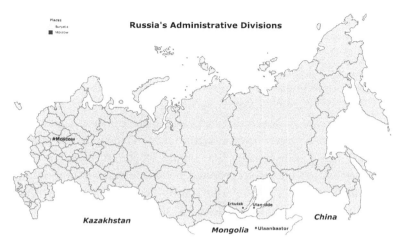

Figure 2. Map with Buryatia highlighted (Created by the author)

invocations of the "ecologically clean" geological features of southeastern Siberia, such as Lake Baikal and the Sayan Mountains, with claims about the therapeutic efficacy of the local flora, mineral waters, and climate.

When Nikolai Kovalev,[1] one of the members of the delegation from the National Institute for the Preparation of Cosmonauts (NIPC) and a guest of honor, bearing the title of "Hero of the Soviet Union" for his numerous space missions, stood up to make a toast, the room quieted, expectant faces turning toward him. In his mid-fifties at the time, Kovalev was a charismatic presence, easily commanding the attention of those assembled in a way that allowed him to speak in an even tone when others had to shout to be heard over table conversations and the clanking of silverware. "It might come as a surprise to some of you that I have been in your area before," he began, pausing for effect. "The last time, however, I was approximately 350 kilometers above where we are currently sitting." After providing a brief description of what the area looks like from this high vantage point—the vast undifferentiated landmass of the Eurasian continent, where geopolitical borders or sociological details were invisible, and only the narrow crescent of Lake Baikal anchored the imagery to Russia—Kovalev proceeded to thank his hosts for providing him with the opportunity to literally set foot on a land he had previously only overseen from orbit.

Shortly after Kovalev's toast, one of the representatives from Buryatia's Ministry of Health Protection followed up with his own announcement, returning the conversation to the main theme of the event—namely, Tibetan medicine in Buryatia and its potential utility for Russia's broader state interests. Although, like many of his colleagues, he affirmed that Buryatia's culture, here embodied in the historical presence of Tibetan medicine, was also Russia's undeniable legacy, he invoked one of the recalcitrant and seemingly trivial problems that had plagued the conference. Before moving forward to a greater institutionalization of Tibetan medicine in Buryatia and Russia more broadly, how should Tibetan medicine in Buryatia be identified? In a humorous proposal, he offered his own solution: "I have suggested that we call it the 'Tibeto-Indo-Perso-Greeko-Mongol-Buryat medicine of Russia,' but I was told that this is too long and isn't catchy enough."

I begin with these two toasts because they are symptomatic of competing geopolitical imaginaries. On the one hand, Kovalev's literally "global" extraterrestrial gaze offered a fantasy of uniformity, a single undifferentiated geopolitical space, identified by a national landmark like Lake Baikal, and yet relegating Buryatia to a remote periphery only accessible through radical deterritorialization, captured in the imputed inference of the astronaut "having been in this region before." By contrast, the medical official's humorous quip emphasized Buryatia's inclusion into identifiably transnational and historical flows of diverse medical, cultural, and religious knowledge, ones that are certainly not restricted by historically fluctuating national borders. This chapter analyzes the competing visions and politics of medical integration for Tibetan medicine articulated in Buryatia and Moscow during my fieldwork in the late 2000s. I argue that visions of medical integration put forth at these disparate sites are not simply about therapy or practical health care, but rather serve to articulate Buryatia's relations with the Russian state and to formulate a peripheral politics that challenges the entrenched center-margin narratives that often come to define relations between Moscow and Siberia.

HEALING THE NATION BY MAKING IT PAY

In the 1990s, Russia began to reform the financing of health-care provisioning while reiterating its commitment to providing medical services free of charge to the population. Introducing Compulsory Medical Insurance (OMS), the government created two monetary funds: the centralized Federal Compulsory Health Insurance Fund (FFOMS) in charge of managing the OMS, and the Territorially Compulsory Insurance Funds (TFOMS) tasked with the distribution of the OMS in Russia's regions (Gordeev, Pavlova, and Groot 2011). In addition to the OMS, a separate structure of health insurance—the Voluntary Medical Insurance (DMS)—is provided by employment organizations and includes additional services, such as a choice of a more comfortable hospital room or the use of resort and sanatorium medicine. Despite the hopes that this new system would rectify the problems of Soviet health-care provisioning, many of the informal aspects of dispensing care under socialism proved recalcitrant. In her analysis of socialist health care, Michele Rivkin-Fish notes that the redistributive top-down economy of the Soviet state and the subsequent shortages and inefficiencies that plagued the Soviet system of services more generally created a space for the proliferation of what Ledeneva (1998) calls an "economy of favors": an exchange of bribes, gifts, and services that attempted to remedy the widespread sense that what the state was prepared to offer fell short of adequate care (see also Rivkin-Fish 2013). These informal exchanges and the expectations associated with them are still present in the restructured health-care sector.

The commercialization and monetization of medical services also entered Russia's network of health-care institutions in a more formal way. Private for-pay medical institutions began to multiply throughout Moscow's urban landscape, especially in the case of dental and walk-in clinics (Boykov et al. 2000), although during my fieldwork I was frequently told that they were too expensive for the average patient. Services at these clinics were not covered by OMS, and rarely by DMS, and therefore most of the time operated on a fee-for-service basis. While it was theoretically possible for an individual to obtain a yearly subscription to a specific clinic, thus bypassing the insurance system altogether, the contractual aspects of such arrangements varied between institutions and remained bureaucratically opaque. In Moscow, clinics that explicitly claimed an affiliation with traditional medicine tended to be limited to this private sector. However, similar services were also offered in state medical institutions, especially in the case of such well-established therapeutic forms associated with "traditional" care as phytotherapy, medicinal leeches, and reflexotherapy. In state institutions, they functioned under the umbrella of rehabilitative medicine and did not advertise themselves as primarily "traditional."

I met with Vladimir Viktorovich in the summer of 2009, at one of the private Tibetan medicine clinics in Moscow. Located on a quiet side street at the heart of Moscow's old city center, "LotusMed" was housed in a beautiful nineteenth-century neoclassical building, with tall windows and an ornate white facade. The interior was perhaps even more lavish than the exterior, gleaming marble tile, and spacious hallways, ornamented in a vaguely "Eastern" aesthetic that occupied two floors of a building that was, by all accounts, prime real estate. As we went up the stairs, Vladimir Viktorovich, the head physician and director of LotusMed, commented offhandedly about the spectacularly high rent. His public persona was a jarring and carefully cultivated blend of unapologetic cynicism, frequently attributed to doctors in Russia, and an impassioned enthusiasm for his professional vision.

What had originally intrigued me about LotusMed was the content of its printed newsletter, which I had come across in another context. Each monthly issue featured on its front page an article in the form of a historical or social riddle, from relatively straightforward ones, such as "Why does Russia need Tibetan medicine?" to more obscure questions, such as "How did Genghis Khan manage to conquer half of the world?" or "How did Ivan the Terrible cure himself?" On the front page, a recognizable image typically associated with Russia, such as Red Square, generally cohabited with a smaller, more discreet one of a Tibetan monk or a Buddhist structure. The answer to most of these historical and social mysteries was inevitably Tibetan medicine's ability to address the relevant historical and social pressures of the moment. Providing a kind of revised history of both pre-revolutionary Russia and the Soviet Union, the newsletter inserted Tibetan medicine at the center of important historical events as the hidden enabler or motivator for their unfolding, much like the photograph of the Buddhist monk seemed to haunt the larger iconic representation of Russia.

The newsletter also did something else—it suggested that the clinic could deliver "the medicine of the future, available *now* at LotusMed." The clever slogan formulated a familiar claim: efforts to recuperate traditional medicine in the private medical sector in Russia typically hinge on collapsing a presumed historical past with a future of perfect therapeutic integration just over the horizon and to reinsert this blended vision of care into the present as a space of exception from everyday life: a new epoch that has not yet fully arrived everywhere, but could be accessed in scattered pockets by those who knew where to look and had the means to afford it.

Vladimir Viktorovich's professional trajectory is somewhat typical of doctors in Russia who specialize in traditional medicine. He was a trained physician, with a specialty in dermatology and venereology, and had finished his medical education in one of Moscow's universities before pursuing an additional specialization in homeopathy, which he had practiced since 1996. In the mid-1990s the market for homeopathic remedies in Russia was still mostly limited to domestic products, and so Vladimir Viktorovich and some of his colleagues worked to organize imports of homeopathic remedies from France and Germany. In the early 2000s he began to work as a practitioner at several "Eastern" clinics in the city, until he was able to open his own clinic in 2007. His integrative vision came from combining Chinese medicine and homeopathy in clinical practice. He explained that Russian homeopathy was already heavily influenced by Chinese medicine, and its efficacy could actually be increased by switching the administration of homeopathic remedies from standard intramuscular injection sites to acupressure points. His dermatology practice encouraged him to experiment with nonbiomedical methods, because traditional medicine, as he explained, afforded him a systemic view of the body, which he felt was missing from standard biomedical approaches. From blending homeopathy and Traditional Chinese Medicine, he became interested in incorporating other methods, Tibetan medicine especially, because it offered an alternative to what he called "the prescription of massive amounts of antibiotics" often practiced in the case of recalcitrant skin disorders. The pursuit of a systemic view of the body and of a systemic form of treatment motivated the ways in which Vladimir Viktorovich understood the possibilities of medical integration:

> The reason I think LotusMed is the clinic of the future is because the main goal . . . our main goal here is to combine European medicine and Tibetan medicine and traditional medicines for one purpose: to help people. Because homeopathy, like pharmacopuncture, we sometimes use only in those cases when it's necessary. . . . Because Tibetan medicine or Chinese medicine taken separately, or Iranian medicine, or Ayurveda, you can't take them as mono-medicines at the present stage

of development, here in Moscow, in Russia—alone, they won't achieve anything in a contemporary society. In chronic pathologies, there's no singular approach possible. Wait, that's not true—there's one approach. [Laughs] "Nine gram injection to the heart," and you get a reliable diagnosis from the crown jewel of all medical science—the forensic pathologist. And even then sometimes he gets it wrong. So really, what we want to do is to crystalize Tibetan medicine, maybe even integrative medicine itself. No one does that.

For Vladimir Viktorovich, the necessity of an integrative medical approach stemmed from a particular understanding of the kind of ailing bodies medical professionals in Russia predominantly face in their everyday practice. Because most illnesses are what he describes as "systemic," a single "mono-medicine," be it biomedicine or Tibetan medicine, is insufficient for addressing all the specific manifestations of these complex failing physiologies. The nature of these bodies is frequently articulated in temporal terms as a particular historical narrative of the peculiarities of the present moment, as we see in Vladimir Viktorovich's invocation of the "present stage of development" in Russia. This temporal argument, I suggest, addresses more or less explicitly a "post-socialist condition," even if the term "post-socialism" is not in fact used in these accounts. While I will explore what treating a post-socialist body means in clinical practice more thoroughly in Chapter 4, here I would like to point out that despite Vladimir Viktorovich's claims that LotusMed is adopting a unique and innovative medical model, it was, in fact, part of a broader rhetoric and practice of medical integration. In other words, that LotusMed was somehow unique in this privileging of an integrative medical approach to treating systemic disorders was an exaggeration—both private and state clinics that claim traditional medicine in Moscow, and Russia more generally, assert an integrative practice and combine different therapeutic techniques and methods to target the treatment of complex, frequently chronic illnesses. Blending different therapies, both biomedical and not, with each other is a widespread way of articulating what is both progressive and timely about these institutions—and what sorts of bodies are at the center of their care.

At another Tibetan medicine clinic in Moscow, Gregoryi Mikhaylovich, the head physician trained in Soviet reflexotherapy who traced his intellectual genealogy to the 1957 collaborations between Chinese and Soviet physicians, explained that in the case of complex disorders, one had no choice but to combine treatments. Sometimes these combinations had unexpected results. Narrating the story of a patient who had come with a severe case of polyarthritic inflammation, he explained that after treatment with acupuncture and phytopharmaceuticals derived from Tibetan medicine the patient's self-reported health (*samochuvstvie*) improved, the inflammation went down, and the clinical symptoms, like swelling and impaired mobility, abated—but the subsequent blood tests showed an unexpected spike in the rheumatoid factor (RF).[2] However, none of the associated biochemical changes were observed: "The alpha 2-protein and c-reactive protein should have gone up, but they stayed normal. So where did this increased RF come from?" he asked rhetorically during our conversation. He speculated that the botanicals and acupuncture had acted upon the affected tissues, causing them to release chemicals into the blood that the blood work identified as the RF factor, but the mechanism of what exactly had transpired had to be investigated more closely. In order to address these unexpected effects, Gregoryi Mikhailovich suggested that this was where integration had to happen: biomedical specialists could work alongside practitioners of traditional medicine in order to determine how each might address the unforeseen consequences of the other's treatment, especially when dealing with complex cases of systemic illness.

Similarly, because most of the patients that came to LotusMed were chronic patients, Vladimir Viktorovich emphasized that in order to adequately treat the complexity of their conditions, one had to draw on all available therapeutic modalities, from biomedicine to Tibetan medicine to acupuncture and homeopathy. The patient's body became a space for combining these different therapies with each other, tracking their reciprocal influence. Like in the case of combining homeopathy with acupuncture, he understood this mutual interpenetration of seemingly distinct therapeutic modalities as the only possible route for medical progress because the imperative of global medicine, in his opinion, was inhibited by a kind of biopolitical reduction to the mean. In an effort to "make live," to reprise Foucault's formulation of the chiasmic tension underlying modern biopolitical arrangements, he seemed to suggest, the state (and the global medical apparatus) were devoting attention to the wrong thing:

Global medical science is really in a bad spot at the moment. The cause of illness, the cause of the pathological process is ignored, but what's happening is an attempt—and this might sound a bit cynical coming from a physician—to try to drag up those who are already in a critical situation, instead of trying to make sure that it doesn't happen. Don't get me wrong, we should try to help them, that's all well and good. Sure, we can try to cure diabetes, we can conduct complex studies, but this is not the way. . . . Where else can medicine go? So, on the one hand we have medicine going toward technological aspects, nanotechnologies, but then again, technology can do what? Stem cells, organ transplant. And so what? We take the liver and replace the hell out of it. So what? I'm willing to bet you that in a year, it'll be back to where it was before the operation. Why? Because the [body's] system remained the same. We didn't regulate it, we have to change the entire person, and even then he'll probably kick the bucket (*zdokhnet*) just as quickly as what would have happened if we didn't conduct the surgery. Why is that? Because his energetics (*energetika*) is the same, and here [gestures toward his head] is the same thing as well.

The reference to *energetika* is suggestive in this case (Lemon 2018).[3] A system view of the body presupposes that there is something uniquely self-perpetuating and recalcitrant about specific forms of embodiment that lead to illness. For Vladimir Viktorovich, his task was phrased as a project of changing the "entire person," not simply of treating an already ailing body. Although Vladimir Viktorovich conceptualized his own professional identity as, first and foremost, one of a biomedical doctor, he emphasized that "modern" European medicine, as it was practiced in Russia, was unable to structurally or practically address the contemporary body in all of its physical, social, and psychological complexity. In Vladimir Viktorivich's account, the Soviet past provided a more desirable model for both the administrative organization of health care and for creating an appropriate culture of health. This was not, however, a proposal for the self-responsibility of the patient, but an overhaul of the state. Health, he explained, was not simply the responsibility of the Ministry of Health, but of every other state structure, from education and sports to culture and the arts. The state had to cultivate a "fashion of health," propagating images of healthy bodies and providing institutional structures that monitored and maintained the population's vitality. Tying his own medical activities to the interests of the nation, he explained that integrating traditional medicine systematically with biomedicine was the only way in which the pathologies of the present could be addressed:

> You know, there are very few procedures I can do that will guarantee that you won't suffer from the same thing in the future. . . . Something goes wrong with your body—too much work, stress, physical, emotional . . . maybe even alimentary. Hypodynamia. . . . Now this is when the system starts breaking down, and comes out as a disorder of the skin, the small intestine, cardiovascular problems. The pathological process starts. It starts to make itself known: you get a pain here, a pain there, you get morning heartburn of some sort, you get irregular stool or something. Little things people don't pay attention to. Sometimes it's almost not noticeable. Until it gets to a clinical picture, you'll ignore it. Since we no longer have professional dispensarization, although the nation would be so much better off. . . . Because seeing something at the early stage is what's important.

Because traditional medicine was more attuned to illness before the revelation of what Vladmir Viktorovich called "its clinical picture," integrating it into practical health care aligned it with the best aspects of what Soviet health care had to offer—namely, its stated focus on prevention. Soviet health care, in Vladimir Viktorovich's account, was not as flawed as it might appear at first. In the process of restructuring and creating a new, more market-based model of medical provisioning, the state had lost one of its chief functions in managing the population's health—namely, what he called "health propaganda": "This isn't new, you know, we had this before. Remember, under the Soviet system we had GTO,[4] we had compulsory physical training, and people cared about how the body looks and might be improved. Now what do we have? Beer advertisements."

For Vladimir Viktorovich, the new system failed to fulfill the health-care needs of the population for another reason as well. Because patients were streamlined through state medical institutions, practicing doctors were not encouraged to consider a systemic view of the body, but limited themselves to their own narrow specialization. This resulted in patients being "bounced" from one institution to another, often with a lack of an established diagnosis because each specialist failed to see the "big picture."

There is perhaps a profound irony to the ways in which Vladimir Viktorovich marshaled claims to his clinic's integrative take on both bodies and medical therapies in the service of national interests. After all, LotusMed and most other clinics featuring Tibetan medicine were private institutions, made possible by the post-socialist restructuring of the health-care system in Russia. His own facility with recruiting allies and enthusiasts in the Ministry of Health and in other federal bureaucratic structures notwithstanding, Vladimir Viktorovich's clinic and medical institutions like it are largely enabled by the very structural problems that he critiqued. When I asked him what he thought of the transition to an insurance system, Vladimir Viktorovich vehemently rejected it as a poorly thought-out solution that only worked to reproduce the problems of Soviet health provision while dismissing its strengths. Doctors, he explained, were still overworked, required to fulfill a daily quota of patients that receive little to no individual attention: "Let's say you come to see me with a sore throat. What do I do? The easiest thing for me is to write out a prescription for antibiotics and send you on your way, then call in the next patient." As a medical institution, LotusMed specialized in patients who had tried the state health-care system, but because they were streamlined through it with no careful, personal attention to their particular case, their systematic ailments remained and got worse.

The inefficiencies of the system could be exploited when doctors and patients still expected an exchange of bribes or gifts to guarantee careful care. This, in turn, led to what Vladimir Viktorovich bemoaned as the patient's woeful refusal to take responsibility for her health, assuming that a financial exchange puts all responsibility back on the doctor. While on one level, Vladimir Viktorovich seemed to advocate for individual responsibility, the argument was in fact more complex and more situational. Making patients pay a rather steep price for a "cycle" of services (each treatment would cost 6,000 rubles, or about $200 per treatment at the time, with a full cycle consisting of ten to twelve treatments) was part of his philosophy of "curing" the nation: "The patient has to *feel* the money he pays, otherwise he won't take his health seriously," he explained. In the absence of proper "health propaganda" on the part of the state and in a context where an exchange of bribes or favors encouraged the patient to relinquish all responsibility, he articulated that steep costs were the only way of impressing upon the patient the responsibility of proper self-care and desirable embodiment. It wasn't about markets, for him—it was about disciplining citizen-bodies.

Despite being the head of a private clinic and stating outright that the institution operated at a profit, he saw his therapeutic practices and hopes as firmly aligned with the interests of a Russian nation in crisis. He moved with ease between imaginaries of a future that recovered the best aspects of a Soviet "culture of the body" and combined them with traditional medicine deployed in the service of maximizing health as the only solution to a current national malaise of perennially untreated chronic conditions. While it is certainly possible to view this approach as a rationalization of the profit-generating practices of his clinic, the formulation he used is suggestive. Vladimir Viktorovich emphasized that the high costs to the individual budget of the patient was as much a method of psychological intervention as a question of financial solvency for LotusMed. He articulated the statement as part of his professional philosophy and vision, stressing the degree to which, in contemporary Moscow, money—or more specifically, the unpleasant experience of parting with it—was frequently the only way to "get through" to the patient. What is remarkable in this philosophy is the fact that Vladimir Viktorovich did not view this as the inevitable or natural effect of the entry of market logics into health-care arrangements, but instead as something very peculiar to the emotional and cultural universe of the post-socialist metropolis. "Of course, we're not going to take a grandma's last 20,000 rubles of saved-up pension money," he said, qualifying his statement. But reforming an aging population's consciousness or treating the inevitable deterioration of the health of the elderly was not his primary professional mission or the object of his political or ethical commitments. He would still do it, he said—he was a doctor after all—but it wasn't enough. Instead, Vladimir Viktorovich was interested in intervening into the minds and bodies of a wealthy Muscovite elite—and, often, their children—to impress upon them the importance of their health. As a more general approach to both what health care should be and to the present state of affairs in Russia, Vladimir Viktorovich argued that the mission of medical professionals should focus on cultivating the subjectivities and bodies of the future generations of Russia's economic, political, and intellectual upper class and not on the recuperation of those who had already found themselves affected beyond recoverability by the turbulent transitions of Russia's post-socialist reforms. In this, a framing that assigns blame for patients' flagging health by blending the problems of modern *biomedicine* as epistemology with the inefficiencies of health-care delivery shifts responsibility away from the day-to-day problems of the state health-care system, welding a vision of a better, integrative "medicine of the future" with the private health-care sector while simultaneously aligning such clinical experimentations and treatment philosophies with the official goals of healing the body politic.

In the various rumors and reviews that circulated about LotusMed and other similar clinics in Moscow, patients' opinions seemed to diverge. Some lauded these institutions as qualitatively superior to anything available in the public sector; others critiqued the exorbitant prices and apparently profit-driven unscrupulous attitudes. Others yet questioned the legitimacy of the practitioners who worked there, wondering whether their frequently ethnically marked identity—*sploshnoy Kazakhstan* (total Kazakhstan), as one patient wrote on a forum—offered sufficiently "authentic" forms of traditional medicine. Welding ethnic identity with traditional medicine, Muscovite patients were suspicious: what sort of qualifications did these "traditional" doctors have, and what did their non-European physical appearance indicate? Were they the "wrong kind" of ethnicized subject?

Private clinics of "traditional" medicine in Moscow are in fierce competition with each other, but they are relatively unconcerned with the patients who prefer to use state services because they cannot afford private care. Institutions like LotusMed attempt to cultivate an "elite" public that can afford their services, although they might offer a rebate on "functional diagnostics"—the first stage of triage for patients, before they are directed to a specialist within the clinic. At the same time, the directors of these institutions that I had interviewed frequently spoke to me of a population of patients that moved unpredictably and haphazardly between medical facilities, spurred on by the sense that new therapeutic fads were constantly erupting in what Vladimir Viktorovich identified as Moscow's "medical El Dorado."

Most of the clinics in Moscow I observed or heard about from local interlocutors operated under a similar formula: they offered a range of services in traditional medicine, listed the kinds of illnesses they were prepared to treat in biomedical terms, and operated an herbal pharmacy that offered a range of predominantly imported products. To return to one of the central themes that has informed this chapter—namely, the ways in which

Tibetan medicine in Russia is recruited into metropolitan projects of medical integration—these clinical sites frequently emphasized in their self-presentation the failures of biomedical treatment and of a biomedical approach to the body. In this sense, the vision of a failing biomedical system and dissatisfied patients attracted by the promise of better care was a discursive genre, carefully reproduced. This rhetoric is consistent and identifiable across clinical sites, although the level of critique toward the achievements and merits of biomedicine varied. Clinics like LotusMed were also places for the generation of popularized expert discourses on the utility of traditional medicine, and their directors often wrote self-help books for a wide audience on healthy living, diet, and exercise, which are frequently implicitly or explicitly critical of biomedical practices. Most of these critiques focus on biomedicine's failure to treat the cause of various illnesses, on its propensity to be predominantly focused on symptoms, and on a tendency to favor hormonal, pharmaceutical, and surgical interventions over more systemic approaches. There is a certain paradoxical element to these claims, since the treatments offered by institutions that identify themselves with traditional medicine were also mainly focused on symptomatic, palliative care—their stated goal was to relieve the discomforts associated with the chronic conditions they set out to treat and to extend periods of remission. Patient testimonies tended to address these questions as well: ultimately, the patient's embodied experience of illness does not focus on the presence or absence of a specific condition, discernible through biomedical diagnostic technologies or an examination performed by a physician, but on "self-experience." I find the Russian term *samochuvstvie* productive to think with in this case. After all, *samochuvstvie* does not index a permanent state of health or its absence, nor does it index any specific disorders, but focuses on the minutia of day-to-day bodily variations, allowing for a wide margin of fluctuation that takes into account the assumption that experiencing the embodied self will inevitably shift over time.

One way to understand why clinics like LotusMed in particular—and the ways in which traditional medicine has entered Russia's post-socialist health-care market more generally—have such wide appeal for patients in Russia is to consider the implications of what is meant under the label of "treating symptoms," when it is inhabited as a critical stance against the biomedical ordinary. There is certainly the reality of failed treatment, or of insufficient relief that patients frequently complain about when faced with state medical institutions, or sometimes with their experiences of care in "traditional" clinics. However, the discursive field within which these pursuits of care operate equates "symptomatic" treatment to the masking of symptoms with "artificial" interventions, which preclude the possibility of experiencing one's body as reliably healthy.

To illustrate this point, it may be helpful to return to a statement by Vladimir Viktorovich. In an effort to explain what he thought was so flawed in the epistemological premises of modern medicine, he equated it to a crutch. Since the statement happened in the context of discussing the reliance on chronically consumed synthetic pharmaceuticals, I asked him whether by "crutch" he meant a sort of prosthetic extension—something that becomes incorporated as part of a habitual bodily experience. He vehemently rejected the analogy, suggesting that a prosthesis was too permanent, too easily signaling an irreversible modification of bodily integrity: "No, a prosthesis means that it's all over." The image of the crutch better captured the kind of relationship he was trying to delineate between the patient and biomedical interventions: while necessary on occasions, the point of the crutch, after all, was that it would enable one to move about and eventually could be shed once the injury had been healed. But, much like the crutch, the relationship with biomedical treatment, in Vladimir Viktorovich's opinion, too frequently morphed into precisely the kind of prosthetic dependency that he was trying to reject as an adequate model for the body's various medical entanglements and extensions.

If *samochuvstvie* is taken as the object of medical treatment, it provides an unreliable index of one's actual physical processes, and yet the only one that is reliably available to the patient, and most immediately relevant, especially in cases of chronic illnesses that one must manage on a daily basis. Taking herbal remedies and undergoing procedures such as massage, acupuncture, or leech therapy while also providing symptomatic relief emphasizes this situated and temporary organismic viability, suggesting that the treatment process in fact works to return the body to its normal, preillness state without permanently modifying it. This pursuit of "natural" treatments—not simply derived from natural substances, but rather as something that does not fundamentally change the body but merely returns it to itself, without setting roots—operated in a semiotic context where biomedical treatment was already understood to be incapable of truly acting upon the "true" health of the patient, precisely because it was synthetic or artificial: limited to reducing or hiding symptoms without fundamentally readjusting the "system" as a whole on the one end or running the risk of creating permanent pharmaceutical dependencies on the other.

What is important about this conceptualization of health is the way in which prevention and adjustment in Moscow's private health-care sector that sought to deploy "traditional medicine" on the model of "medical integration" were not formulated in relation to patient's engagement with personal health risks as part of the neoliberal sensibilities of patient self-responsibility and personal management (Dumit 2012) but, rather, invoked organismic viability as a way of addressing a body conceptualized as a "system" of interrelated processes that is simultaneously relatively stable, yet in perpetual flux, always open and permeable, and always the product of uncertain and shifting historical forces. To return to Vladimir Viktorovich's account:

> You know, they say the Soviet system this . . . the Soviet system that . . . that we didn't have anything to eat, we had no choice. That's rubbish. I was born in 1970, grew up at the peak of Soviet stagnation. We ate just fine. Maybe we didn't have fifty choices of sausage, but is that really the point with health care? You can have ten bedrooms, you can still only sleep in one [at a time]. . . . The same with health care, you can have all these new technologies—we all have cars, we all have mobile phones, so I don't know what's left, implanting microchips into your brain? But all of this is no longer interesting. What we need to try to do is to heal the nation. . . . This is where the East matters, you see—the East tells us that we might have one diagnosis, but there can be many causes. But this is something you can't prove to an insurance company, that one patient needs an enema and another needs surgery, even if your diagnosis is the same. You can't invent a single "Kremlin pill" for everything, a universal panacea. Or if that's what we want to do, then fine, but then who needs medicine at all?

In an odd, refracted echo of Pyotr Badmaev's arguments about how medical symptoms, accrued into the wrong clinical picture, might impede the alleviation of suffering, Vladimir Viktorovich argued that an integrative model that incorporated Tibetan medicine offered a way to reform the current health-care ideologies that imperiled the body politic—but without the universalizing ethics of care that both Buddhism and Communist ideologies share. At the same time, he was perfectly cognizant that symptoms might accrue in all manner of ways, mostly mediated by the particular specialized therapeutic optics a patient would encounter while moving through the topographies of Moscow's medical "el Dorado." From this perspective, practitioners and medical administrators working with nonbiomedical therapies are perfectly cognizant that their medical institutions are only one stop on patients' spatially and temporally diffuse trajectories of self-care concerned primarily with maintaining an adequate *samochuvstvie*—a state of functional health where experiences of a fluctuating vitality and the search for treatment are always primarily a matter of day-to-day embodied experience and not so much configured in relation to biomedical metrics.

RECENTERING PERIPHERIES

The politics of deploying traditional medicine in Moscow are quite distinct from the ways in which they play out in Buryatia, although the rhetoric of integration was pertinent to both sites. For Moscow-based practitioners and administrators interested in traditional medicine, the problem of integrating different techniques seems to be ultimately a question of managing one's clinical practice. That different therapeutic traditions and methodologies were easily available for incorporation was never in question, nor were there discernible ethical stakes to the process beyond the problem of how to retain patients, how to best organize therapeutic tactics appropriate for each patient, how to acquire a specialization in a new therapeutic methodology, hire qualified specialists, or establish lasting relationships with suppliers of phytopharmaceuticals and homeopathic remedies. By contrast, the kinds of body politics that were at stake in Buryatia's integrative vision of health care—and in its effort to promote Tibetan medicine—often complicated and unsettled metropolitan assumptions about an easy and frictionless co-optation of traditional medicine in the service of a utopian "medicine of the future." Ultimately, it opens up the question of *whose* futures were at stake.

Scholarship on the globalization of "traditional medicine" has made several important points that challenge assumptions about the self-containment and homogeneity of different medical systems. Scholars of Asian medicines, for example, have pointed to the heterogeneity and plurality that result from the long histories of cultural borrowings and

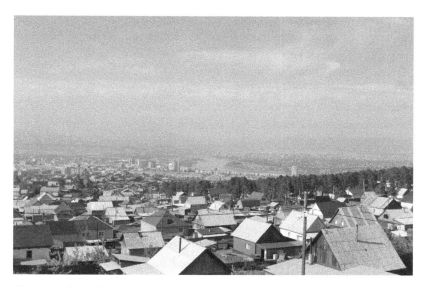

Figure 3. Ulan-Ude, 2017 (Photo by the author)

encounters at the intersections of trade routes, military conquests, colonial projects, and religious expansions, as well as to the contingent processes of formalization within therapeutic traditions that are internally plural (Scheid 2002; Pordié 2008; Hofer 2018). In other words, "traditional" medicines are never singular homogeneous formations. Indeed, it was precisely this very point that Buryatia's health-care administrator, cited previously, highlighted during his toast. The establishment of "national" medicines tethers specific medical traditions to the national histories and present political ambitions of states, where a focus on homogeneity and continuity makes the claims to uninterrupted traditions firmly contained within singular national pasts more convincing and authorizing (Farquhar 1994; Alter 2005). Medical anthropologists who focus on the global circulation of practitioners, methods, and therapeutic materials suggest that "traditional" medical practices are transformed and adapted to the cultural contexts they enter, affected by authoritative regimes of knowledge such as the "gold standards" of evidence-based medicine, as well as local moral economies of care (Adams, Schrempf, and Craig 2011; Zhan 2009). Conversely, as "traditional" medicines enter national and transnational therapeutic markets, their links to readily identifiable points of origins, ethnic groups, or cultural formations are inseparable from their ability to function as commodities (Janes 2002; Kloos 2010; Saxer 2013; Kloos et al. 2020). In Russia's vibrant domain of nonbiomedical, "natural" care, which includes a variety of institutions, therapeutic methodologies, and products, Tibetan medicine is only one of multiple therapeutic offerings identified as "traditional." Several conceptual contrasts operate in this field of therapeutic distinctions, where "Eastern" modalities of care and forms of knowledge are almost automatically identified as simultaneously "traditional" and "natural," in distinction to biomedical (and, implicitly, "Western") approaches equated to essentially "synthetic" or "artificial" interventions. In western Russia's urban metropolitan centers, Tibetan medicine simultaneously draws on an orientalist aesthetic of the mysterious East while referencing the internal diversity and "multinational" (*mnogonatzional'naya*) composition of the Russian Federation. At the same time, it is discursively linked to an ecological imaginary of distinctly *national* biological and ecological diversity. Despite the fact that medical practices identified as Tibetan medicine are certainly found in other Buddhist regions of the Russian Federation besides Buryatia, such as Kalmykia and Tuva, as well as in private clinics throughout the country's metropolitan centers, local medical professionals and administrators insist that Buryatia has achieved a level of formalization and clinical integration for Tibetan medicine far greater than in any other region in Russia and, some argue, in any other place in the West.

Tibetan medicine in Buryatia is co-opted into a practice of what I label here "peripheral visions"—hopes and strategies on the part of the region's administration, medical professionals, and scientists to establish Buryatia as its own center of gravity, both in Russia and more globally, but one that works to derive new forms of value from its very distance and marginality in relation to the nation's recognized cultural and economic centers. I find the term productive for thinking about the future-oriented aspects of the rhetoric surrounding Tibetan medicine in Buryatia, where it is invoked to articulate the region's anticipated economic and social developmental trajectories.

Over the last forty years, since the original project of investigating the legacy of Tibetan medicine in Buryatia was instituted at the local Academy of Sciences, the vision of what Tibetan medicine is understood to be has undergone significant changes. Since the early 1990s, it progressively became tethered to and bounded within a local geography of institutions and resources. In invoking the World Health Organization's repeated calls for a greater incorporation of local "ethnomedicines" into public health care, local scientists and medical practitioners interested, either intellectually or financially, in the potential of traditional medicine frequently insist that Buryatia, unlike other regions of Russia, in addition to having inherited Tibetan medicine with the spread of Buddhism, had the time to develop its own unique school: an established body of research and clinical deployment within the public health sector, unique in and to the Russian Federation. In addition, Tibetan medicine in the region is both discursively and institutionally aligned with a network of health resorts and sanatoriums that tend to derive their efficacy from assumptions about the curative properties of certain ecological features specifically, and of the therapeutic efficacy of an "untouched" environment more broadly.

Establishing Tibetan medicine as a recognizably Buryat form of care depends on scaling practices of place-making that unsettle entrenched national center-periphery imaginaries. By this I mean that local efforts to make Buryatia into a center of Tibetan medicine in Russia and, concomitantly, to define what makes Tibetan medicine in Buryatia unique and different enough from other forms of Himalayan medicine elsewhere to warrant these claims to centrality, challenge a national rhetoric that casts Russia's nonmetropolitan, non-Western frontier as simply a natural resource annex for Russia's "Western" federal centers. This chapter follows arguments about the self-enclosure or open-endedness of Tibetan medicine in Buryatia and tracks discussions of its hybridity and derivativeness as they become uneasily aligned with the therapeutic and political imaginaries of the Russian state.

GEOPOLITICS AS SORE POINT: CENTER-PERIPHERY LOGICS AND BURYATIA'S "BRAND"

The astronaut's unearthly vantage point seemed to haunt the mood of the informal social interactions at the conference. After participants eventually relocated to the shores of the aforementioned lake to relax and enjoy "being in nature," some of them gathered around a portable amplifying system brought by the conference organizers. Two songs were especially popular, drawing guests and hosts into an enthusiastic singalong. The first one was Aleksandra Pakhmutova's 1963 *"Glavnoe Rebyata Serdtzem ne Staret'"* (The Most Important Thing Is to Stay Young at Heart), which invokes the story of young geologists, dropped off in the middle of the Siberian taiga, in an area that can "only be reached by plane," and bravely setting up a new settlement in order to "take all the riches from under the earth." The song's refrain, articulated from the vantage point of an airplane window, wonders what the "green sea of the taiga" under the plane's wing might be singing about. The second song, entitled *"Trava u Doma"* (Grass Near the Home) was a much later (1983) Soviet pop-rock arrangement about an astronaut's nostalgia for Earth. Despite the lure of the vastness of space, the song suggests, the Earth, viewed from the remote perspective of a spacecraft porthole, invokes an aching sense of longing for the "green green grass near one's home." This nostalgic invocation of an extraterrestrial Soviet frontier seems especially provocative. Sometimes referred to as a "deep province" (*glubokaya provintzia*) both by local inhabitants and by those situated in Russia's more immediately recognizable centers, Buryatia rarely figures in the state media beyond its association with Baikal or, even more rarely, as a region defined by the prevalence of Buddhism. Most typically, and much like other "provincial" regions, it is neither heard nor seen outside of reports on wildfires and other ecological challenges, relegated to national imaginaries of an evacuated nature that blankets "Asian" Russia. These asymmetries sometimes percolate into vitriolic debates about the relationship between Buryatia's local administration and the federal government, which, in turn, express broader concerns with Russia's federal arrangements aimed to cope with the country's territorial gigantism and multinational composition.

I use the term "periphery" as a translation for a set of terms deployed interchangeably in Russian, such as *"okraina," "glubinka," "provinzia,"* and the calque *"periferiya."* Peripheries, margins, frontiers, and, more generally, places defined by their distance from recognizable centers are especially fertile ground for the proliferation of hybrid discourses that reflect on and recenter claims to global incorporation (Tsing 2005). While in Russia those regions that are actively identified as removed from the centers of economic and political power are often understood in relation to a single center—everything that is not Moscow is construed as the "periphery"—Buryatia finds itself in a kind of gravitational relationship to multiple "elsewheres." These multiple spheres of influence are not necessarily delimited by predetermined state formations and national borders, but instead span different kinds of geographic and social arrangements and encompassments, including the pan-Buddhist world and Eurasianist politics of pan-Mongol ethnicity. While Buryatia's inclusion into the Russian Federation is rarely publicly contested, people's individual strategies for education, health care, career advancement, and business look as much, and as critically, toward the Russian "West" as they do toward the Russian "East," as well as to China, South Korea, and Japan. But beyond these individual decisions and preferences for how to "make a living" outside and inside the region, this chapter is concerned with the ways in which a politics of marginality in a province at the periphery of Russia's national imaginary lays claims to unique forms of global and national relevance and inclusion.

Anthropology has classically critiqued center-periphery models for their inability to account for the complexity of cultural and economic circulations and flows (Appadurai 1996). Alternatively, anthropologists and historians of South Asia have different models of statecraft and a different vision of the distribution of power between center and margin, such as the Mandala-inspired "galactic polity" model developed by Stanley Tambiah (1976) and reprised by Geoffrey Samuel (1993; see also Hevia 1995). In the context of Russia, it is worthwhile to reflect on how center-periphery models operate when they are locally taken to authoritatively describe current political and economic arrangements. Distinctions traced along a "center"/"periphery" (or "center"/"regions") axis are part of a colloquial geopolitical mythos, frequently invoked in everyday conversations to account for Russia's geography of internal differences and inequalities.[5] The actual political and fiscal organization of the Russian Federation is a complex matter, however, with multiply defined tiers of administrative and territorial units. One dimension of differentiation between regions is whether they derive their political identity from a particular ethnic group that inhabits them—such as Buryatia or Tatarstan (Busygina and Taukebaeva 2015)—with the caveat that there is no one-to-one correspondence between ethnic population and eponymous region, and not all ethnic minorities have an associated territorial unit. Regional identification is thus articulated laterally (a regional identity that is distinct from Moscow), but not "vertically." As an analytic, "center-periphery" is not limited to describing

Russia's internal affairs. It also informs Russia's perceived position in a global economy. Thus, for example, thinking with Wallerstein's "world system" model, neo-Marxist sociologist and activist Boris Kagarlitsky suggested that post-socialist Russia found itself playing an economically and politically peripheral role in the global capitalist order as an extractive economy for the export of fossil fuels and other natural resources (Kagarlitsky 2002, 27).

The tendency to pin the center and periphery in a relationship of mutual confrontation also emerged in scholarly debates about Russia's possible territorial and political disintegration following the 1998 fiscal crisis. In the late 1990s, the possibility that the Russian Federation might cease to exist as a single entity was high on the agenda of political analysts, both in the country and abroad; ethnonational separatist rhetorics, as well as the attempts by local administrations to institute regional currencies and economically isolate themselves from the rest of the country, made the fracturing seem inevitable, a simple matter of time before Russia followed in the footsteps of the Soviet Union and ceased to exist as a single entity (see Alexseev 1999). That this did not happen is sometimes attributed to the rise of Putin's "strong state" in the early 2000s. For Russia's central government, balancing local elites' desire for autonomy with a promise of political allegiance to Moscow, on the one hand, while taking into consideration a region's economic solvency and bargaining power, on the other, involves some complicated political maneuvering that facilitates the entanglement between power and capital (Ross and Turovsky 2015; Sulakshin et al. 2013).

It may be helpful to consider the center-periphery logics in present-day Russia in terms of the semiotic interplay between marked and unmarked poles (Waugh 1982) of two mutually calibrated, but nonetheless distinct axes: Muscovite identity opposed to undifferentiated provinciality and ethnic Russianness versus other types of ethnic identification. The precarious work of aligning these two sets of distinctions occasionally spills out into aggressive nationalist rhetoric along the lines of slogans like "Russia for Russians." What I would like to note here is not simply that Russia's public sphere and public life have, to a certain degree, normalized racist and xenophobic sentiments, but that what characterizes the relationship of the ethnically marked to the ethnically unmarked is laminated over the opposition between center and periphery, which finds itself in a state of unstable equilibrium, always threatened by a figure-ground reversal of what comes to stand for the abstract, general category.

One example of this figure-ground relationship is expressed in a common and politically heated discourse, which articulates that Moscow is rather an exception when compared to the rest of the country. Pithily captured in a phrase that by now has acquired a kind of proverbial authority—"Moscow isn't Russia"—the sentiment gives rise to debates in the media and the political sphere around the necessity of greater decentralization. Sometimes critically referred to as "the state within the state," Moscow frequently incurs accusations from other metropolitan areas within Russia that it "lives at the expense of other regions," draining them of their natural resources and capital, and reinvesting it solely in Moscow's development, a view further buttressed by the eighteen years of Moscow mayor Yuri Luzhkov's "reign," which ended in 2010.[6]

Like other regions within Russia that derive their status and identity from being home to an ethnic minority population, Buryatia is marked as a kind of internal cultural "other," even though the extent of this difference is never set in stone and is always open to reevaluation. This markedness is also not necessarily, or at the very least not always, laminated over ethnicity, but rather is expressed in an opposition between "Western" or "European" Russia and the rest. It should be noted that the epithet "Russian" was not used as an ethnonym at the time but instead references national affiliation that occasionally comes to the surface of public debate and works to animate local political discourses about the nature of provinciality and the necessity and effectiveness (or, more typically, the lack thereof) of federal oversight, since "Moscow" comes to stand in for the federal government. Tensions sometimes come to the surface around scheduled visits by heads of state or other prominent outsiders, where preparations made on the part of the municipality and host institutions to receive honored guests are read into the region's uneven and superficial development, aimed only to signal to the remote metropole the regional administration's successful management.[7] In this vein, I frequently heard complaints from Ulan-Ude's permanent residents that the cosmetic changes to the city made in anticipation of these visits only served to throw into greater relief the self-serving nature of the local administration and its failure to cultivate a properly urban (and urbane) cityscape.

On the other hand, it is precisely Buryatia's markedness and distance that work as value added for local imaginaries of the region's future economic and social development. The following section thus explores the ambiguities that arise from efforts to transform the marked into the marketable. While processes that convert ethnic and cultural distinction into a form of regional capital have been documented elsewhere (Comaroff and Comaroff 2009; Lindquist 2005), the local administration and experts in Buryatia express concerns about a set of limitations that make the task of distilling a specific regional "brand" that would act as a source of value for Buryatia's identity difficult.

Expert RA, Russia's largest credit rating agency, tends to assign rather low estimates to Buryatia's investment potential according to most metrics. In 2009–2010, the region was placed into category 3B2, which translates to "lowered potential, moderate risk," a rating that has since dropped to 3C1, "lowered potential, heightened risk" (RAEX 2019). The ecological tourism sector presents a notable exception to these rather bleak evaluations. As such, Buryatia's administration pursues investment strategies that emphasize the region's suitability for developing ecological, pharmaceutical, and tourism industries.

Debates about branding began very visibly in 2008, with an initiative by the republic's administration to create a regional image-developing unit as part of the presidential council. Buryatia's "brand" featured regularly in the local media and became the focus of several conferences, as well as the basis of a genre of news articles that speculated about whether some local phenomenon might become Buryatia's new (and definitive) symbol.

On February 3, 2007, Russia's federal government passed legislation that declared the "Prebaikal region" of Buryatia a "Special Economic Zone" (SEZ) to bolster international tourism in the east of Russia, develop Russia's domestic sanatorium and health resort industry, and improve the economic prospects of the region (Sanzhin 2010). Tibetan medicine featured prominently in furthering this project. However, in 2008, Buryatia's president at the time, Vladimir Nagovitsyn, pointed out that before Buryatia could be turned into an attractive destination for domestic and international travelers, the administration ought to focus on raising general awareness about the region's very existence, suggesting that outside of Buryatia most people still confuse Ulan-Ude (Buryatia's capital) and Ulaanbaatar (the capital of Mongolia). By 2010, the debate had shifted. During a conference on the image of Russia and its regions conducted in Ulan-Ude in June 2010, the participants had recognized the relative success of promoting Buryatia's association with Lake Baikal, although they bemoaned the fact that "Irkutsk"—a synecdoche for Irkutskaya Oblast', the administrative region on the Western side of the lake—was still more readily associated with Baikal than Buryatia. The conference participants thus reaffirmed the necessity of furthering the region's attractiveness as a recreational and ecological destination. At the same time, some of the non-local participants cautioned that any brand development would be taking place in the context of Russia's broader geopolitical reputation, which gave little cause for optimism.[8] In response, one of the local experts on regional branding expressed his concerns that banking on Buryatia's "otherness"—Buryatia as the "the Heart of Russia in Asia," as the title of the report declares—drew attention to Buryatia's inherently ambiguous marginality:

> The geopolitical question for the Russian Federation is a sore point. The Far East is under threat of Sinification, which is something that worries Russian geopolitical analysts. The fact that Buryatia is part of the Mongol world within the RF is something that they feel ambivalent about: strong connections with Mongolia, Asia, China, and Tibet give some analysts reason to talk about separatist tendencies in Buryatia. To reduce these tensions, it would be correct to signal to the federal government that we consider ourselves one of Russia's regions, that we guarantee Russia's interests. (Kuzmin 2010)

A political geography defined in terms of oppositions between center and periphery is thus both part of local analytical categories and of everyday imaginings of what it means to live in one of Russia's "regions."[9] In the case of Buryatia, its status is further complicated by the fact that, as an ethnic minority republic, its relation to Moscow—and to Russia more broadly—frequently moves across degrees of inclusion as people distinguish, for example, between "Western Russia," "Siberia," and the "Far East" as different geopolitical and cultural entities that include smaller divisions. This mapping is also not necessarily aligned with ethnic identification, since ethnic Russians in Buryatia frequently insist on an inclusive

Siberian identity—"Sibiriak"—distinct from "Western" Russians (see also Quijada 2009).

In "European" or "Western" Russia, which typically refers to the territory to the west of the Ural Mountains, Buryatia is known mostly for its claims to Lake Baikal, one of the world's largest reservoirs of drinkable water and a UNESCO world heritage site. Concurrently, its details are curiously invisible to the gaze of Western Russia's metropolitan centers, beyond concerns about the ecology of the lake, such as the "MIR" diving expeditions undertaken from 2008 to 2010 or the regular protests, both local and national, against the operation of the technologically outdated and toxic Baikal Cellulose Paper Combine (BCBK).[10] Beyond the ecopolitics of Baikal, for people in Moscow, the mention of Buryatia seems to evoke a pure geographic blankness, the familiar image of the frontier equated to a potentially rich, mystical nature.

Curiously resonant with these images of "pure nature," local official discursive formations cast Buryatia in a markedly feminized register that emphasizes an emotional link to the local environment, praising its ecological diversity and unmarred purity and underscoring the population's geographical attachments to place and space.[11] In contradistinction, the more self-deprecating voices that rarely make it into the official media, but frequently permeate everyday conversations, frame Buryatia as one of Russia's ambiguously depressed margins that uncomfortably blends "premodern" rural landscapes with (post) Soviet, postindustrial decay. For example, my interlocutors frequently responded to my questions about what they thought about branding and the possibility of turning the region into a thriving tourist hot spot with disparaging and ironic critiques about the lamentable state of the local infrastructure. Despite the ecological and cultural potential of the region, I was often told, Western tourists would expect basic comforts in places understood as resorts.

At the same time, from the vantage point of Buryatia itself, Moscow is certainly not the only or the preferred center. The gravitational pull of Russia's capital is frequently displaced, in practice, in favor of other centers, depending on the closest metropolitan hubs, historically established patterns of migration for labor and education, and perceived ideas about how open to ethnic minorities any given large city in Russia might be. These choices are further impacted by Russia's laws carried over from the Soviet system of internal passports and household registration, where residence in any given city, and therefore employment, as well as social services dispensed by the state, are contingent on local household registration. Many of my Buryat friends and interlocutors chose Novosibirsk over Moscow to send their children to university or to seek out professional contacts, not only because the city is perhaps one of the largest and most developed metropolitan regions in Siberia and much closer geographically, but also because its everyday culture was perceived to be more friendly toward Russia's citizens who were not identified as ethnic Russians. In a sense, the image of Moscow in Buryatia frequently carried the aura of an alien other, with its overtones of colonial oversight, xenophobic anxieties about "Asianness" fueled by an ignorance of Russia's internal ethnic diversity and citizenship laws, and impersonal and commoditized social relations. At the same time, for most local projects of development, and especially for the development of an "integrated" medical system that recruits "Asian" medicine into its fold, Moscow (and, more specifically, various institutions of the federal government, such as the Ministry of Health) are practically the sole, or at least the most substantial, source of external funding. Most grant applications written by local researchers and medical administrators in Buryatia attempt to fit their understandings of Tibetan medicine to the current goals of these centrally issued programs.

In addition to these more practical limitations, establishing a recognizable and distinctive image for the region encounters conceptual problems, ones that have to do with claiming a cultural icon that is identifiably local rather than already co-opted by other, more recognizable entities. Much of the culturally distinguishable features to which Buryatia might lay a claim, for the purposes of self-presentation, have already been claimed by other national entities. Debates around Tibetan medicine in Buryatia make these difficulties especially visible. While Buryatia has unexpectedly found itself at the forefront of Russia's institutional experimentation with nonbiomedical healing, the semiotics of regional self-presentation betray a constant slippage between Tibetan medicine as part of Buryatia's claims to a Buddhist heritage, and therefore the region's inclusion into a broader Buddhist world, and its incorporation into the republic's health-care system and the academic efforts of scientific research centers as part of a more broadly defined "traditional"—and, therefore, localized—knowledge and skill.

In other words, attempts to produce and stabilize the "Buryatness" of Tibetan medicine open up the question of what is identifiably Buryat in the first place and how practices of Tibetan medicine in Buryatia are to be differentiated from those in neighboring Mongolia, which is understood locally to have a more authentic claim to an immediately recognizable cultural identity. Medical practitioners who use Tibetan medicine (and "traditional" medicine more broadly) in their professional practice often wistfully mentioned to me Mongolia's ability to "nationalize" Himalayan medicine by making it Mongolian, on the model of TCM in China. Institutionalizing Tibetan medicine in Buryatia along the same national medicine model is patently impossible, in part because of the tenuous claims Buryatia might have to an authentic and uninterrupted medical tradition, but more importantly because this kind of nationalization would run against a model of medical integration that recruits a variety of therapeutic forms. Despite the fact that different modalities of traditional or nonbiomedical healing are widespread in Russia and that Tibetan medicine has a degree of visibility and institutional recognition in Buryatia unmatched in other regions, once it is scaled up to a federally recognizable level, it is only allowed to enter public health provisioning as one of many elements in a system of fungible, self-similar modules.

TIBETAN MEDICINE AS INNOVATIVE TECHNOLOGY

The conference "Development of Traditional Medicine in Russia" brought together local administrative officials, directors of the city hospitals, and head physicians, as well as a number of participants from other regions, including Moscow, St. Petersburg, China, and Mongolia. As has been typical of previous conferences organized by the East-West Medical Center around the same theme, the 2010 meeting was defined as a "scientific-practical" dialogue, aimed at sharing research results and providing a forum for a wide variety of practitioners who identify their clinical practice with traditional medicine. Spanning three days of intense scholarly activity, where a variety of presentations ranged from general historical assessments of traditional medicine in Russia and abroad to very specialized reports on the efficacy of specific botanical remedies or physical procedures in treating concrete medical conditions, the conference was a cornucopia of everything and anything pertaining to nonbiomedical practices. The resultant assembly brought together a wide variety of specialists, from doctors to inventors of diagnostic and therapeutic machinery to professional medical practitioners. Among these guests were the vice president of the NIPC specializing in space medicine and a number of leading medical professionals working in the fields of restorative medicine. The conference had successfully united them in Buryatia's capital to delineate a therapeutic horizon that would effectively draw "traditional" medicine into the "therapeutic arsenal" of Russia's official health care.

As the idea for the conference was first fleshed out in the spring of 2010, one of the goals for the East-West Center's organizing committee was to establish an "exchange of experience" (*obmen opytom*) concerned with the incorporation of traditional medicine into domains of health care that dealt with recovery, prevention, and health optimization. Specialists at the center were especially excited to see what achievements in the domain of integrative health care were happening in other regions of Russia, as well as in Mongolia and China. Historically, the East-West Medical Center has successfully presented itself as an integrative medical institution in its own right, where different therapeutic modalities were seamlessly blended together. The East-West Center was systematically invoked as the main symbol of Tibetan medicine in Buryatia, specifically because it claimed to offer an integrated medical practice, one that brought together, under the single formula of "rehabilitative medicine," "Eastern" and "Western" care. Claims to integration functioned to differentiate it from other possible sites where Tibetan medicine is deployed in the region, such as temples or private clinics. Conversely, on a federal scale, it was the only site where Tibetan medicine found official endorsement by the health-care administration. In other words, for the purposes of its regional brand, Buryatia became the only region in Russia where Tibetan medicine was said to be practiced under full recognition from the Ministry of Health, although what is typically omitted in these claims is the fact that this state of exception was enabled through Buryatia's status as a minority republic with certain aspirations to a cultural and religious autonomy, and Russian federal law leaves regional health-care organization, including the deployment of traditional medicine, to the discretion of local governments. From the vantage point of the federal health-care administration, "East-West" was a state institution of health protection (GUZ) specializing in rehabilitative medicine (*vosstanovitel'naya meditzina*), much like a health resort or a sanatorium, and therefore was expected to use an armamentarium of typical rehabilitative techniques, such as reflexotherapy and massage associated with "traditional medicine."

In terms of its public self-presentation, East-West tended to bank on the concept of medical innovation, and its administration narrated it as a progressive medical institution that might eventually become a model for integrative medical care throughout Russia. In her introductory speech at the conference, the director of East-West emphasized the innovative approach espoused by her institution in particular and Buryatia more broadly, arguing that traditional medicine was itself an "innovative technology" (*innovatzionnaya tekhnologiya*). After all, she explained, "everything that pertains to promoting human health belongs to the domain of the highest [most important] of technologies." Representatives from the Buryat Ministry of Health emphasized that because of East-West, Buryatia might serve as an example of successfully deploying traditional medicine to address current concerns that are most relevant for Russia's health care, thus furthering the health-care priorities of the state. Signaling a recuperation of a therapeutic past—longstanding cultural traditions embedded in the region—into a nationwide therapeutic future is a common strategy in Buryatia among medical professionals and institutions interested in traditional medicine. Furthermore, the desirability of this seamless collapse between the "past" and the "future," between the "traditional" (and implicitly Asian) and the scientific (and implicitly European) were further buttressed by the presence of representatives from the NIPC, who had used the services of East-West in previous years and were working to secure future collaboration.

Although the presence of astronauts at a conference on traditional medicine might appear somewhat counterintuitive, this juxtaposition shed light on some of the ways in which technologies of traditional medicine are currently recuperated into an imaginary of future medical progress. The medical director of the space flight institute, whom I will here call Doctor Sidorov, and his entourage of stone-faced and mostly military-trained pilots were paying homage to their previous collaboration with the East-West Medical Center, where astronauts from the program had undergone rehabilitative treatment to compensate for the physiological transformations that accompany the return to Earth after a long sojourn in space. Visiting the conference was also an occasion to renew a commitment to collaborating with the center and to establish a more formalized and permanent relationship that would enable post-flight astronauts to "rest" on the shores of Lake Baikal and to undergo treatment with Tibetan medicine as part of a rehabilitative regimen. In his own report, illustrated through an image of the Yin and Yang symbol, which he allegedly derived through complex mathematical manipulation of the I-Ching, complete with an illustration of equations and formulas, Sidorov argued that the picture represented the path to properly integrating "Eastern wisdom" and "Western science" in the service of rehabilitative medicine.

The welding of traditional medicine to restorative medicine, which tended to be the dominant professional identity for most medical specialists present at these public events, merits an explanation. In Russia, the concept of restorative medicine (RM) (*vosstanovitel'naya meditzina*) as a separate branch of both practical health care and medical accreditation is typically traced back to the formation of a department of restorative medicine at the Sechenov Moscow Medical Academy in 1993. The goals of RM were closely linked to national anxieties about the health and demographic structure of the Russian population, and they were originally formulated in terms of "protecting the health of healthy people" (Bobrovnitzky et al. 2012; Razumov and Bobrovnitzky 2008). Throughout its development, RM progressively expanded beyond health protection, and it is now focused on "restoring" the "functional reserves" of bodies affected by illness or nefarious environmental conditions by acting on the "adaptive capacities of the organism" through the "integration of diverse health-promoting and rehabilitative technologies" (Razumov and Bobrovnitzky 2008). In this sense, despite being cast as a "new medical technology" in the professional medical literature, the language of RM echoes older logics. It invokes hidden potentials for recovery locked inside the human body, situating the body proper at an intersection with environmental and social conditions. Because RM focuses on noninvasive, nonpharmaceutical interventions, it aligns "natural factors" (such as climate and water therapies) with "techniques of traditional medicine" to achieve recovery.

As an "integrative" medical project, RM is a self-evident administrative classification for those institutions and therapeutic sites interested in mobilizing traditional medicine. It is precisely on these grounds that the collaboration between East-West and the NIPC was made possible. Starting in 2008, when a team of astronauts underwent post-flight rehabilitation at the East-West resort facility, the development of Tibetan medicine in Buryatia (and the future of East-West more specifically) was firmly tethered to imaginaries of futuristic bodies in space and maximized athletic performance. The long-term goal of the center's administration (later thwarted through the center's restructuring in 2016) was to create a "Zvezdnyi Gorodok" ("Star Town")—a kind of total rehabilitative institution catering to post-flight rehabilitation and treatment. Despite the fact that, in practice, the center tended to treat an aging patient population for various chronic conditions, its aspirational goals for the future were systematically articulated in relation to "rehabilitation" more broadly, including a turn to the optimization of athlete's bodies in preparation for future Olympic competitions. When China won gold in the 2008 Olympics, much of the discussion among medical professionals at East-West cited Vladimir Putin's speculation that the reason for their overwhelming success was the athletes' use of TCM. More broadly, Russia's sports medicine, much like space medicine, tends to be articulated in terms of harnessing the "hidden reserves" of the body for increased performance. In her opening speech at the conference, the director of East-West emphasized that it was precisely these potentials, locked away in the human body, that Tibetan medicine—and traditional medicine more broadly—were uniquely suited to access.

It may be useful, in this case, to reflect on how traditional medicine and space medicine could be imagined as naturally in dialogue. Much like sports medicine, "space medicine" is understood to optimize, rather than treat. Unlocking and mobilizing "the hidden reserves of the human organism" has a long history in both Soviet psychology and medical practices, especially in the domain of space medicine and athletics (Krippner 1986). It is interesting, then, that Tibetan medicine in Buryatia linked future visions of integrative medicine to a plurality of different "peripheries" or "margins" that made them meaningful. Insofar as the Space Age was rife with metaphors of a colonial frontier, one that invited imaginaries of human expansion beyond the confines of earthly lived place, it also exploded bodily boundaries, relativizing the concept of "earthly" health as something that is already, inherently, local. Focusing on space medicine in the U.S., anthropologist Valerie Olson has suggested that the body in space unsettles typical biomedical assumptions about healthy "baselines," forcing medical practitioners to imagine a different way of understanding and conceptualizing human vitality and human health (Redfield 1996; Olson 2010).

For his part Dr. Sidorov's report regrounded this deterritorialized health through a cosmic detour. The maintenance of health in space, he argued, and the necessary period of post-flight rehabilitation both presented unique challenges peculiar to the nature of space flight itself and spoke to the nature of modern life on earth. "Cosmic health," he reminded his audience, is a prerequisite of an astronaut's body, a state that goes above and beyond normal "earthly" functioning, and its detection qualifies a human body for deterritorialization. This image of a body stretching the limits of the typical presupposes a greater reserve of vitality, one that will allow an astronaut to withstand the wear and tear of prolonged time spent in orbit in conditions of zero gravity. The members of the astronaut training institute present at the conference equated traveling above the Earth's atmospheric periphery to moving forward in time at a faster pace. Bodies exposed over time to an environment of zero gravity eventually develop the same characteristics of bone loss, hypotension, and muscular atrophy that are typical of the aging process. Dr. Sidorov thus emphasized that the same physical deteriorations, albeit not quite as rapid, could be observed in modern city dwellers. He articulated the process of rehabilitation in terms of "anti-aging" (*omolozhenie*), arguing that because space flight prematurely ages the body by metaphorically accelerating time, the efforts to restore the astronaut's health to its pre-space mission state can eventually be extended to age-reversing procedures aimed at regular civilian patients afflicted with living in conditions of "modernity." In these articulations, the contrast between "tradition" and "modernity" in medicine did more than simply rehash a logic of geographically distributed social evolutionism (although it certainly did that as well). Instead, it also seemed to suggest, albeit implicitly, an aspirational collapse of temporal qua physical horizons. If, as Susan Buck-Morss has argued, Soviet imaginaries of progress sought to conquer time by accelerating it toward a communist utopia (Buck-Morss 2002), then Dr. Sidorov and his colleagues were in the business of pulling the brakes by appealing to medical traditions carefully maintained as outside of the pathogenic temporalities of modernity. Because the pharmacopeia of Tibetan medicine includes a variety of anti-aging formulas, locally referred to as "*zhudlen*," Dr. Sidorov argued that it was uniquely appropriate for counteracting these processes of senescence, accelerated through the stresses (and immobilities) of modern life. In other words, space flight and space medicine were quickly mapped onto the ills of modernity, which the techniques of "traditional" (and implicitly pre-modern, non-European) medicine would be uniquely suited to remedy.

COMING TO TERMS WITH TIBETAN MEDICINE

Anticipations of complementarity and fusion across multiple temporal imaginaries and scales of emplacement and displacement were haunted by a constant sense of unease at the idea that, as long as Tibetan medicine in Buryatia eluded easy categorization, its place within a national health-care future might be compromised. In 1998, when the founder of the East-West Medical Center gave a presentation of his work at the now disbanded State Scientific Research Institute of Traditional Treatment Methods in Moscow, the stated goals of his research were formulated as follows:

> [Our aim] is to show that traditional medicine in Buryatia is Tibetan, that [the kind of] Tibetan medicine that had spread on Buryat territory has a number of characteristics that distinguish it, and allow it to call it that. It is to single it out among other Eastern medical systems, and to consider it a Russian phenomenon. It is to find and formulate approaches for the further successful development of this branch of medicine.

If the task at the end of the 1990s was to demonstrate that traditional medical practices in Buryatia were recognizably Tibetan, by 2010 this concern had shifted. Administrators, scholars, and medical professionals were more concerned with the second part of the research goals stated earlier. In this sense, demonstrating that Tibetan medicine in Buryatia was properly Buryat and that it was therefore the legacy of a multinational Russian state had come to the forefront of public debates. It is then unsurprising that the hoary problem of labeling Tibetan medicine in the region introduced the conference proceedings. In his introductory address, the vice minister of Healthcare and Social Development for the republic began by drawing attention to this seemingly trivial issue: what should Tibetan medicine in Buryatia be called? Discursively staging a debate with one of the region's most prominent researchers on Tibetan medicine, also present at the honorary panel, but conveniently unable to object or intervene during the official speech, he formulated the problem as a recalcitrant impasse that impeded further development and frustrated the possibilities of adequate integration:

Dear friends, the fact that the conference on the development of traditional medicine is happening here in Buryatia is deeply logical. After all, Buryatia is the only region of the Russian Federation wherein the culture for many centuries so-called traditional Tibetan medicine is used. By the way, we call it different things. Some time back, I have proposed to Sergey Matveevich to establish a unified term, and I proposed the term "Tibetan medicine of Buryatia" but it just won't take root—right, Sergey Matveevich? Or were you simply ignoring me? In fact, there is a problem in identifying the medical system that concerns us. And, there are reasons to say that since the middle of the seventeenth century, on the territory of Siberia, Russia, Buryatia, this medicine lives and develops, and we can say that in the same way that there is Tibetan medicine, there is also a Tibetan medicine of Buryatia, although if someone has a better, more exact formula, we have no objections. Before moving forward, we really must come to some kind of term, no?

This statement uniquely captures a conceptual paradox that informs much of the efforts at institutionalizing Tibetan medicine in the region. Tibetan medicine in Buryatia is caught between two imperatives, derived from the local administration's desire to articulate it as part of Buryatia's regional identity. On the one hand, in order to legitimately become part of Buryatia's national offerings to the state, it must be presented as compatible with the Russian state's health-care objectives. Because of its legal status, or rather lack thereof, Tibetan medicine, insofar as it is to be used in Russia's official health sector, must lend itself to easy disassembly into alienated medical "technologies"—therapeutic modules recognizable within Russian mainstream public health categories, such as massage therapy, acupuncture, moxa, "traditional diagnostic techniques," and phytotherapy. From the perspective of this modular and atomized view, different "medical technologies" cannot be overtly "marked" as culturally or ethnically specific, or, minimally, they must be detached from their philosophical or conceptual underpinnings to be deployed discretely. This is not simply a conceptual problem, but a practical one at the level of the clinic. Thus, for example, the head of an important homeopathy clinic in St. Petersburg present at the conference eagerly explained to me and a group of doctors from East-West that he had been successfully combining homeopathy with diagnostic techniques derived from "Asian" medicine. This practitioner used traditional pulse diagnosis, presumably derived from Traditional Chinese Medicine, and subsequently prescribed homeopathic remedies in accordance with his diagnoses. Later, one of the doctors from East-West grumbled privately: this was truly a bizarre hybrid, in his opinion. Such combinations were unproblematic only if each therapeutic approach is completely detached from its broader philosophical assumptions and reduced to the level of "technique." Most jarringly, whereas homeopathic remedies were based on the principle of *similia similibus curantur* (like cures like), Tibetan medicine followed an allopathic logic, such that diagnosing the excess of a particular illness in most cases would be followed by a medicine that works to counteract it. Yet, the combination of homeopathy and Tibetan medicine is also practiced at East-West, in the same manner—pulse diagnostic leads to the prescription of a variety of procedures that are not limited to Tibetan medicine formulas, but because it is practiced by doctors who identify as Tibetan medicine practitioners, it is the Western roots of homeopathy that are conveniently and felicitously erased.

On the other hand, the appeal of "traditional" medicine for the main therapeutic domain where it was deployed—namely, rehabilitative medicine—was derived from its claims to being a "system"—a total form of care, both principled and internally coherent. Systematicity, in turn, mapped onto claims to distinctions between ethnically and culturally identifiable (textual) medical traditions and empirical and unsystematic folk practices. To reconcile these tensions between the impetus to view Tibetan medicine as efficacious precisely because it is systematic and constitutes an epistemological totality, mediated through its "Buryat" identity, and the necessity to align it with the interests of national health care seen as an assemblage of alienable modules, local scholarly voices began to argue that what made Tibetan medicine distinctively Buryat is that it was not *singularly* Buryat. In other words, Tibetan medicine is already always integrative, and especially so in Buryatia, these discourses claimed. If Buryat–Tibetan medicine is in reality an assemblage of different medical cultures and techniques—Russian, Mongolian, Persian, Greek, Indian, and so forth—then what makes it Buryat is that it is, like Buryatia itself, always emerging at the crossroads of a variety of traditions, that it is simultaneously derivative and hybrid by default, incorporating local and remote forms of knowledge and practice, and adapting them systematically to regional ecologies and the needs of local populations—figuratively, rooting them in place.

It is useful to contextually situate these claims in relation to broader discourses on the history of medicine in Russia. Russian scholars of medicine and medical professionals tend to divide different therapeutic approaches along three principal types: folk medicine, traditional medical systems, and scientific medicine (Mirskiy 2005; Muzalevsky 2007). In this literature, folk medicine is understood to be an unsystematic miscellany of empirically established therapeutic techniques that may or may not have a scientific explanation. By contrast, traditional medicine, understood as the next evolutionary step on the path to medical progress from folk medicine, is interpreted as a system, where philosophical and religious epistemologies undergird and tie together different empirically established therapeutic technologies. In more popular usage, folk medicine typically refers to "esoteric" healers, whereas Tibetan and Chinese medicines are more likely to be classified as "traditional." As a collection of methods and techniques whose efficacy is empirically established, culturally marked therapeutic practices might thus scale up to being seen as a total system for manipulating the body's vitality or be disarticulated into separate components, or modules, and recombined into new systematic approaches to health within a modern health-care system. In this sense, Tibetan medicine in Buryatia was caught between two contradictory descriptive regimes. Thus, claims to systematicity were deeply political ones—a gloss for whose claims to epistemological authority counted more.

One view, most often espoused by those practitioners with strong Buddhist allegiances or those whose training in Tibetan medicine followed a more classic, apprenticeship-like pattern, posited that, because of the systemic nature of its Buddhist philosophical underpinnings, Tibetan medicine could not be parsed into separate components and recombined with other, non-Buddhist approaches without losing its efficacy or potentially becoming harmful. In other words, without an understanding of the cosmological principles on which Tibetan medicine was founded, a practitioner would be unable to properly diagnose and treat her patient. On the other hand, medical administrators and biomedical practitioners seemed to view Tibetan medicine as inherently a combination of alienable parts— separate techniques, capable of being effectively recombined and integrated into new systems of health restoration.

This approach has specific ramifications for the establishment and recognition of a distinct "Buryat-Tibetan" medicine. Earlier works published in the late 1970s and up until the 1990s equated Tibetan medicine with the "ossified" canon of "Indo-Tibetan medicine" (cf. Khundanov, Khundanova, and Bazaron 1979; Khundanov et al. 1993; Bazaron, Aseeva, and Nazarov-Rygdylon 1984; Bazaron 1989; Nikolaev 1998). These works were mainly concerned with primary sources and much less with lived practice. Although these scholarly accounts point to the ways in which Tibetan medicine had borrowed from both Ayurveda and Chinese medicine to constitute its literary canon, they also presented it as a self-enclosed and finished product. They rarely emphasize a distinctly Buryat inflection of the medical knowledge and practices labeled "Tibetan medicine," noting only in passing that local practitioners had adapted some of the original formulas to fit with the local flora, especially when medicinal components were endemic to warmer climes and difficult to obtain.

Certainly, writing about traditional medicine under late socialism came with its own ideological pressures, such as the necessity to emphasize the materialist nature and possible practical application of traditional medicine for modern science and public health and framing its religious cosmologies and principles as belonging to a previous stage of historic development. However, for the purposes of this discussion, I am less interested in how scholars justified the validity of studying Tibetan medicine than I am with the ways in which they thought of Tibetan medicine as a largely bounded, "complete" medical system. Most of these accounts framed medical knowledge through an evolutionary model, as moving from disparate "folk" techniques to self-enclosed medieval religious-based knowledge "systems" to, finally, modern "scientific medicine." As a result, these accounts appeared to reinforce the idea that the object they studied was static and complete and largely relegated to a previous historical phase.

By contrast, a different way of framing Tibetan medicine in Buryatia became widespread in local scientific discussions and publications in more recent years. These works pushed against the imagery of ossification, emphasizing the ways in which Tibetan medicine in Buryatia, while still an expression of its "original" Indo-Tibetan formulations, dynamically adapted and changed, absorbing the traditional folk techniques of local nomadic people, and incorporated the local flora and fauna into its *materia medica*. In a sense, this is more a change of emphasis than a radical reconceptualization of what Tibetan medicine is. The capacity to find local botanical equivalents and substitute them for the ones in "original" recipes has changed valence from simply a matter of expediency to the proof that there is a distinct, Buryat tradition of Tibetan medicine, one that is uniquely adapted to local bodies and to their particular environmentally inflected physiologies. Local scholars thus argue that Tibetan medicine in Buryatia is at once dynamic and changing, yet distinctly local, unfolding along its own recognizable "branch."

Practicing *emchi* in Buryatia certainly do not limit themselves to using only local botanicals when preparing medicines, nor are they strictly limited to the region, often relocating to Moscow for part of the year, for those "out of season" periods when the collection and preparation of medicines are impractical. Assembling medicines from scratch requires, among other things, the capacity to mobilize vast networks of suppliers, often straddling the political and legal boundaries that regulate the traffic of seeds and plants across borders and geographic distances, from packing houses in India, China, and Mongolia to the botanical gardens of Moscow and St. Petersburg. They also require an intimate knowledge of local geographies—the ability to track, from year to year, the capricious life of scarce and ecologically sensitive plants. They demand an extensive knowledge of geology or at the very least an access to qualified geologists capable of recognizing, for example, different types of calcite that are "extinguished" differently in processing.[12] It is easier, I was frequently told by my *emchi* interlocutors, to simply go back to the original recipes, replacing the Buryat botanical substitute with something that one could order online or ask a friend to bring from his or her next trip to India or Mongolia, where plantations of medicinal botanicals were more common and the industry more developed. While making one's own medicines is still taken to be the sign, par excellence, of an authentic *emchi*, practitioners of Tibetan medicine in Buryatia are certainly not bound in practice by an ecology of local plants and bodies in the same way that the ideal type of Buryat–Tibetan medicine articulated in scholarly and public discourses seems to suggest.

My point here, however, is not that there is a chasm between ideology and practice, but that the rearticulations of Tibetan medicine in Buryatia, as a form of knowledge that should be recognized as characteristic of the region, recreates a sense of closure and encapsulation that echoes earlier understandings of Indo-Tibetan medicine as a complete and self-enclosed system, frozen in time, that long ago achieved its maximal development. In other words, the historical trajectory of Tibetan medicine is now being redefined as a knowledge practice that has adopted local techniques and methods in order to adapt to its new context and that treats situated physiologies with available means, understood as de facto appropriate (because naturally preadapted) to local biologies. However, in the contemporary moment, it is again seen as static, implicitly incapable of creativity and change outside of the next moment of "encounter" with a different therapeutic form—namely, integration with biomedicine.

In this respect, current debates around the integration of Tibetan medicine in Buryatia have a teleological quality. Although an emphasis on its previous historical plurality works to actively subvert earlier definitions of Tibetan medicine as an ossified, purely textual system belonging to a previous stage of historical development and to a social and religious geography that does not include contemporary Buryatia, new forms of objectification and stasis are emerging. Even when it is seen as a therapeutic assemblage at the intersection of multiple flows of knowledge and practice, Tibetan medicine in Buryatia is still spoken of in relation to an evolutionary view of medicine, which moves from the empirical to the cosmological to, finally, the scientific. Integration with biomedicine thus becomes the next obvious step in the development of any form of nonbiomedical practice. However, it is here that its ascribed capacity for absorption and innovation is dismissed because the grounds for integration are envisioned on the basis of the only remaining systematic medical knowledge, which is to say biomedicine. Such visions of development elide the lived forms of knowledge and practice that, although they are not necessarily systematic, do not easily fit a modular view of alienable medical technologies, and, by extension, those practitioners who know how to use them. It also ignores the inventiveness of day-to-day medical practice. Practitioners who are outside the official medical sector are thus doubly marginalized by these articulations—first, because their practice has at best a tenuous status under Russia's system of medical licensing, and second, because reframing their activity as a series of "techniques" obscures and devalues the knowledge and expertise necessary to appropriately deploy them.

THE "WE" OF INTEGRATIVE MEDICINE

Unsurprisingly, discourses on integration generated resistance. The following section draws on the debates taking place at another conference, organized in July 2010, and entitled, "The Convention of World Mongols," a recurrent event envisioned as a cultural exchange between representatives from different areas of Inner Asia united by a loosely defined common Turko-Mongol cultural, religious, and ethnic heritage. Unlike the medical conference discussed in the previous sections, the convention offered a platform for framing Tibetan medicine in Buryatia not as a source of alienable therapeutic techniques, to be integrated into a system of state health care largely defined by biomedicine, but as a total system of local care that might address the issues specific to a region defined by its political and geographic ambiguities. In other words, the conference presented a different therapeutic future for Buryatia, one that challenged the discourse on standardized national rehabilitation. It also challenged the kinds of "center-periphery" imaginaries that informed the medical conference described earlier, offering a different take on Buryatia's political and geographic encompassments and relations.

The roundtable on traditional medicine brought together a variety of participants, from local Buddhist lamas to representatives of Buryatia's government to scholars and medical professionals. Unlike the previous conference, this event did not exclude temple-based practitioners, but instead encouraged their presence. While the speeches began with the typical enumeration of Buryatia's achievements in the domain of traditional medicine and its study and the potential for furthering Buryatia's "brand" as the "Heart of Asia in Russia," the optimistic tone was quickly offset by voices that drew attention to the political underpinnings of the conversation.[13] Focusing on the ecological challenges to the region, problems of public health, and an absence of a reliably salubrious "lifestyle" among the population, speakers attempted to mobilize Tibetan medicine as a potential source of solutions to social problems. However, much like the conversations described in the previous public event, these discussions were plagued by the apparent instability of the object under scrutiny.

Ayuna, one of the pediatricians from East-West Medical Center with whom I attended the event, who was also interested in nonbiomedical practices, noted with a degree of amused frustration that the introductory speech that was meant to clarify the goal of the roundtable and to set the terms for its subsequent unfolding had taken the shape of a typical conceptual muddle. She charged the speaker with a lack of epistemological clarity, saying he lacked a firmly established framework that could guide the desired integration between "Eastern" and "Western" medical practices, the formulation of which had admittedly been the goal of the session. In my many conversations with Ayuna throughout my fieldwork, this problem had become a theme for her, a concern that she, an ethnic Buryat and a practicing Buddhist, as well as a biomedical doctor by training who was avidly interested in traditional medicine more broadly and in the possibility of an integrative approach to health more specifically—the lack of clear definitions and boundaries was a source of professional and intellectual frustration. The discussion at the roundtable was the archetypal expression of a conceptual *kasha*, to use her own vividly coined analogy. This *kasha* of loosely mixed entities reflected, in her opinion, both her institution's medical philosophy and her own place within it. In fact, the deterioration of medical integration into *kasha* or other equally unwieldy and unsystematic assemblages was a common source of anxiety for many of my informants who, as medical practitioners, attempted to navigate on an everyday basis bodily ontologies and medical principles that resisted conceptual commensuration, even when they managed to coexist peacefully, and even productively, in clinical practice.

The main source of Ayuna's irritation had been the remarks delivered by Dr. Badaraev, the head of a local medical vocational college and the chair of the session. While Ayuna's professional training drew her attention to the speaker's failure to volunteer any practical or substantial content about the nature of traditional medicine or the principles that should organize its incorporation into practical health care—when and where to use it, under what conditions, in combination with what sorts of diagnostic techniques, to replace which synthetic medications—my own sense of confusion with the speech centered on my inability to determine who Dr. Badaraev meant by "we." Rather than viewing our respective confusions as existing in two separate conceptual spheres or motivated by entirely different intellectual concerns, I would like to propose that they were, in fact, mutually illuminating. I do not mean to suggest here that the ethnographer's lens provides a privileged point of access to what really organizes the epistemological muddle that both my interlocutors and I often experienced when trying to make sense of integrative medicine. Instead, I suggest that what made nonbiomedical therapies in Russia such a conceptually elusive object was the work that went into maintaining a tension between claims to their potentially universal (because broadly medical and hence humanist) relevance and applicability and their situatedness and cultural markedness. Ayuna's *kasha* and my confusion at the elusive indexes of Dr. Badaraev's "we" pointed to a single political conundrum for Buryat-Tibetan medicine: namely, the layered and contested politics of its inclusions.

Dr. Badaraev's use of "we" switched creatively between categories. It alternated between pointing to his professional alignment with a biomedical community on the one hand and to his identity as Buryat on the other, which is to say, multiple geographic, cultural, and religious encompassments within differently defined social fields. The first self-identification presupposed the existence and ready availability of two separate domains— European medicine and Asian medicine—and the desirability and feasibility of combining them in practical health care. The second laid claims to traditional medical practices simultaneously articulated as part of an identifiably Buryat cultural heritage and located in a broader Asian way of thinking about and treating bodies and their vitality. He motivated the necessity for the roundtable by pointing out that, while the theme of developing traditional medicine was in no way new, it remained exceptionally timely and relevant for Buryatia's prosperity. Because Buryatia was a potential "branding point" for Russia and Buryat-Tibetan medicine was a "branding point" for Buryatia, formulating the proper way to incorporate traditional medical practices with the existent health-care system was, according to Dr. Badaraev, a matter of both medical and political importance:

> We have managed to conquer a multitude of diseases, . . . but how do we develop standards for using traditional medicine? How can we teach our students and workers traditional medicine, so that the person knows its foundation, can use the herbs on our territory for treatment?

The referent for his "we" was exceptionally elusive throughout his speech, shifting from his fellow medical educators, the republic's health-care workers, to Buryats writ large within a bigger world of Mongol cultural identity, to, finally, a civic alignment with the interests of the Russian state. In a striking formulation, where these different levels blended, Dr. Badaraev declared, wistfully, "The more Western we become, the more we forget traditional medicine." Shifting effortlessly to Buryatia's geopolitical place in Russia's broader health-care crisis, he continued:

We see on this slide that we spend a lot of money on health care, something like 145 billion rubles. The Russian people have encountered a problem: socially significant diseases are prevalent, and people can't afford the expensive drugs. We have 12,000 medical workers in RB [Republic Buryatia]. That's a big army. Why can't we use traditional medicine to address some of these issues? . . . Unfortunately, our population is becoming older. We lose one small village every year. Lately, our birth rate has become higher than the death rate, but our life span is decreasing. . . . The problem is quality of life, and this is a political, economic question. Can we not use our traditional methods to improve the situation? . . . Our European medicine has always developed, and has been doing so very fast, lately. Nanotechnologies are becoming widely used. But with the technologies of traditional medicine, we could influence European medicine. Our drugs are effective, but they don't heal the reason behind the disease. We heal one thing, and harm another. We must heal the person, not the disease. We already have integrative medicine, and we must emphasize those results we have already obtained, and show the problems we have solved, so we can get recognition for it.

As Dr. Badaraev's speech unfolded, the use of "we" extended to include Russia's federal government: "Our government expresses respect for our religion and our culture, it accepts the significance of the Mongolosphere. Buryatia is the Center of Asia in Russia."

The speeches and conversations that followed the keynote address can be read as efforts to articulate and stabilize the groupings and alignments that Dr. Badaraev's ambiguous "we" had left open-ended. Most of the speakers who were firmly situated within official health care tended to remind the participants that the medical integration of traditional medicine in Buryatia had already, by and large, been achieved. In part, this sense of accomplishment exists as the result of the progressive decentralization of Russia's health-care system, where the organization of local health provisioning is left to the regional governments and exhibits significant variation (Danishevski et al. 2006; Gordeev et al. 2011).

Proposals on how to reach this goal varied, from suggestions that the development of each region's unique brand of traditional medicine ought to be incorporated as a mandatory element of the school curriculum to more practically minded proposals that medical students should learn the techniques of traditional medicine in parallel with their primary biomedical training. Some of these suggestions were met with concerns. How, for example, could students be taught the principles of Western anatomy and physiology alongside the logic of meridians, "biologically active points," and the flow of Qi without becoming confounded by seemingly incompatible claims to distinct bodily ontologies? Some of the members of the audience raised concerns that such juxtapositions would needlessly confuse students, who would be stumped as to what they should believe or take seriously.

Badaraev's predominant orientation toward a "Western" Russia as the main audience, source of legitimacy, and important consumer of traditional medicine also elicited critiques. As the discussion became progressively more heated, one of the participants, a representative from the regional ministry of health, cut in with an irate pronouncement:

> We are talking about integration here, but the integration of what? Officially, we know of Tibetan, Chinese, Indian medicine. Which one are we talking about here? What specific technologies are we supposed to be introducing? We must study these technologies first. There was a proposal to petition the health ministry to incorporate our [botanical] medicines, but they've heard about that already [and done nothing]. We have a lot of medicines here, but you know, on the other side of the Urals, they just think of them as weeds. This is relevant to Asian geopolitics. China is developing very quickly, including in the domain of traditional medicine and health care. Maybe the Western part of Russia doesn't need our medicines? So let us try instead to institute it in those regions that are genetically close to these [therapeutic] technologies.

The most forceful protest against the idea that combining "Western" and "Eastern" medicine was a desirable future for the republic came from speakers who were institutionally affiliated with Buddhist temples. In his speech, the head of the Aginsky Tibetan Medicine Academy, Babu Lama, inverted the terms of the debate, suggesting that the moral economies and underlying philosophical orientations of biomedicine were inherently incompatible with Buddhist philosophy and profoundly insufficient to address the social needs of the region:

What is traditional medicine, how does it get integrated—well, that's a controversial question. Each disease has its own name in different languages, but the [fact] of illness is always the same. I am not a doctor, I am a priest and a philosopher. But I would like to note that Western medicine might not be integrative. Before the Revolution, we had what I call Russian-Tibetan medicine, widely used by the population. There are many formularies written by local lamas [using local botanicals] and standardization might in fact not fit. A formulary, after all, is personalized, it is the lama's personal creation. And there is a significant problem, in addition to that. We need to prepare doctors who don't have spiritual evil. But science has no capacity to counteract it. In all of Eastern medicine, we have an anthropological approach. It's all good and well to think of the body as something that you can go fix, like a nice new car. But how are you going to fix it, if its owner insists on filling it with diesel when it's meant to run on 98 gas?

I understand Babu Lama's rather condensed car analogy to be more than a critique of poor lifestyle, something that became clearer in the broader context of his discussion. I suggest that it is, instead, grounded in a Buddhist understanding of health as an extension of a certain kind of ethical behavior. Like other Buddhist practitioners I spoke with, he did not see scientific and biomedical knowledge as concerned with or capable of addressing the body as the expression of moral, cognitive, and physiological habits, which, in the logics of a Buddhist bodily phenomenology, constitute the basis of physical existence. According to Babu Lama, the biomedical gaze understands bodies mechanistically and thus fails to see the root of the problem, which, in this case, is the same sort of ethical ignorance manifested by the patient, who insists on using the wrong kind of "fuel" to power her body. In his conclusion, he repeated a similar distinction:

> The object—or the subject—of medicine is the same—the human, right? China has been doing this [developing traditional medicine] for forty years. Does this mean that Chinese medicine will work here? I doubt it. Just the temperature spectrum here is over 100 C, to give you an example. What does that mean? In terms of methodological recommendations, what we actually need is a survival guide (*posobie po vyzhyvaniyu*), and a resource center, based on the principles of traditional medicine.

There is a demand for that. How can you tell the quality of a person? It's in the difference between education and upbringing, and that's where traditional medicine can help.

To follow Babu Lama's provocation, if the human is the universal object of medicine, what sort of human is at stake? In his commentary, Babu Lama drew on a widespread distinction that pins education (*obrazovanie*), which is to say, a set of knowledge and skills one is expected to acquire as part of schooling and upbringing (*vospitanie*) meant to define a set of moral attributes and behaviors that define a person's ethical being. The Buddhist underpinnings of Tibetan medicine are here reconfigured as the missing and necessary element for the creation of ethical medical subjects, both healers and patients. Reorienting the usefulness of Tibetan medicine in the region from Dr. Badaraev's discussion of its potential for solving Buryatia's public health problems and to further address the national health crisis, Babu Lama proposed a different assessment of its necessity. The image of the survival guide and of the resource center suggests extraordinary and unlivable conditions, a situation whose rules have changed so suddenly and so radically that those who find themselves in the grips of illness have no technologies of coping. It also suggests a certain lack of universality or broad applicability. It was there, in his opinion, that Tibetan medicine could help—precisely because it provided a philosophical basis that extended beyond the state's concerns with public health or individual concerns with their personal physical well-being. Similar to previous speakers who argued for the development of Tibetan medicine in the region as something that is essential for Buryatia—and perhaps nonessential or irrelevant for the rest of Russia— Babu Lama was carving out a separate space of exception, one that emplaced Tibetan medicine in a specific regional ecology and linked it to cultural and religious traditions that would be irrelevant elsewhere. For Babu Lama, medicines might travel—which did not mean that they *should*. Much like Chinese medicine, which Babu Lama felt would not be as effective for Russian or Buryat bodies, transplanting Buryat–Tibetan medicine to other parts of Russia or the world characterized by a different set of ecological and social conditions would impede its efficacy.

Toward the end of the roundtable, one of the moderators, a high-ranking official from the local Ministry of Health, attempted to calm the tense atmosphere in the room by suggesting that, instead of framing the problem of medical integration and development in terms of coherence or incoherence, one had to consider it in relation to broader cultural processes: "We should remember that what is happening currently is globalization. I think no matter what we do, what will happen in the future is that we all will end up incorporating bits and pieces from here and there." In other words, for the health-care administrator, in a "contemporary" globalized moment, the coherence and philosophical underpinnings of medical practices no longer mattered. Globalization, for him, was already defined by a piecemeal incorporation of different "bits and pieces," and therefore the hybrid nature of Buryat–Tibetan medicine would lend itself perfectly to this process.

"SITTING ON A GOLD MINE"

Riding at the back of a rickety Soviet-era SUV along a dirt road, crammed together with several local Buryat doctors and scientists, I asked one of the Muscovite conference participants—a well-known phytotherapy expert and activist for the greater recognition of phytotherpy in Russia—why he so insistently wanted to go gather *badan* (*Bergenia*) root[14] on an early morning after a busy and long conference day. "For small business purposes," he laughed in response. His mood suddenly turning sullen, he proceeded with an impassioned and patronizing critique, addressed mostly to his silent local colleagues: "You people are sitting on a gold mine, and don't know how to use it, or how to present it." To the Muscovite phytotherapist's now quite grounded, yet still curiously metropolitan gaze, Buryatia remained an intensely peripheral culturally and socially evacuated frontier—by the end of the conference, he had not been convinced that there was anything to recuperate from Buryatia other than its remarkably biodiverse array of medicinal plants. Tibetan medical formulas did not hold much intrinsic interest for him—Russian phytotherapy, he suggested, already had a theory and didn't need a new one. At most, the region provided an interesting collection of medicinal substances, useful for expanding Russia's official pharmacopeia. For the Muscovite expert, local plants were certainly not weeds, and he could perfectly recognize their medical and monetary value. Similarly, local therapeutic infrastructures were legible as sites of rehabilitative medicine, much like any other sanatorium or health resort in the rest of the state. He admitted that Lake Baikal provided an attractive backdrop for bolstering their popularity. However, there was no particular value to be found in Buryat–Tibetan medicine as a system. His vision of the region's future was limited to the export of *dikorosy* (wild medicinal plants), the establishment of a phytopharmaceutical industry, and the further development of medical tourism associated with Lake Baikal and the region's ecology.

In this chapter, I have outlined competing visions that recruit Tibetan medicine into a projected future of Buryatia's development. These articulations hinge on claims about the epistemological systematicity of Tibetan medicine, the potential for its disassembly into separate methods and its subsequent incorporation into national and regional health care, and the terrain on which such incorporations are made possible. Much like the debates around Tibetan medicine in the late nineteenth and early twentieth centuries, the discursive practices on the part of local scientists and health-care administrators aim to define and stabilize Tibetan medicine in Buryatia as a distinct, recognizable entity, commensurable with other forms of traditional care. Such visions of national therapeutic integration often generate forms of exclusion, making only certain kinds of knowledge and practice visible and relevant, and open for institutional uptake and circulation.

The argument that Buryat–Tibetan medicine is grounded in a Buddhist cosmology frequently became eclipsed in rhetorics that viewed Tibetan medicine as nothing more than an assemblage of useful therapeutic techniques to be cherry-picked for the clinic and for research. Claims that Tibetan medicine in Buryatia is distinctly Buryat because it was able to incorporate folk practices and adapt to local ecologies troubled assertions that it is a systematic, yet stagnant way of knowing and treating the body— but whether it offered an epistemological terrain for integration was in contention. Once incorporated into discourses and projects meant to address a national scale, plants and other resources that constitute Tibetan medicine in its Buryat inflection were easily imagined as parts of circuits of medical commodities, entirely divorced from the ways in which Tibetan medicine understands their efficacies or from the ways in which local practitioners deploy them and make sense of them.

Temple-based practitioners and *emchi* practicing privately were often overlooked in these conversations and definitions. For their part, these practitioners argued for the inutility or impossibility of uprooting Tibetan medicine to other regions and expressed concerns about its incorporation into mainstream medicine, suggesting instead that it is better suited to treat ecologically circumscribed populations and address specifically local situations. While both positions worked to ground Tibetan medicine in Buryatia, the conclusions they drew were different. These competing visions mapped separate ways of conceptualizing political relationships and geographic encompassments and articulated a competing knowledge politics and temporalities. The administrators and medical officials in the official health-care sector tended to orient themselves toward Western Russia and the federal government, tying the development of Buryatia to the interests of the Russian state. Local practitioners working outside of the official medical sector, many of whom had strong Buddhist affiliation, imagined the region as part of a cultural and religious world that had its own set of unique and inherently local connections.

4

"TREATING NOT THE ILLNESS, BUT THE PATIENT"

Integrative Medicine for Dislocated Bodies

In October 2009, I began fieldwork at the in-patient clinic of the East-West Medical Center in Ulan-Ude. Established in 1989, East-West was conceived as a radically innovative medical institution—one where cutting-edge future-oriented medical practice would deploy Buryatia's Tibetan medicine archive and the research that had gone into decoding, translating, and testing the medicines listed in the formularies and compendia of Tibetan and Buryat pharmacology. Officially supported, yet uniquely regional in that it aimed to incorporate Buryatia's tradition of Tibetan medicine into clinical spaces, East-West began as a collaboration between some enterprising doctors from the local Ministry of Health, scientists and researchers from the Siberian Branch of the Soviet Academy of Sciences, a Chinese firm making medical equipment, and a local food manufacturer interested in producing phytopharmaceuticals. In the 1990s, the Chinese firm became embroiled in a scandal for providing faulty equipment and was evicted from Russia, and the food manufacturer gave up on the idea of making botanical remedies, focusing its production line on the more lucrative regionally branded liqueurs and herbal tinctures. Despite these perturbations, East-West persisted and grew.

While the original idea behind the center focused on Tibetan medicine specifically, at the end of the first decade of the 2000s the therapeutic techniques and resources used in its various divisions were no longer limited to or solely dedicated to institutionalizing Tibetan medicine, but also drew

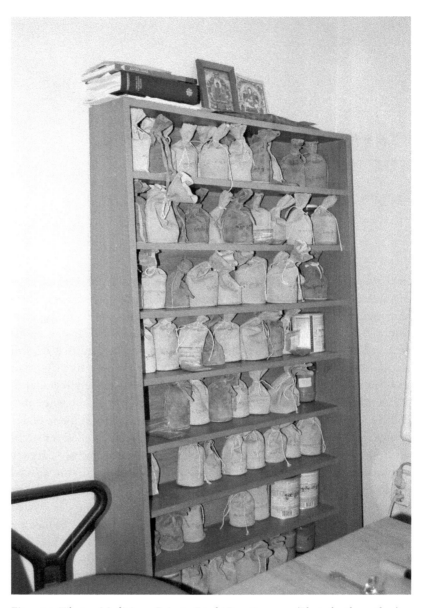

Figure 4. Tibetan Medicines, Private *Emchi* Practice, 2017 (Photo by the author)

on many other forms of nonbiomedical care. The center also offered a variety of standard biomedical tests, from ECG to bloodwork, and an array of more or less mainstream biomedical interventions. Officially under the aegis of Buryatia's Ministry of Health, the center was linked to the city's main hospitals and polyclinics through a standard referral system. Yet, though it was still endorsed and up until 2011 was largely funded by both the local government and by grants from the federal government, at the time of my fieldwork East-West was an administrative hybrid. Neither unambiguously a hospital nor a straightforwardly rehabilitative medical facility such as a health resort, neither for profit nor fully covered by the universal medical insurance (OMS), its shifting status appeared to reflect the difficult work of administratively classifying the vision of integrative care deployed within its walls.

While most doctors and administrators at East-West felt that the clinic did not need any publicity—that it was already well known and required only minimal PR work—the administration had put a lot of thought into telegraphing the center's mission. I was struck by the prevalence of two apparently unrelated slogans recurring throughout the center's various textual self-representations. My original ungenerous suspicion was that the public relations staff simply could not decide which phrase more accurately captured the center's philosophy and therefore had chosen to reproduce both utterances as a kind of dicephalus motto. Both statements circulated beyond the walls of the clinic itself, albeit in different domains. The first phrase, "to treat not the disease, but the person," is attributed to a variety of sources, from Hippocrates to Sergei Botkin, the nineteenth-century Russian physician and reformer considered one of the founding fathers of Russia's clinical experimental medicine and a pioneer of a systemic approach to disease. The slogan was featured on the informational posters hanging on the walls of the center's clinic and polyclinic and constantly resurfaced in patient brochures and other promotional materials. The other slogan, a rephrasing of a well-known utterance by the painter, explorer, scholar of Buddhism, and mystic Nicholas Roerich, was printed in calligraphic letters against the rich burgundy canvas of the permanent Tibetan medicine history exhibit adorning the main lobby of the center's polyclinic, and it was repeated in the same dark burgundy on the institution's website: "Preserving the past, we look to the future."

While I was initially perplexed at the apparent unrelatedness of East-West's two mottos, especially considering their historical origins, the center's staff, whom I questioned about them, felt that both phrases not only encapsulated the center's medical philosophy, but were also self-evidently complementary. Both statements aimed to directly address the reason behind the center's therapeutic strategies and approaches to patient treatment. Drawing on familiar articulations about the human body's internal reserves, East-West's mission was described as follows:

> Eastern medicine sees the person from the perspective of the total organism, located in a state of mutual interdependence with the external milieu. The methods of Eastern medicine are directed to the restoration of the internal milieu and the development of a human's own reserve capacities. This is why a combination of contemporary and traditional methods enables one to carry out the most effective prevention of illnesses, and to reach the highest expression of therapeutic efficacy in case of disease treatment.

Medical treatment at East-West promised to "rationally deploy traditional medicine" in conjunction with the "achievements of contemporary medicine" to "effectively restore the adaptive mechanisms of the organism, . . . and uncover the body's own reserve capacities." According to the center's administration and medical staff, the recuperation of traditional medicine techniques into a biomedical therapeutic present would enable medical progress to move away from some of the shortcomings of Russia's system of public health care. Most importantly, the center's administration prided itself in refusing a model of routinized, "assembly-line" treatment of patients in conventional biomedical institutions that applied standardized procedures without taking into account the particularity of each patient's medical and social biography. "Integrative medicine," according to East-West, replaced the shortcomings of conventional biomedicine with a vision of more individualized, catered care. In line with the claims about reclaiming the "past" to further medical progress, the center's head doctor insisted on presenting Tibetan medicine as one of the institution's "innovative technologies," meant to address both the shortcomings of biomedicine itself and its implementation in official state health care.

In this chapter, I use East-West's two slogans to interrogate the apparently natural connection between the promise of personalized, patient-focused medicine and the recuperation of "traditional medicine" into a therapeutic future in Buryatia. How is *individualized* medicine practiced at East-West, and why is *traditional* medicine posited as the ideal path to achieving it? In other words, how does the slogan "preserving the past" help practitioners visualize and treat particular persons and bodies, and what sort of "pasts" are being preserved, and which are disavowed? Conversely, what is the promissory valence of a medical care that claims to integrate a plurality of approaches while striving to keep them on equal footing, and on what epistemological and practical grounds are such pluralities imagined?

To explore these issues, this chapter follows the concepts and ideas that inform the shifting meanings "person" of "personalized medicine." I argue that the bodies East-West set out to treat were conceptualized and experienced, by both clinicians and patients, as distinctly post-socialist physicalities, characterized primarily by a failure to adapt over time to the historical, social, and geographic circumstances of their physical existence. This, I suggest, might be read as a reflection of a broader, longstanding concern with the living body's situatedness characteristic of both the pre-Soviet medicine of late Imperial Russia and its Soviet re-imaginings. The first section of this chapter situates "integrative" medicine in relation to current anthropological discussions of biomedicine and medical pluralism. I suggest that some of the approaches and categories used to understand what constitutes medical individualization emerging from this scholarship may not be entirely portable for exploring the stakes of what an individualized qua integrative medicine at a place like East-West sets out to achieve. Put simply, not all individualized bodies are made into the unit of medical treatment in the same ways, and these differences have implications for their political, social, and therapeutic encompassments. The second section traces the genealogy of the two slogans used by East-West to tease out some of their implications in order to locate the place of traditional medicine in Russia's medical imaginaries. Grappling with the problem of bodily variation has a long and specific history, both in Russian and Soviet medicine and in public health, with the problem of individual "adaptability" emerging at the heart of these debates. The last section of the chapter follows ethnographically what individualized integrative medicine comes to mean in the clinical spaces and everyday practices of East-West. I argue that for patients and doctors at East-West, the deployment of plural therapeutic modalities seeks to suspend and partially mitigate geographic, social, and temporal encompassments experienced as distinctly *pathogenic* and that "scientific" medicine is no longer thought to adequately address.

LOCALIZING THE BODY

If, as I have argued in Chapter 3, the integration of modern and traditional medicine in Russia is locally understood to be the next necessary step in the development of medical care—traditional medicine *as* "innovative technology," as the administration of East-West suggests—it becomes useful to ask what sort of present it attempts to intervene in and remedy, and what kinds of bodies it takes as its object and site for manipulation and redress. Drawing on the insight that the meanings and natures of bodies themselves tend to pluralistically multiply and proliferate and that a great deal of work goes into stabilizing them as bounded *things* (Lock and Farquhar 2007; Mol 2002), the following discussion is concerned with understanding the post-socialist body and its medical entanglements. I argue that, taken as the unit of integrative medicine in Russia, this post-socialist body comes into view through a unique set of frames and practices that unsettle the received distinctions between "biomedicine" and "traditional medicine" or "Western" and "non-Western" therapeutic cosmologies on which the very project of integrative medicine relies for distinguishing itself from the medical mundane.

Envisioning what integration might signify is additionally complicated by a certain lack of consensus in anthropological writings about which therapeutic contexts should be characterized as plural. Studies that use medical pluralism as an analytic typically put in tension modernity and tradition, where one pole is defined by the hegemony of a single medical modality while the other is characterized by multiplicity and polyphony. While these categories have been extensively problematized, the question of whether pluralism is an attribute of tradition or modernity has shifted over time. For example, anthropologists Charles Leslie and Arthur Kleinman have classically argued that the syncretism of non-Western therapeutic practices—especially of Asian medical systems—stands in contrast to the hegemonic tendencies of Western biomedicine (Leslie 1980; Kleinman 1980). Other scholars draw attention to the pluralisms inherent in and alongside biomedical practice itself and, writing on the use of alternative and complementary medicine in the U.S., have suggested that non-Western medical systems are characterized by a greater degree of coherence than the diverse and often antagonistic therapeutic forms that coexist in "complex societies" (Lock 1990; Scheper-Hughes 1990. Cf. Baer 2004).

Scholars working in situations where biomedicine exists alongside other state-sponsored medical systems have suggested that the concept of pluralism neither adequately captures the complex mutual imbrications or the power differentials between biomedicine and other forms of treatment nor serves to elucidate patients' decision about what kinds of treatment to seek and when (Scheid 2002; Lock and Nguyen 2010). In spite of (or, perhaps, because of) these multiplying definitions, medical anthropologists now take pluralism to be the inalienable characteristic of any medical practice at all, which diminishes its usefulness as a theoretical analytic (Lock and Nguyen 2018; Biehl, Good, and Kleinman 2007).

In part, these apprehensions of coherence, incoherence, and multiplicity are differently produced depending on what is taken to be the primary focus of anthropological examination. To be sure, there are important differences between the utopian visions attributed to biomedical and technoscientific imaginaries and those implied in the recuperation of practices associated with biomedicine's geographical and temporal "others," as one might see in the popularization of yoga, Ayurveda, Chinese medicine, and other nonbiomedical forms of therapeutic self-management in a Euro-American context. Rather than creating prosthetically mechanized or densely biological beings modified through scientific and technological manipulations, appropriations of traditional medicine purport to offer the reanimation of the body's own preexisting, but ossified potentials. Yet, both promissory futures operate in the spaces of a universal and portable human body, already delinked or easily extricable from its temporal, geographic, and social encompassments. By contrast, the co-optation of traditional medicines into a Russian medical mainstream, while also framed in relation to the body's "hidden potentials," takes for its unit an intensely local and situated physiology, excisable from its social and ecological milieu only at great cost to its vitality. Although, as I argue in Chapter 5, practicing *emchi* often critique medical integration on the basis that Russia's "official medicine" is frequently blind to the ways in which concrete, local bodies are produced, the treatment of uniquely emplaced physiologies is very much at the center of the clinical practices of East-West.

I situate the appeal of integrative medicine in relation to the criticisms leveled against both biomedicine and the organization of health care in Russia. Both patients and doctors at East-West often expressed to me the same sentiment: that contemporary medicine, while effective and unavoidable in certain acute, and especially infectious, cases, was liable to cripple the body as much as it was to provide a cure. By targeting the symptoms of a specific pathology, they argued that it frequently caused collateral damage without necessarily removing the cause. This sentiment is often captured in Russian through a number of pithy aphorisms, such as "It cures one thing while maiming another" or, alternatively, one lifted from a Soviet joke about doctors—"So, dear colleague, shall we treat him, or let him live?" Conversely, patients and practitioners at East-West frequently argued that traditional medicine could properly detect and address the "real" causes of illness by "treating the person, not the disease," as one of the East-West slogans suggests. If traditional and modern medicine are posited in Russia's contemporary medical discourses as at best complementary and at worst antagonistic, what makes their integration desirable or imaginable in the first place? The following section explores the conceptual common ground that enables projects that bring together and align the disparate therapies East-West draws together into the same clinical space.

"PRESERVING THE PAST, WE LOOK TO THE FUTURE"

As I have mentioned, the slogans East-West uses to define itself are in fact modifications of two widespread and familiar citations that circulate far beyond the walls of the center, albeit usually in quite separate domains. By drawing out the history of both slogans, I aim to situate the relationship between body and environment as a site of individualization in the historical context of Russian and Soviet medical care, on the one hand, and the deployment of traditional medicine, on the other. This section argues that the way in which traditional medicine at East-West is framed subsumes it into an already circulating logic of bodily individualization that takes health to be a function of contextual viability.

"Preserving the past, we look to the future" is a modified version of a well-known statement taken from the writings of Nikolai Roerich (1874–1947), Russian traveler, painter, philosopher, mystic, and scholar, often considered one of the most influential "Western" popularizers of Buddhism in

Russia. Conversely, "to treat the patient, not the disease" is a statement most typically attributed to the medical philosophy of Sergey Botkin (1832–89), a famous Russian clinician, social activist, and researcher. Within Russian medical historiography, Botkin is taken to be one of the founding fathers of Russia's experimental clinical medicine and of the modernization of medicine in prerevolutionary Russia more broadly. The rise of the laboratory in Russia's nineteenth-century medical teaching and practice owes a great deal to Botkin's efforts to merge experimental physiology, on the one hand, and bedside therapeutic practice, on the other. Botkin's clinical laboratory, created in 1860–61, was the site where Ivan Pavlov did the first ten years of his canine research.

At first glance, Botkin, methodical clinician, supporter of Pavlov, and father of the "materialist" approach in the history of Russia's medical modernization, and Roerich, propagator of Agni yoga and of a universalist spiritualism inspired by "Eastern philosophies," have little in common. My goal in this section is to trace a kind of history of "echoes" that allows us to see how Botkin and Roerich are transformed into discursive allies in the center's efforts to articulate what is intended when this institution labels itself "integrative." I draw on Foucault's concept of genealogy and on the insights of linguistic anthropology that suggest that while texts never quite lose their previous indexicalities, their recontextualizations are always productive of new meanings (Silverstein and Urban 1996; Gal 2003; Hrycak 2006; Briggs and Mantini-Briggs 2003). The following discussion reflects on how the two slogans are actively reimagined to frame the integration of traditional medicine as a particularly useful modality for treating specifically individualized and emplaced physiologies.

The philosophical writings of Nicholas Roerich and his wife, Katerina, are perhaps best known for inspiring the theosophical movement, both in Russia and the U.S. Roerich's philosophy is often placed within the school of Russian cosmism, also notably forwarded by the late writings of V. I. Vernadsky (1863–1945), credited with developing the theory of the biosphere. Much like Roerich, Vernadsky viewed human activity as inextricable from and deeply transformative of the geological and biological processes that constitute what is typically thought of as inanimate and nonsentient "nature." Although Roerich's original utterance is perhaps one of his most famous statements, it is entirely unrelated to medicine in his original writings. Its metamorphosis into a slogan has also made it lose some of its flourish: "From the ancient and wondrous stones of the past, construct the steps of things to come" (Roerich 1995, 58). A more expanded version used to serve as the introduction to East-West's promotional pamphlet circa 2006 and added a clarification that was not in the original source: "Today is yesterday, today is tomorrow." The utterance is locally taken as a call for the recuperation and study of traditional medicine. The exact same phrase is frequently mobilized in the scientific and scholarly publications produced by researchers at the local research center of the Siberian branch of the Russian Academy of Sciences to describe and justify the usefulness of their efforts to "decipher" Tibetan medicine. Roerich is, of course, not a random choice. Following their many expeditions throughout the Himalayan region, the Roerich family founded the Urusvati Institute of Himalayan Studies, where, among other scientific endeavors, they undertook research into Tibetan medicine. Roerich's two sons became involved with the documentation and translation of Tibetan pharmacopeia, although Nikolai Roerich himself thought that the arcane language of the Tibetan medical canon should be scientifically rationalized (Grekova 1998). Much of the translational work undertaken by Roerich and his sons and, notably, the Tibetan-Russian-English dictionaries they produced together, are widely used and cited in the publications of the research center.

The original remark is found in a diary entry, written sometime between 1936 and 1941, in which Roerich reflects not on medicine, but on Russian art. The statement is a lament on the incredible disjunctions between the glory days of civilizations past (Rome, Byzantium, Kiev Rus') and the present-day scanty remnants of their artistic and aesthetic expressions. In this sense, the statement does indeed reflect one of the most important aspects of Roerich's work—the formulation of the first heritage preservation treaty, the "Roerich Pact," or the "Treaty on Protection of Artistic and Scientific Institutions and Historic Monuments." The agreement, signed in Washington in 1935, later served as a foundation for UNESCO's regulations for the protection of heritage sites. In the quote's recirculation, Roerich's original wistful tone is replaced by one of reserved optimism, where it serves to motivate the translation of canonical texts of Tibetan medicine and suggests the possibility of accessing and confirming the validity of the pharmaceutical knowledge contained within for the future of medicine and science (Khundanov, Khundanova, and Bazaron 1979; Bazaron 1992;

Nikolaev 1998). In this sense, East-West's use of Roerich's statement has more to do with these anticipated discoveries and present-day applications than with the preservation of legacies past.

The second statement—"To treat not the disease, but the patient"—should be situated in relation to Sergey Botkin's modernizing activities. By following the history of this statement, I hope to show certain continuities in the logics that characterize Russia's medical modernization. The utterance provides us with a vantage point to see one of the features that distinguishes Russian medical modernization from a strictly European biomedical trajectory. In the remainder of this section I follow the persistent concerns with the body's "emplacement" in a surrounding environment, characteristic of nineteenth-century, Soviet, and contemporary medicine in Russia. This emplacement, be it social or ecological, consistently informs contemporary theories of pathogenesis in Russia, but also motivates the attractiveness of traditional medicine techniques and approaches. Yet, the sense that bodies are, first and foremost, local, embedded, and temporally situated entities consistently troubles the possibility of effective and consistent treatment for specifically those physiologies traditional medicine is supposed to best suit.

Efforts to modernize the medical system, perceived as symptomatic of a broader stagnation within Russia's autocratic, hierarchically rigid, and excessively bureaucratized government in the second part of the nineteenth century, arose against a background of social unrest and political movements that called for social change. They were also undertaken partly in response to the incredible losses of the Crimean War, which incurred more casualties because of epidemics of cholera and dysentery than to the fighting itself (Kichigina 2009). Two especially important reforms were, in 1861, the abolition of serfdom and the creation of *zemstvo*.[1] *Zemstvo* medicine, implemented in the 1860s, significantly departed from previous models for providing medical care to rural populations, both in Russia and in Europe. Historians of Russian medicine argue that *zemstvo* medicine was perhaps the first significant and, at the time, pioneering departure from the developmental trajectory of medicine in Western Europe in that it combined a strong emphasis on general hygiene and disease prevention with the notion that medical care was neither a private for-profit venture nor charity, but a form of social service (Mirskiy 2005; King 2005). The double emphasis on disease prevention and on the social service nature of medical care later became central to the ideology of Soviet medicine (Graham 1993; Gross Solomon 2004).

More generally, Botkin's school of clinical medicine is now remembered and cited for three principles: all pathologies are closely related to the functioning of the nervous system (what Botkin and his followers had labeled the "nervism" theory of pathology); a disease is never confined to a small area of the body, but rather affects the body in its totality; and the environment plays a central role in pathogenesis.[2] In this sense, for Botkin, the individuality of the body—and hence its different responses to what therapeutic medicine classifies as the same disease—are conditioned by, on the one hand, the body's own internal vitality, and, on the other, its situatedness and connection to the environment. Botkin defines all organic life (from cell to complex organism) as the capacity for autonomy of the unit of life from the external milieu, which is to say, its ability to adapt to the external world such that it is able to maintain itself over time (Botkin 1886).

The focus on the body's emplacement in a surrounding environment was also characteristic of the logics of Soviet medicine. This attribution of pathogenic qualities to the body's immediate social conditions was in line with the ideological tenets of Marxism-Leninism, since it emphasized the social origin of illness, which is to say it grounded illness in the social conditions of life and labor, as was articulated by Soviet social hygienists (Gross Solomon 2004). Both Western and Russian scholarship tends to define the uniqueness of the Soviet medical system in relation to its emphasis on prevention, derived from what Loren Graham has called "an environmentalist theory of disease" (Graham 1993). Both Graham and Gross Solomon note that the focus on the relationship between body and social milieu was not an entirely new theoretical orientation that defined the early formulations of Soviet health care, indebted solely to communist ideology, but an extension of, on the one hand, *zemstvo* medicine, and, on the other, a borrowing of German social medicine (*soziale medizin*). A prophylactic or preventative turn was a defining characteristic of the system from early on. Nikolai Semashko, who became in 1918 the first People's Commissar of Public Health, wrote in 1919 that "the prevention of illness is the main task of Soviet medicine" (Semashko 1934, quoted in Starks 2008). Sanitizing social conditions meant improving the health of the population at large.

If social hygiene was primarily concerned with removing epidemiological threats from everyday life and labor, other emergent Soviet medical disciplines focused instead on the body's ecological surroundings. The notion that the human body is inextricably linked to its ecological and social milieu and that diseases are primarily derived from the interactions between the body and the outside world reoccur systematically in professional texts on resort medicine and medical geography. While medical geography evaluated pathogenic environmental factors, resort medicine (*kurortologiya*) was interested in mapping and harnessing the therapeutic properties of the Soviet Union's diverse ecology. At its inception, resort medicine aimed to rationalize workers' rest in order to increase productivity, educate the population in the principles of socialism, and collapse the capitalist dichotomy between rest and labor. In the end, as G. M. Danishevskiy, the director of the Central State Institute of Resort Studies, wrote in his *Problems of Mass Recreation in the USSR* (1934), the goal was to fully realize the dialectic nature of labor and rest such that labor became productive rest and rest became joyful labor. The administration of health resorts was the domain of professional unions, and for workers to gain access to the benefits of these therapeutic natures, they had to undergo medical evaluation and be issued a referral to a specific site that would fit their diagnosis (Davydkin 2002). For their part, "natural factors"—from mineral waters and muds to climate, amount of solar radiation, air, and landscape—came to figure as important, quantifiable, and therefore "prescribable" elements of medical treatment.

These early Soviet-era efforts to formally theorize the relationship between the environment and the body's vitality reverberate in latter efforts to formulate a new theory of health. Definitions of health emerging in the 1980s and 1990s in Russia tended to draw on these older assumptions that physical functioning can be mitigated through various "exposures" to nature. This is to say, while the body of the Soviet worker could be placed, quite literally, *inside* a therapeutically harnessed nature, as in the case of Soviet medical tourism, these new logics suggested that introducing various "natural" agents into the body could fine-tune its "life." While Soviet medicine was certainly not unique in trying to harness "nature's" salubrious qualities, the ways in which this kind of therapeutic efficacy was framed is important for understanding the place of traditional medicine in current projects of medical integration.

A later attempt at theorizing an ecological understanding of health, one that has both historical and conceptual bearings on the models of medical integration in present-day Russia, was made in the 1980s and 1990s by proponents of an emergent interdisciplinary orientation dubbed "valeology." The term "valeology" was coined in the 1980s by Soviet physician Israel Brekhman. Brekhman himself was a student of Nikolai Lazarev, a prominent Soviet physician and toxicologist who did most of his work in the late 1940s and 1950s in the Russian Far East. Lazarev's work involved experimenting with bendazol, a chemically synthesized drug prescribed for its neurotropic vasodilating properties, by asking whether it might also have immunity-boosting effects. Lazarev's research, which focused on oncology, was part of a broader push in Soviet medicine to develop ways of mediating the effects of nuclear radiation on the body. Short on bendazol, Lazarev and his students eventually switched to investigating the pharmaceutical properties of *Eleutherococcus senticosus* (Siberian Ginseng), which grew in the region and was used in TCM, with which the researchers were familiar. As a result of this work, Lazarev coined the term "adaptogens" to describe plant components that increased what he defined as the body's "state of nonspecific heightened resistance" to external stressors and harmful influences (see Zabrodin 2005; Apanasenko 2012).

Expanding the theories of his mentor on plant adaptogens, Brekhman suggested that health was not simply the absence of diseases but a state that allowed the person to optimally fulfill his or her social and professional functions, while simultaneously adapting to a constantly changing external milieu (Brekhman 1987). Brekhman's project was one of practical ambitions: advocating for a serious study of what he called "Oriental medicine" and its focus on cultivating health, Brekhman suggested that the next pharmacological frontier would be to make "medicines for the healthy," designed to increase the body's adaptability and curtail the risks of environmental pathogenesis.[3]

A vocabulary of adaptation as something that is central to thinking about health has a broad circulation in Russia. "Adaptogens" is in fact a product category, an officially endorsed designation referring to a wide and profitable line of commodities on the Russian pharmaceutical market aimed at increasing, as the name suggests, the body's ability to adapt to "external nonspecific stressors" (see Barnaulov 2001; Studentsov et al. 2013). Adaptation is defined broadly—it ranges from fighting off infections, decreasing the iatrogenic effects of harsh pharmaceutical treatments, and mitigating environmental exposure and social stressors to improving overall "functioning"—from increased energy levels to better concentration and memory. Most pharmaceuticals based on plant and animal extracts are in fact labeled as adaptogenic.

Brekhman and his followers argued that valeology was distinct from social hygiene because it was not concerned with the health of populations and with developing a generic "healthy lifestyle" theory. Instead, it focused on understanding the health of the *individual* and developing a theoretical apparatus capable of gaining insights into what constitutes health in the first place. The history of valeology as a formal discipline is relatively short and scandalous, interesting both for the ideas it attempted to introduce and for the panics its "pluralist," ontologically decentered position caused. Valeology gained significant popularity in the late 1990s and early 2000s, such that the Ministry of Health of the Russian Federation began to include "physician-valeologist" as an official specialization in the registry of medical professions. Shortly after, the specialization of "educator-valeologist" was introduced by the Ministry of Education. The discipline was to be taught in schools as part of a civics course aimed to educate schoolchildren in the principles of healthy living. Yet, as valeology-related publications and manuals proliferated in the late 1990s, it came under attack from both medical professionals and the Eastern Orthodox Church for its introduction of "irrational" and "mystical" content—from "Agni yoga" to what was deemed inappropriate sexual education for children. As a result, by the year 2000 the Ministry of Education had removed the specialization of valeologist from its list of higher education options, leaving stranded a number of students seeking a degree in valeology.

Like many of his contemporaries in the Soviet Union, Brekhman was influenced by cybernetics and thus deeply dissatisfied with a reduction of human life to simply an energetic exchange with the external world. Invoking, notably, Shrödinger's "What Is Life?" (1944) in trying to convince his audience that metabolism is not simply a matter of energy exchange, Brekhman proposed to view the body through the cybernetic idiom of information. "Structural information" for Brekhman is an umbrella term that unites the different necessary chemical and biological components that pass through the body. How else, he asks, can we explain that diseases take on different shape and gravity in different individuals, depending on what they have been exposed to? "Nature," for Brekhman, is thus the bearer of information locked in the complex structures of matter (Brekhman 1980, 31), and human life is a constant exchange of not simply matter and energy, but information between the body and the environment.

At the mercy of these semiotic flows, the body becomes radically open and malleable. If therapeutic efficacy is not limited to the substances one injects, but expands to include all those one ingests, bodily health becomes a temporally and environmentally entrenched balancing act with indeterminate contours. Brekhman called this "the third state" (Brekhman 1980, 1987). Health and sickness, he suggested, are not two mutually exclusive binaries, but a spectrum, with most people falling into an in-between limbo (Brekhman 1980, 56). Most importantly for this discussion, the "third state" would also include various conditions of bodily "disadaptation" to the environment, mostly articulated in terms of literal dislocation (change of place), as well as the physical state of populations with lifestyle risk factors (exposures to harmful chemical from work, alcohol, tobacco consumption, and "irrational diet"). It is this third state—the state of disadaptation—that lies, according to Brekhman, at the origin of all illnesses, yet is insidiously elusive, since official biomedicine is incapable of diagnosing it.

A concern with adaptability and with the insidious bodily deregulation invisible to a clinical eye informs much of East-West's claims. Indeed, detecting and intervening into the preclinical manifestation of illness was one of the ways in which the center presented the usefulness of the various "traditional" diagnostic techniques it offered. Practitioners, researchers, and state officials in Buryatia interested in Tibetan medicine—and in Eastern medicine more broadly—frequently claim that traditional medicine holds the keys to anticipating and correcting the subtle deregulation of internal processes, invisible to standard biomedical diagnostic methods (Kozhevnikov et al. 2010). My point here is that arguments made in favor of traditional medicine already incorporate it into a preexisting logic of adaptability—an environmental view of health that imputes to traditional medicine a privileged access to the body's "adaptive reserves" and "potentials." The environmental and psychological stresses of everyday life are then understood to deplete the body's adaptive reserves, to make it more "rigid" in its ability to respond to the external world in which it is situated—disadaptation becomes seen as the root of all illness. Unlocking the body's potential for greater adaptability in order to harness a kind of "total" health motivates the possibilities of medical integration and reframes "traditional" therapeutic approaches as uniquely suited to the task.

Considering its promise of personalized preclinical therapy, one aimed at realigning the body's "content" and "context" before more serious deregulations take place, it is both revelatory and deeply ironic that most patients at East-West seek treatment for long-term chronic illnesses. The remaining part of this chapter explores how the chronically sick body becomes articulated in terms of disadaptation to social and historical conditions experienced as pathogenic. In the daily life of the clinic, the rejection of the "disease view" in favor of the "person view" does not simply come to signify that the ailing body should be taken holistically as a system or individually as a uniquely manifested physicality rather than a series of co-present, but independent disorders—what, in Russian, is sometimes ironically referred to as a "bouquet of illnesses." Despite the horizon of ever more precise customization that the center's integrative model promises—one that would take into account not simply an encapsulated bodily totality but a body with fluid and indeterminate boundaries, an ever-shifting life form adapting (or failing to adapt) to its environment—in the daily practices of East-West bodies are not so much individualized as they are typified. Even when they attempt to therapeutically address concrete patients, the medical staff at the clinic tend to talk about their patients as sharing fundamental similarities—a typification that is not the result of epidemiological commitments, but of a practical orientation that tries to coordinate between therapeutic needs and administrative requirements. These typifications are not necessarily, or exclusively, articulated around the patients' medical histories. Instead, the pathologies from which they suffer are taken by the doctors—and by patients themselves—to be symptomatic of a certain kind of geographically, socially, and culturally embedded being, a product of socio-biographic time that is neither entirely personal nor unproblematically collective.

"OUR ILLNESSES ARE THE ONE THING THAT'S DIFFERENT"

On one particular Monday, I sat with a group of patients in the lobby of the East-West inpatient hospital as they waited for their turn to go through the admission process. As I asked patients about their previous experiences with traditional medicine and with treatment at the center, Yelena and Katerina, two sisters in their early sixties, entertained the somewhat anxious crowd with loud and occasionally ironic answers to my prodding. "We're sisters, as you probably can see." Katerina, the heavy-set brunette, smiled, nodding toward her reed-thin blonde companion. "She's a year younger. We grew up together, we had everything in common. Same mom, same home . . . and those were difficult times you know, so we even had the same bed for both of us, for lack of space." While some of the other patients, most of them women of about the same age group, nodded approvingly, one interjected, "And now, here you are, with the same *bolyachki* (Rus. col. "boo boos")." The comment was met with uproarious laughter from the group, including Katerina herself. Suddenly turning serious, Katerina retorted, "Why, no. Our illnesses are the one thing that's actually different."

I suggest that in order to understand Katerina's sudden insistence that she and her sister did not, in fact, share the same experiences of illness (as well as to unpack the humor of the quip), it is important to keep in mind that the sense of individualized embodiment is by no means a priori in the Russian medical context and that the logics of shared, collective conditions frequently override the experience of a distinctly personal form of suffering. In other words, the forms of collective identity that Paul Rabinow has termed "biosociality" (Rabinow 1992) and Rose and Novas and Adriana Petryna have described as "biological citizenship" (Petryna 2002; Rose and Novas 2005) for patients at East-West are already a *given*, but their collectivity does not derive from the experience of a common biological or somatic denominator, such as a shared diagnosis, genetic marker, racial or ethnic identity, or exposures to a single catastrophic event. Instead, it is the collective and prolonged experiences of a Soviet and post-socialist life often simply described as being a "pensioner" or as the product of living at the geographic and political "margins" of the state, a bodily history that includes, but is not limited to, mismanagement at the hands of a fraught medical system that makes up the corpus, both literally and figuratively, of East-West patients. Cumulatively, these living conditions and shared temporalities converge for both patients and doctors in a generalized sense of patients' "un-health," accumulated over time, a broad state of disorder that might be offset by the therapeutic temporalities of the clinic.

An example might illustrate this point. In December of 2009, a wide panic erupted in Buryatia concerning a possible outbreak of the H1N1 influenza virus. Local pharmacies were rapidly depleted of their stock of antiviral medications, and all public institutions instituted a "mask regime"—the requirement of wearing a protective mask whenever entering a public building, from cafés and stores to institutional spaces like libraries and hospitals. The swine flu panic also led to deficits in the availability of these masks and to soaring prices on those drugs, like the popular "Arbidol," that were labeled "adaptogenic." As cases of swine flu diagnosis multiplied in local hospitals, informal discussions began to center on the possibility that this was not a regular yearly flu outbreak but a "super bug," with likely origins in the U.S. military complex.

Discussions about the possibility of a swine flu pandemic among doctors in the clinic were, at best, skeptical. Most believed that the panic was the product of the media and that the sense of fear among the population was maintained exclusively because it benefited the pharmaceutical industry. At the same time, conversations around the swine flu enabled a different kind of discussion—namely, one centered on the ethics of communicating risk. As the clinic doctors met over their usual morning coffee in the break room, a lively conversation broke out between Zhamso Sayanovich, the head neurologist, Aleksandra, a practitioner of Tibetan medicine, and Nadezhda Maksimovna, the head nurse. To my surprise, they were largely in agreement that certain kinds of prognoses were simply irrelevant to the actual life of the patient. Aleksandra articulated this sentiment as follow:

> This swine flu diagnosis, it's similar to telling someone that they might have a risky pregnancy. What's the point of doing that if there's nothing that can be done about it? Does the woman really need to know this? Besides, there's never any way to be sure. It might happen, or it might not.

When I asked whether there were other occasions when communicating risk might be appropriate, especially in light of the center's claims to treat illness before its clinical manifestations, Zhamso Sayanovich volunteered a counterexample. He recently had a patient whose ultrasound results could not reliably establish the absence of gallbladder stones. The patient's clinical symptoms suggested that it was a possibility, but neither the clinical exam nor the ultrasound was conclusive. Zhamso Sayanovich explained that his approach to the case, as a doctor of rehabilitative medicine, was to consider the person to be in the "preclinical" phase of gallbladder disease. In other words, it was possible that gallbladder stones could develop in the future, and his task was therefore to change the conditions that might lead to this development, and it was in this modification of conditions that the clinic truly specialized. Although Aleksandra seemed to agree with the latter point, she bemoaned the fact that, outside of the walls of the clinic and its interruption of the accumulation of pathogenic times of a patient's life, things would revert back to "business as usual":

> When we try to tell someone to change their lifestyle, to change what they eat, to quit smoking or drinking, or what have you—patients aren't going to do this. In Russia, people have this mentality, you know. We can do this here [in the clinic], but outside they'll do what they always do.

Beyond questions of lifestyle, there was a certain sense of inevitability about what the recurrent health problems treated at the clinic would look like. For Aleksandra, who tended to first establish a diagnosis based on Tibetan medicine, then translated it into "biomedical" terms, these tendencies became acutely visible:

> You see cold in the kidneys all over the place. It tends to underline many other conditions with which patients come to get treated. It's because of Buryatia's environment and climate—there's really no getting around it.

For the doctors that I interviewed and shadowed, thinking about this diffuse "health deficit" characteristic of the clinic's patients became a matter of understanding a set of bodily states seen as the result of habits and exposures accumulated over years of a geographically and historically situated life, one that wove together the effects of a specific ecology and climate, the "natural" dietary proclivities of a Siberian population, and the attitudes and mentality cultivated by the Soviet state. To be sure, patients at East-West do share many demographic and medical similarities, produced both through a cohort effect and through the specialized training of the physicians employed there, most of whom were neurologists with an additional training in reflexotherapy (*iglorefleksoterapia* [IRT]—the Russian term for acupuncture), massage therapists, and practitioners of Tibetan medicine.

Against the background of this expected typification, practitioners at the East-West clinic demanded of their patients the kind of inward-focused attention that would unsettle the default sense of "natural" collective convergence of suffering. The practices of self-accounting and bodily habitus institutionalized at the clinic worked to replace and thus throw into sharp relief this sense of collectivity. Through a distinctly personal, day-to-day accounting of biographic-pathogenic time temporarily suspended by treatment-time, patients were called upon to experience *personalized* illness and convalescence. Yet, the very practices of maximized self-attention that doctors at East-West encouraged from patients mapped in complex and occasionally contradictory ways onto patients' own embodied experiences and daily strategies of self-care, as well as their sense of sharing a collective experience of ill health.

"WE DON'T KNOW WHAT HURTS"

New patients arrived early on Mondays to stay at the East-West Clinic from one to two weeks, and the admission stage was often marked by nervousness. The waiting time for one of the hospital's thirty-six "cot-spaces" (*koy-komesto*) averaged at around three months but could extend for longer periods during the more desirable summer months. Identified as a space of rehabilitative medicine, the clinic offered post-operation treatment as well as more general "finishing" treatment (*dolechivanie*) after a stay at the hospital. In practice, many patients checked into the clinic for chronic illness as an alternative to treatment at a nonintegrative state institution. While a reservation almost certainly guaranteed a spot, unpredictable events had to be taken into consideration: there was always a sense that new admits could potentially be turned back. Because the clinic hosted a heterogeneous mix of patients, from the aging parents of well-connected local administrative and business leaders to regular middle-class pensioners who saved up their pensions over time to secure a spot to younger patients with chronic conditions who used it as a kind of health resort, the hierarchy of priorities was never entirely predictable to the doctors working there or to the patients seeking admittance. Even with reservations and a long waiting list, some patients arrived spontaneously with the hope that a spot might open up at the last minute. Sometimes, new arrivals had to be sent away: for those who came from other regions of Russia or from rural parts of Buryatia, this meant a long trip home—several days by train or shuttle bus. The uncertainty of admission added to the overall sense that staying at the clinic was a privilege and an exception—not simply a medical necessity prompted by illness, but a conscious act of doing something "for oneself," an opportunity to rectify a body made fragile by the onslaughts of everyday life. Although this was in part mediated by the fact that patients are often middle-aged and older and defined as pensioners, this was not a site of end-of-life treatment. According to Russia's labor laws at the time, which decreed that state pensions can officially be received from age fifty-five for women and age sixty for men, most patients at the clinic were either close to the "pensioner" status or were already "on the pension," although the younger cohort in the early to mid-fifties was often still employed. With a variety of financial and social obligations that precluded or interfered with retirement—from supporting their families and paying for their children's now often expensive university education to the endless apartment remodeling that people in Ulan-Ude often jokingly refer to as the country's "national sport"—most still tried to supplement their state pensions with salaries from their work, in dire cases resorting to unskilled labor once they were made "redundant" in their previous employment, or sometimes by selling the produce from their vegetable garden. "You can't survive on just your pension," patients often explained to me, especially when trying to account for the complex networks of monetary flow between kin and the convoluted living arrangements that sometimes meant that at least three generations lived in the same household, sharing the same apartment that had been issued to one of the older members by the Soviet state. The word "pensioner" itself carries a complicated and contradictory symbolic load and, in the medical context, often comes to signify a special kind of vulnerability, one that balances precariously between financial destitution and flagging health as a distinct consequence of a shared "post-socialist" condition. Many of the women patients I have interviewed during my fieldwork at the clinic felt squeezed by these financial demands, on the one hand, and on the other by the sense that their aging physiologies were no longer up to the task, that the stresses of work and social obligations had condensed within the materiality of their bodies into pains, fatigue, various chronic illnesses, cognitive or nervous disturbances, and physical unattractiveness.

For most patients at East-West, the clinic was only one stop on itineraries of care that ran both longitudinally in time and laterally through the therapeutic landscapes of Ulan-Ude and Buryatia and, occasionally for some of the wealthier patients, spanned much broader geographic regions, bringing them to other areas of Russia as well as China, India, Mongolia, and South Korea. Most patients I spoke to did not narrativize these trajectories as efforts to treat or manage a specific condition but described much more diffuse and momentary tactics undertaken to mitigate a proliferation of symptoms and bodily processes that did not necessarily emerge or accompany those diagnoses listed in their medical histories. Many of these narratives expanded beyond the strict limits of disease-centered symptomatology to include both everyday life events and the by-products of diverse health-related endeavors ranging from self-healing practices to the iatrogenic effects of different medications and therapies. They were also tightly woven with experiences of historical and political state transformations.

Katerina and Yelena described themselves as veterans of the center— at the time of my fieldwork, their stay at the clinic was the third time they had made the journey from Yakutsk, some 430 kilometers to the north of Ulan-Ude, to undergo treatment. Both were diagnosed with multiple chronic illnesses—from bronchial asthma to arthritis—which treatment at the center allowed them to rein in and manage, for a time. When I asked Katerina why she found the center's use of traditional medicine appealing, she began her answer by discussing the state of official health care in Russia.

> Doctors nowadays don't know what they're treating. You come in, and they barely look at you, they don't have time for you, so they can't figure out what you have, or how to treat you for it. You're forced to give them suggestions—why don't we try this, something you hear about [independently]. Here, most doctors are attentive, they really listen to you.

I heard this critique repeated time and again by the patients at the center. Patients frequently contrasted their experiences in the clinic to those in biomedical state care, listing attention (*vnimanie*) as the main differentiating factor between treatment at the center and treatment elsewhere. Attention, or rather its absence, characterized both the relation doctors had to their patients and the self-relation patients had to their own body. Katerina further explained that she was always trying to manage her symptoms with traditional medicine anyway—and at the center, she had the opportunity to expand this practice in a more formally medical, yet caring environment. This section explores what patients mean by "attention," beyond the performance of a kinder, sympathetic affect by doctors widely experienced as lacking in both Russian present-day medical care and, more broadly, in the practices of modern biomedicine.

I was first alerted to the importance of attention during a conversation with Dmitry, a former woodworker in his early forties who was receiving disability benefits for his arthritic knees. Several years prior, he had been exposed to severe cold (-50 C) for a prolonged period of time. As a result of this, he explained, he developed knee pain that progressively grew more and more crippling until he could no longer walk. When I asked Dmitry how he had become aware of the center, he explained that because of his doctors' lack of attention, he could not obtain a diagnosis and had become caught in an endless loop of referrals. Making light simultaneously of his own debilitating condition and his treating physicians' inability to diagnose or comprehend it on a purely practical level, Dmitry explained:

> Doctors couldn't establish a diagnosis [without which Dmitry could neither obtain a "*bolnichny*"—a paid leave of absence—nor get treatment in a state institution]. The rheumatologist kept sending me to the general practitioner, the general practitioner sent me back to the rheumatologist, and back and forth I went, until I simply couldn't walk anymore. I couldn't work. Eventually, they sent me to the hospital for treatment for arthritis, and put me on medication for twenty-five days.

Dmitry explained that, at first, his symptoms seemed to get better, but then, in February of the previous year, he experienced an acute relapse. He speculated that if he could only receive a firm diagnosis, then he could begin to manage his condition, but because doctors are overwhelmed with the number of patients they have to see daily, there is little incentive for them to really try to get to the heart of the matter.

> My wife heard about this place, and we finally decided for me to come here. I barely limped in here. We don't have traditional medicine in my area [*Irkutskaya oblast'*]. We have a few sanatoria, and they do have massage therapists there, but they didn't help.

For Dmitry, who was receiving acupuncture treatment, massage, and paraffin compresses and was drinking anti-inflammatory teas based on Tibetan medicine recipes, the treatment felt effective "in complex," although he voiced a certain sense of anxiety about how long the reprieve would last:

"What will happen when I leave?" he asked. At the same time, for the doctors treating him, the question of his diagnosis—that is, establishing whether his knee pain in fact was arthritic in nature—wasn't the primary concern. Instead, they were maximizing treatment for a variety of possible disorders that would result in the inflammation of the joints. Their primary task was to restore mobility and decrease pain, not to actually look for the underlying biomedical cause.

Similarly, Alla, a patient in her late forties who had experience with both the center and other traditional medicine institutions in Mongolia, reflected on why the treatments at East-West helped her manage her chronic polyarthritis flare-ups. A businesswoman running her own tourist firm, Alla often complained that in present-day Russia, the pace of her life demanded a new kind of ability to ignore her body because time wouldn't stop just on account on her being ill. The difficulty of convincing treating physicians to issue a doctor's note encourages patients to ignore their illness, she argued. Doctors, she explained, sometimes suspect the patient of being lazy, of trying to skip work, and take it upon themselves to withhold a diagnosis and thus a paid leave of absence. The patient is thus faced with a choice of taking a leave on her own time and money, which many cannot afford, or to ignore her symptoms. It is telling that Alla did not blame the institutional insufficiencies or bureaucratic pressures put on general practitioners that might lead to this sort of withholding of diagnosis. Instead, she found fault with "modern medicine" and with its use of synthetic pharmaceuticals on her present suffering: she had contracted a severe case of tonsillitis in her late twenties, which she "withstood on her feet" (*perenesla na nogakh*), and instead of treating its cause, the treatment she was prescribed allowed her to function and ignore her symptoms, but the illness never went away. As a result, she had developed complications:

> If they had treated me properly when I was twenty-eight, I wouldn't be having these problems now. Instead, I was eating antibiotics by the handful. The pain was gone, but not the disease, so now I'm in the state I'm in. This is why I have an enlargement of the liver, an ulcer, and so on. . . . I have a crappy body.

Contrasting her experience at East-West to these previous forms of treatment, she explained:

I think in part it's the procedures [that are effective], but in part it's because you are treated like a human being (*k tebe po chelovecheski otnosiatsia*). Our bodies are not touched for so long that you don't even know anymore how you feel, or if something hurts or doesn't.

The sense of bodily alienation that Alla describes, of the inability to "know" or "feel" the body, was frequently a source of frustration for patients. Because doctors at the clinic rely on palpation and self-report to cross-check the incoming diagnoses contained in patients' medical histories, doctor-patient interaction demands careful practices of accounting for one's symptomatology. On one occasion, Valerie, one of the neurologists and acupuncturists I shadowed during my fieldwork, noted the frustration of a patient who was trying to explain that she could not answer her questions for lack of a frame of reference. Valerie had asked her patient whether she felt any pain during abdominal palpation, but after a few minutes, the patient simply shrugged. "We are so used to pain, that I really couldn't tell you whether something hurts or not," she explained.

Physicians at the clinic worked to offset this estrangement by exacting from patients a careful and constant self-scrutiny and asking them to report their most minute symptoms and bodily changes. The ritual of the admittance interview, as well as every subsequent day a patient spent at the clinic, were punctuated by the same series of questions. In the mornings, doctors went from room to room with a clipboard, introduced themselves or greeted their patient, and began a questioning that seemed to frequently ignore patients' previous diagnoses, obliquely grazing the surfaces of a body framed in terms of a diffuse phenomenology that never quite condensed into illness. For new patients, the onslaught of seemingly unrelated questions did not, in fact, match the expectations they had of a therapeutic interaction. The first question was almost inevitably, "What are your complaints?" Patients who had not previously stayed at the clinic systematically gave the "wrong" answer by invoking their medical file. Subsequently, the physician would demand more specific information: "What hurts? Does your liver feel heavy? How's your digestion? How's your stool? Are you getting headaches? How's your blood pressure? How is your sleep? Do you ever get dry mouth? Do you get heartburn? Do your feet get cold? Do your limbs feel stiff? Do you cough in the morning? Do you feel like you sweat a lot? Does it hurt here?" One patient, especially flabbergasted by the implications of this mode of attention to his body, eventually asked one of the doctors, "Wait, should I tell you everything?"

This questioning was an unexpected point of convergence between those practitioners trained in Tibetan medicine and those with other specialties, but they led to different conclusions. For the neurologists and acupuncturists, a question about cold feet might suggest that the patient has poor peripheral circulation. For the Tibetan medicine practitioners, it will likely suggest a deregulation of the *rlung* bodily constitution. On one occasion, I stood in the patient's room as Aleksandra, a trained GP and Tibetan medicine practitioner whom I shadowed during her shifts at the clinic, began to interview a new patient.

S: What are your complaints?

P: Osteochondritis. It's all in the medical history file.

S: I don't know what that is. What are your complaints?

P: [pause] Well, my eye hurts, and my neck hurts. [pause] I've done IV therapy for it, and it's helped.

S: So when was the last IV treatment?

P: In July. It's in the medical history.

S: When did it [the symptoms] begin?

P: About ten years ago.

S: Don't you get massage for the neck?

P: Why, yes, I do, but not since last October, since I've been at the center.

S: Do you take medications?

P: Yes, "Kavinton" for blood pressure, I always drink it.

S: What have you been ill with?

P: Nothing.

S: Nothing at all?

P: Well, I've had pneumonia. Haven't had any operations.

S: Anything else?

P: [after a pause] Pyelonephritis, but that was a while ago.

S: Any other complaints?

P: My mouth is dry, and my throat is scratchy.

S: Ok, good. But can we not do this in bits?

P: [the patient shrugs] We're used to it that way.

After Aleksandra palpated the patient's stomach, the patient was surprised to find that the palpation was painful.

P: It hurts.

S: Hmm, why does it hurt . . . ?

P: I don't know. [pause] We don't know what hurts, we don't know why it hurts. We don't know how to complain.

S: Do you ever cough? Any phlegm? Shortness of breath?

P: Yes.

S: So why aren't you telling me all these things all at once?

P: [pause] Because we don't know how to be examined by the doctor anymore.

Knowing how to talk about one's body is an important element of being a patient at East-West, but this practice of daily accounting is built around a set of occlusions and asymmetries. The sense that patients' bodies are alienated objects to which they have no immediate access obscures the fact that the self-accounting required of them is a highly mediated and hierarchical process. Certainly, patients do not suspend their efforts to mitigate the various bodily phenomena that make up what they describe as their health when they are outside of the clinic. But the economies of attention that are deployed in the clinical spaces of East-West make these strategies and forms of bodily care invisible in the daily routines of the center. Patients' apprehensions of their bodies outside of the clinic and their efforts to manage a variety of symptoms and problems are not directly addressed in the clinic itself, precisely because of the kind of unusually minute attention doctors ask of their patients.

In part, the forms of questioning that doctors at East-West appear to favor is a by-product of the internal institutional hierarchy of the center and its relationship with the Ministry of Health, rather than the result of a particular "personalized" medical philosophy. When I asked physicians whether patient admission interviews were formulated in relation to the center's focus on traditional medicine, I was told that they were, in fact, primarily a response to administrative pressures. "The problem here is that we have to fill out these forms for Minzdrav, and we're filling out forms at the beginning which we really ought to be filling out at the end [of the patient's stay]," one of the senior physicians explained. Being accountable to the local Ministry of Health, East-West had to record and report patient improvement. However, because of the constant turnover of patients, the long backlog of the admissions waiting list, and the deadlines for turning in paperwork, physicians had to anticipate the eventual effects of their therapies even before the treatment was finished. Through a detailed yet loose collection of patients' symptoms, doctors were able to create reasonably vague predictions about patients' improvement and meet the deadlines for submitting the paperwork. Yet, I would like to suggest that reducing the doctor-patient interactions to the prosaic necessities of an institutional bureaucracy is insufficient for tracking the implications of a focus on the phenomenological body in the clinical spaces of East-West. The *vypiska* (medical discharge) document doctors had to produce before releasing a patient was highly personalized. Valerie explained that this also served to create an enormous backlog of paperwork. Each document had to be carefully crafted for each individual patient, and there was no standardized form doctors could fill out. "With each one, you start from zero," she explained. Personalized medicine meant personalized bureaucracy. In other words, doctors were responsible for narrating the therapeutic time patients spent at the clinic in such a way as to create a sense of continuity and orderly treatment in response to the patient's multiplicity of seemingly disjointed symptoms and complaints.

On the other hand, for doctors at the clinic, writing out a diagnosis and treatment report was frequently already an approximation, a matter of bureaucratic formality that failed to capture patients' complex forms of embodiment and the therapies that doctors mobilized—a fact that most of the doctors were perfectly cognizant of. This was especially the case for those practitioners who were trained in Tibetan medicine and were working with a different set of diagnostic categories and criteria. Aleksandra would frequently ask the senior neurologist what "biomedical" diagnosis she should write out on a patient form, not simply because she was deferring to his expertise, but because translating patients' diffuse symptoms into a diagnosis was a generalization that had little relevance to her therapeutic practices or to the actual processes of a complex body and its internal phenomena. Within the constitutional logics of Tibetan medicine, a "heart wind" or an "increase in phlegm" worked much more effectively to describe the minute bodily variations patients experienced from one day to the next as their treatment unfolded, but such diagnoses could not be captured in bureaucratic medicalese, only approximated.

During my fieldwork at the clinic, my role, as far as the doctors I shadowed were concerned, was to "entertain" patients with my questions and prodding, the usefulness of my presence to the physicians partly articulated as a function of the peculiar isolation of the clinic itself and partly as yet another element of the economy of individual attention the clinic prides itself in. Such practical considerations aside, the building is, somewhat self-consciously, a space of confinement. Located some ten kilometers north of Ulan-Ude, it stands in isolation on the grounds of an old brucellosis sanatorium formerly owned by a local collective farm that went bankrupt in the turbulent 1990s. Access is difficult, and most patients leave the building only for short walks around the complex or to undergo additional testing at the center's polyclinic, transported there on the center's shuttle bus. Sometimes, patients leave the clinic for short periods, such as a weekend, a practice that doctors jokingly refer to as patients' attempt at "jailbreak." For the treatment to be maximally effective, both doctors and patients tend to agree that one needs to remain in reverse quarantine, refraining from letting the outside world and its concerns inside treatment space. "Of course, patients are bored," Zhamso Sayanovich, the senior neurologist, frequently intimated, when I asked him about some of the difficulties of his work—many are older, most are seriously ill, they are cut off from their everyday lives, their relatives, their jobs. However, he saw this seclusion as the only guarantee that treatment would be maximally effective, and conflicts over interruptions of the treatment cycle often erupted between patients and doctors when the former felt the pull of their everyday obligations. Because most patients are themselves self-taught "experts" on different forms of care, including knowing a variety of sites where they can obtain traditional medical treatment and not simply state-provided biomedicine, they were far from being a docile or pliable population, their bodies a site of authoritative and unquestioned medical interventions. Decisions about treatment frequently took the form of negotiations, either with the patient or with her caretaker when the patient was in no condition to make an informed judgment. In addition to their medical history file—the written records of their passage through various official medical institutions—patients at the clinic often invoked an informal bodily history: the sum of their experiences with various doctors and medical treatment, their continual efforts to learn about, manage, relieve, and medicate their own conditions and symptoms—all inextricably woven with the social relations and biographical events that punctuated their lives. The center was only one stop on their therapeutic itineraries.

These informal histories became only partially visible during the doctor-patient encounter as patients focused on selecting treatment. Patients would often request specific procedures—leech therapy, for example—because they had read about their merits in a newspaper or magazine, had heard about it on television or the radio during one of the many health programs that are abundant in the Russian media, or simply were told about it by friends or acquaintances. Alternatively, some patients refused certain forms of treatment if their previous experiences with them had been unsuccessful or negative or if they suspected the treatment of having adverse side effects. Many patients at East-West relied on constant self-medication, both with over-the-counter pharmaceuticals, which up until the 2009 health reforms included many drugs regulated elsewhere but available without prescription in Russia, and various herbal remedies, some bought at pharmacies, some made at home. For example, Katerina proudly mentioned to me that she was mostly capable of managing the symptoms of her asthma by making tisanes and vodka tinctures, using several botanical manuals for guidance. In part, these forms of self-care were invoked in relation to a distinct lack of care from doctors at state institutions. In a logic that stated that unless they helped themselves, no one would help them, patients avidly collected medical recipes, recommendations, and advice, sharing them with each other and occasionally with the clinic's staff.

For many patients, traditional medicine was synonymous with ingesting plant-based or food-based medicines, and the collection and passing on of recipes are central topics of conversation between patients. The center also takes the use of herbal medicines—whether derived from "classical" Russian phytotherapy or from Tibetan medical compositions—to be one of its main therapeutic modalities. For patients, "Tibetan teas" were a source of great interest and of a kind of theoretical pleasure, at least up until the moment of having to ingest some of the more unpalatable ones. Unlike "synthetic" pharmaceuticals, patients saw botanically based medicines as more gentle, more natural, or, as the clinic's own official brochure explains, "more physiological," which is to say, more closely approximating the body's rhythms and processes. However, they were also widely considered slower-acting, requiring long-term ingestion, repeated medication, and careful attention to preparation and timing and could potentially cause the symptoms to become more acute in the initial phase of the treatment.

These discourses on botanicals shed light on the kinds of anxieties biomedical treatment and synthetic pharmaceuticals appear to invoke for patients in Buryatia and in Russia more broadly. Pills are often taken to have an excess of effect—fast-acting and potentially causing iatrogenic harm, synthetic medicines, or pills, are taken to be appropriate only for acute diseases, but not chronic ones. Concurrently, herbal medicines are seen as ideally suited for chronic illness, both because their action is distributed over time and because, according to the popular descriptions of traditional medicine and especially Tibetan medicine, they are taken to act on the root cause of illness and not only on its symptoms.

The efforts to collect health advice, recipes, and, on occasion, ingredients resonate with an expression I heard time and again from patients who attempted to provide a pithy description for why they kept returning to East-West. They referred to their primary therapeutic strategy as "stocking up on health" (*zapastis' zdorovyem*). In a logic that suggests that health can be accumulated or spent, the perceived distinctions between the therapeutic efficacies of Western and traditional medicine become salient factors in a personal economy of maintaining a functioning body. In other words, while biomedical interventions allowed patients to avert imminent disaster, only those medicines labeled "traditional" or "natural" were considered an effective means of health accumulation.

"You have to keep coming back regularly, because the illness doesn't go away really, this is just a temporary fix" (*vremennaya pochinka*), Natalya, one of the return patients, explained when I asked her about whether she planned on coming back to the clinic in the future. "Is this because you can't remove the cause of illness?" I asked, drawing on the popular critique of biomedicine that circulated among Tibetan medical practitioners in Ulan-Ude, a critique that argued that unlike contemporary medicine, Tibetan medicine can actually address the root cause. "Of course you don't remove the cause—how can you if the disease is chronic?" Natalya retorted. "But you feel better for a while, and then you can come back for another round in a year. Until then I can maintain myself with herbs, but after treatments here, for a while, I don't have anything to complain about (*mne ne na chto zhalovat'sia*)."

While some patients blamed the individual doctors in state hospitals for the medical failures they experienced, others invoked more systemic problems. In a conversation between Aleksandra and two of her patients, one of the women recalled a story about her treatment in her local polyclinic:

> P1: I've been to the polyclinic, to see the doctor who treats veterans. There's a line of dozens of people sitting to see her. By the end of it, it's over, she doesn't even look [at you] anymore. That's the system, so that you can get Putin's 150 thousand [rubles], you have to see all these people. The medical files have to be filled out. You have to lie, or to ignore the patient.
>
> A: I don't work in that system.
>
> P1: You folks, don't, that's true. But in general. It's because doctors don't get any satisfaction from their job. They look at the patient like an object.
>
> P2: Like a source of income.
>
> P1: And we're pensioners—we toiled away, building communism, survived *perestroika*. To beg for money—it's demeaning. But at the same time, everything rises, the prices are constantly rising. . . . In general, in Russia, there is no middle class. What are we choosing? Even if we don't show up, they'll still choose for us.

Treatment at the clinic was always layered over a lifetime of managing a body that is increasingly made more permeable through repeated exposures to environmental, social, ecological, and historical assaults. One patient spoke of her fluctuating health as something that periodically got better or worse, depending on where she was, and depending on the weather. "We are all meteo-sensitive," she remarked. Spending the summer at the dacha relieved her aching joints and allowed her to breathe more easily. Returning to the damp cold climate of the city, she felt her symptoms return.

Lillia, a patient with hypertension and painful varicose veins, interwove her narrative of illness and therapy with questions of both personal and social grief and loss. She blamed her husband's death on the medical system, suggesting that even though he was the most responsible person she had ever known, someone who took treatment very seriously, he still died of a heart attack. When I asked her about her own choice of treatment, Lillia explained that she had very negative experiences with "classical" medicine (biomedicine), and began to rely on East-West for health maintenance:

> I've been here ten times. In complex, the "charge" (*zaryad*) you get is enough to get you through seven months without health complaints. See, it all depends on the person—how do you understand yourself? No matter what the machine is, you have to take care of it, right? We don't have education anymore—hygiene, ethics. You have to know that you only live once. That way, a person would know their body—that's what physical education is for. We study math, but why do we need it? In Japan and Korea, there is traditional education, and traditional medicine. In the Soviet Union, it was a question of discipline, people were doing "GTO." At least, it was a minimum. And now, all stadiums are closed, and to care about your health (*zabotitsia o zdorov'ye*), you have to pay money. Workers used to go to sanatoria and health resorts, but now everything has been transferred into private hands. Professional unions necessarily had a sanatorium. None of this exists anymore, it's all commercial structures. See, my son is a boxer, and from bringing him up [as a professional athlete] I see that it all depends on proper education. But we used to live—you know, "here is this, here is that"—and now, that's all gone. But then, it became clear that the state never gave back in full anyway. We fell behind so much. You know, I remember, my husband was a diplomat, went to Korea—it was his dream—and saw how people lived there. This was in the late '80s, the Soviet Union still existed. For the first time in his life, he felt ashamed [for us]. He used to tell me, "How we live, us, with our huge resources!" It still vexes me to the point of tears (*Mne do sikh por obidno do slyoz*). When he came back, he turned in his party card.

In Lillia's account, bodies become machines that are neither properly cared for by the state nor sufficiently self-aware to be capable of self-maintenance. Her own therapeutic strategies consist of receiving a "charge" of health that will last her a little over half a year before her symptoms return. The temporality of illness is never divorced from other life events, both traumatic and chronic. As Katerina said in relation to her health worsening over the last two years, she noticed some of her symptoms—migraine headaches and knee pain—becoming more acute after the death of her son and daughter-in-law in a car accident. She blamed her flaring symptoms on the additional stress of having to raise her grandchildren and on the sense that there was something deeply amiss about the way her personal biographic time had failed to properly unfold. She extrapolated this to a more general failure of the state to take care of its retired population:

> This is the age when I am supposed to be taken care of, and instead, I am still taking care of others. Pensioners have a bad life here. They're supposed to make medicine affordable for us, but they give us such a pitiful bonus that you can hardly afford anything with it. I receive 700 rubles a month to buy medicines, but you can only use it at certain times, and I can't always make it to the pharmacy at these times. Or if you do, the lines are terrible. And someone is lining their pockets with our pensions.

Shifting from her frustrated account of the state to a more enthusiastic account of her own success at surviving in it, she explained that she was able to stay at the clinic from time to time and relied on the circulation of medical advice and recipes for maintaining herself in the interim. Staying at the clinic was a temporary reprieve from her life and a luxury she was willing to assiduously save her pension for, if only for the fact that her stay allowed her to "save up some health" and get on with her life until the next period of treatment.

CHRONIC DISADAPTATIONS

"I can't stand this work," Aleksandra huffed one morning as we were both entering the clinic's building. Puzzled by her sudden emotional outburst, I asked her to clarify. "I'm a pediatrician by training, I work with kids," she explained. Aleksandra had a fairly active clientele at East-West's polyclinic, where she received mostly young patients and their parents. During her shifts at the clinic, she was frequently on the phone with one parent or another, sometimes running out of the building for better cell phone reception to quickly hammer out recommendations and suggestions. As her shift ended around four, she would speed off in her car to meet with her walk-in patients at the polyclinic, often staying until eight or nine in the evening to provide them with another batch of medicines. She used Tibetan medicine exclusively whenever she could—for children, she explained, it was perfect because there were never any allergic reactions, and the recovery was practically instantaneous. "You know, you give them something in the evening, and the next day the parent calls completely happy, because the kid's doing just fine. Children are so responsive. Everything works quickly and works as it should." By contrast, working at the clinic with an aging, chronically sick population, Aleksandra often felt that her efforts were futile or at least produced very limited and very temporary results. The contrast she was drawing was striking in the way it teased out the logics of accumulated disadaptations—children, after all, did not yet embody much history.

In this chapter, I have suggested that the therapeutic imaginaries of integrative medicine in the East-West Clinic, as in other integrative institutions, inherit and build on logics of bodily adaptation developed by Russian and Soviet medical experts concerned with the optimization of health. Yet, despite the horizons of maximized health and personalization, propagated by such disciplines as valeology and recuperated into the clinic's self-presentation, patients' day-to-day experiences in the clinical spaces of "East-West" tell a different story of recalcitrant disadaptations. Co-opted into mostly chronic care, the therapeutic modalities of East-West do not offer a kind of "super-adaptability" to a practically healthy population. They serve, instead, to remedy the chronic lifetimes of accumulated exposures of patients whose physiologies become a site for articulating a nefarious relationship between local bodies and their living conditions. These misalignments, traced in the critiques of state medical care, the economic difficulties of aging populations, and the harshness of regional spaces, are experienced as hindrances to the forms of adaptability through which good health is understood.

In its own way, the integrative clinic intervenes into this pathogenic unfolding of time through its practices of attending to lived bodies. Patients were encouraged, from day to day, to list the minutiae of everyday pangs and pains, a narrative of suffering circulating in a body that constantly generated new symptoms, nested in certain areas only to transmute later into different spaces and experiences—a dry mouth, a morning cough, a stiffness of limbs—without ever permanently settling into a single medical diagnosis. For patients, these practices of paying attention were sometimes understood as true "care" (*zabota*) on the part of the doctors, a concern with a health always situated at the intersection of biographic, physical, and historical lifetimes. For doctors, their therapeutic efforts frequently felt insufficient—only partially actualized through what they took to be one of the clinic's primary sources of efficacy—namely, the temporary suspension of the pathogenesis of everyday life. The qualities of that attention were, in some ways, a felicitous coarticulation of entirely different needs. Patients' desires for a form of care that recognized the person over generalizing optics—both those of the disease category as a medical abstraction and those of a population at large that shared similar conditions of life, labor, and history—were accidentally amplified not only by East-West's mission, but also by the bureaucratic requirements to make its activities legible to the Ministry of Health. For both patients and doctors, care at the East-West clinic rotated around an individual body deliberately left open-ended—a site where attentiveness to embodied experience could be performed and encouraged in the day-to-day, and where it textured doctor-patient interaction.

But here, I want to loop back to East-West's dual slogans: the one that promised attention for individual patients and the one that saw the future of medicine in the carful preservation of the past. In patients' experiences and narratives, the past was already all too present: it accumulated in an accretion of pathogenic and therapeutic episodes "in real time," experienced collectively but resolved into individual conditions that required specific kinds of attentiveness during the clinical encounter.

5

"WE ARE NOT IRON THAT WE NEED TEMPERING"

The Contingencies of Mixing Medicines

"WHERE DOES MODERN MEDICINE COME FROM?"

The question was first posed to me by Sergei, one of the radiophysicists who worked on developing the electronic pulsometer. Sergei and I sat on a bench outside the university building where he worked, and as I attempted to interview him about the goals of his research and about his participation in the project of integrating Tibetan medicine into clinical and laboratory practice, he matched every question I posed with his own. The interaction was awkward. Turning the questions back on me, Sergei demanded an exegesis on the history of medical science. His provocation, which I first mistook for the physicist's penchant for a Socratic method of communication or for skepticism about a U.S.-based researcher's intellectual credentials, slowly came to reframe my own questions. Sergei's answer was unique to him. At my fumbling response, he traced the genealogy of what he called "scientific medicine" to nineteenth-century European military expansion, the discovery of the anesthetic properties of chloroform, and the development of field surgery. Tellingly, his question was not unique. As I sought to grasp what my interlocutors in Buryatia thought of the Russian state's efforts to formalize the region's therapeutic traditions, I was repeatedly asked, in turn, what I meant when I invoked biomedicine.

The term *integratzia* (a Russian calque of "integration") was a popular shorthand to describe what a number of medical institutions and proponents in the health-care administration and professional medical communities were attempting to achieve. As I have discussed in the previous chapters, it figured prominently in the discourses and goals of a relatively recent medical field, labeled "restorative medicine," that aims to "restore" the health of the nation through noninvasive, "natural" medical technologies. However, what is meant by "integration" is neither entirely clear nor understood as a particularly innovative borrowing from outside Russia's therapeutic context. Certainly, articulations of integrative medicine have by now a level of global circulation, as well as many concrete loci of articulation. For example, the U.S. National Center for Complementary and Alternative Medicine of the National Institute of Health links integrative medicine with CAM therapies and defines it as a patient-centered approach to health that selects techniques from "conventional" and "alternative" medicine (at least, those that have concrete scientific backing) to maximize the body's capacity to heal itself. For its part, WHO tends to focus on integration as the degree to which local traditional medicines are incorporated into the dominant health-care system. But the relationship between these two understandings of the term is not self-evident. In Buryatia—and in Russia more broadly—*integratzia* maps onto longstanding but fraught national discourses about the country's (and, recursively, the region's) cultural uniqueness as a place of transition and translation between the cultures and histories of East and West.

This chapter outlines the ways in which post-socialist politics of medical knowledge in Siberia might illuminate the dynamics of tradition in global discourses on traditional medicine in its relationship to biomedical practices. By paying attention to the relationship between modern and traditional medicine in Russia, I would like to take Sergei's challenge seriously.

Certainly, critical histories of medicine—and science more generally—show the internal plurality of biomedical knowledge and practices, tracking their conceptual transformations, dead ends, and internal polyvalence, frequently forgotten in a posteriori narratives of unidirectional scientific progress (Latour 1987, 1993; Mol 2002; Stengers 2003). For biomedicine to be recognizably operating at a global scale, albeit, as anthropologists have often noted, with different local actualizations and entanglements, it must constantly mask the particularities and origin points of its practices. The stability of biomedicine as discrete object—but also, its implied efficacies in producing and disciplining subjects—rely on the constant normalization of its claims to truth. I take "normalization" in its double meaning, in the sense of appearing as the default form of knowledge about collective and individual bodies and in the sense of being made regular and consistent by obfuscating its internal variations and contradictions.

Sergei's question pushes the classic anthropological insight that biomedicine too is multiple in a slightly different analytical direction: it seems to suggest that while all of its varied, yet recognizable, incarnations retain a connection to a stable form, apprehensions of its many avatars as always manifesting a recognizable totality (however fractured) allow us to speak of therapeutic practices that fall outside of biomedicine's realm as if such lines of distinction were something one would be able to identify without much discussion. In contexts where tracing boundaries between different kinds of medicines is never divorced from questions of how things travel and how they are made to settle, descriptions of therapeutic encounters between biomedicine and nonbiomedical modalities tend to imply, for the sake of drawing the analytical contrast, a consensus about what biomedicine is. It was this consensus that Sergei was reestablishing on new, fraught, and what to me had felt like socially antagonistic grounds—not so much that there *was* a biomedicine, but that we could agree (or agree not to argue) about what we thought it was. It is in this sense that the term "official medicine," as a local gloss for biomedicine, seems especially productive. In Russian, at least, "official" offers more than unquestioned recognition, it implies a kind of doublespeak that brings into the frame its constitutive outside.

Accounts of Soviet science and medicine are sometimes haunted by Cold War legacies—in excavating the uniqueness of Soviet knowledge projects, broadly speaking, it becomes remarkably difficult not to decenter their authority or claims to truth by invoking Soviet political ideologies and institutional configurations as the determining factor for the ways in which they came to be. Conversely, conflations between, on the one hand, a history of Soviet and Russian therapeutic practices and ideologies and, on the other, of "Western" (European, North American) approaches to both biomedicine and traditional medicine miss the subtle and not-so-subtle differences.

If, following Latour, purification is always an important, although never perfectly realized process through which modern scientific knowledge is (co)constituted vis-a-vis those practices it excludes, then what happens when an acknowledged hybridity stands at the crux of what it means to achieve medical and scientific progress? These dynamics in Russia displace the expected locus of tension between a global circulating authoritative biomedical discourse and local understandings of bodies and health. In fact, as I will argue, the oppositions between global and local, as well as between traditional medicine and biomedicine, became analytically limiting in a therapeutic context where the questions of scale, points of origin, and the nature and locus of medical efficacy and adequate care are constantly worried and interrogated. Scholars have argued that Soviet notions of progress had silenced a variety of actors in the name of a modernist project of rapid technological and social development founded on scientific rationality—a project, moreover, that was understood as simultaneously universal, yet uniquely manifested (Field 2000). For its part, as we saw in Chapter 1, Soviet engagement with Eastern medicine in general and Tibetan medicine in particular were integral to claims about what it means to practice medicine as a scientific discipline—and offered a contrast set on which articulating a programmatic relationship between medicine and the modern state became possible. If, as historian Susan Buck-Morss (2002) has argued, the Soviet project's aspirations to its own version of cosmopolitan universalism was centered on intervening in a dialectical unfolding of time, then leaving the "medicines of the past" in the past in the hands of appropriate experts (such as historians and ethnographers) offered a way to adjust the Soviet Union to a vision of medicine's universal and explicitly European history. The resurgence of once silenced modes of healing as audible, tractable, and manageable agents under late socialism and in a "post-socialist" moment is as much a resignification of political histories as a ground on which Soviet ideologies of health were being remapped and reconfigured in the present, shifting the goalposts of what might count as universal and what counts as particular. We might therefore ask, along with Sergei, "whose" universal, and "whose" particular?

Integrative medical projects in Buryatia coalesced around two focal points: first, what is to be counted as "traditional" care, and to whom do such traditions belong? Second, how can these traditions be systematized and integrated into a state-prescribed division of therapeutic labor that identifies and maximizes their therapeutic efficacies? This chapter looks at the ways in which the relationship between modern and traditional medicine is formulated at different sites that bring these complex and contradictory stakes to the surface. I am concerned here with a version of therapeutic interventions that simultaneously strive toward a totality of care but are frequently troubled, or, in the words of Isabelle Stengers, "slowed down" by the juxtapositions between multiple ontologically and epistemologically distinct "takes" on bodies and health (Stengers 2005, 995). The therapeutic bundles that medical integration enacts are inflected by a sense that in a context where biomedicine does not (or no longer, or not fully) hold a hegemonic, authoritative monopoly, new ways of imagining totalities emerge, but remain suspect for all involved.

The first section discusses what counted as traditional medicine in Russian legislative documents and officially sanctioned expert discourses in the first decade of the 2000s. Focusing on the instability of the term "traditional," it engages with the politics of differentiation between traditional and modern medical practices in Buryatia. The second section of the chapter focuses on the spaces defined through practices of medical integration proper. By tracing the scandals of integration—the institutional difficulties of incorporating nonbiomedical practices and the frictions of epistemological incompatibility, I suggest that it is precisely the localization and de-universalization of biomedical practice that allow practitioners (and patients) to experience a multiple and ontologically open-ended therapeutic landscape.

PRECARIOUS LEGALITIES

Scholars looking at the global distribution of traditional medicine and its state regulation often use a shorthand to articulate a contrast between East- and South-Asian state health care and "Western" approaches. In these analyses, Asian medical practices are characterized by a tendency toward the nationalization of traditional medical systems alongside biomedicine in a distribution of health-care practices along a model of more or less orchestrated medical pluralism (Lock 1990). By contrast, Euro-American approaches divide therapeutic knowledge and practice into biomedicine and everything else, under the umbrella term of "complementary and alternative medicine" (for an account of this contrast set, see Scheid and MacPherson 2012). It should be noted that these accounts of different medical systems describe classificatory logics that tend to posit dual or triple contrast sets: biomedicine vs. traditional medicine, or, alternatively, biomedicine alongside a national medical tradition, alongside "folk" or "indigenous" practices (Kayne 2010). Certainly, these are generalizations—in practice, the relationships among different therapeutic forms are both more complex and more subtle (Scheid 2002; Hardiman and Mukharji 2012). However, the ideological efficacy of presenting different medical modalities as if they were self-contained, separate, and identifiable entities, developed over time in a continuous accretion of knowledge and techniques into a unique "system," is what enables different actors—official health-care bureaucracies, international organization, professional associations—to mobilize therapeutic forms in the service of political arguments about the nature of the state, national identity, and history.

For their part, international organizations like WHO base their assessment of the vitality of traditional medicine in different regions primarily on state policies that locally regulate health-care possibilities. The resulting "bird's-eye view" of the global distribution of traditional medicines visually maps a division between the "Global North" and "Global South," where the Global North is primarily defined by its lack of regulation of nonbiomedical care, discursively equated to traditional medicine's relative absence from the therapeutic field. In other words, the relationship between biomedicine and traditional medicine is cast as a zero-sum game, where traditional medicine tends to be understood to fill the lacunae of unevenly distributed biomedical care or to remedy the "lack of success" of "available medical care."

Certainly, careful ethnographic case studies of different spaces of encounter and translation, as well as attention to the ways in which "tradition" becomes commodified and circulates in an international market, complicate these generalizations (Adams, Schrempf, and Craig 2011; Alter 2005; Cohen 1995; Janes 2002; Farquhar 1994; Langwick 2008; Pordié 2008, 2012). It is then not surprising that integrative approaches that propose therapeutic hybridization can make the stakes of welding medical practices to national ideologies apparent. The Russian case offers a lens into these questions, primarily because it remains unclear what sort of medicine might map on to the Russian state and whom its traditional "roots" might belong to. If, by virtue of its historical development, Russian discourses on national identity, *pace* the recent rise of nationalist sensibilities, are always haunted by claims to geographic and cultural exceptionalism formulated in terms of their hybrid, cosmopolitan history, then the politics of tradition in labeling and identifying nonbiomedical practices reveal the fragile sutures between biopolitical purposes and the imaginaries of a multinational state (Laruelle 2009; Bassin 1991).

Over the period of my fieldwork in this region, the Russian state's attempt to discipline a multiplying therapeutic pluralism had cycled through multiple phases, often several times over, toggling between top-down and grassroots efforts to formalize, systematize, and cultivate and their opposite—a tendency to scatter, ignore, or let grow in the cracks, unattended, a variety of different therapeutic practices and logics. Over the years, most *emchi* I have met have worked across the institutional, administrative, and ethical divides between legal and illegal, visible and invisible, officially recognized and barely tolerated.

In practice, *emchi* are not, in fact, incorporated into the local healthcare system in any straightforward way, and Tibetan medicine in Russia often takes the shape of what Hardiman and Mukharji have termed "subaltern therapeutics"—the modalities of care that fall outside of what is deemed by the state as recognizably medicinal (see Hardiman and Mukharji 2012). No clear-cut way of authorizing Tibetan medicine exists in Buryatia or in Russia more generally. As such, Tibetan medicine suffers from a kind of Schrödinger's Cat legality: it is *potentially*, contingently legal at the same time as it is *potentially*, contingently illegal, depending on the position of the observer.

To understand the nature of this legal precarity, it helps to illustrate some of the linguistic and organizational conundrums of Russia's medical legislature. Tibetan medicine's alegality, in the sense of being aside rather than outside the law, has to do with the terminological confusions and internal inconsistencies of Article 50 of Russia's Federal Law "On the fundamentals of health protection of citizens in the Russian Federation." The confusion stems from a kind of linguistic artefactual amalgamation to the regulatory framework. Older iterations of Article 50, in charge of regulating medical activity, drew a distinction between traditional medicine and folk medicine, in part in an effort to comply with WHO's resolutions on traditional medicines as a matter of indigenous sovereignty and in part in the hopes of getting a handle on a distinctly post-socialist therapeutic multiplication—namely, the effervescence of magic and healing that began in the 1990s against the backdrop of protracted and difficult health-care reforms. Folk medicine is defined as "those convalescence (*ozdorovlenie*) methods that have been established through people's experience, at the basis of which lies the use of knowledge, know-how, and practical skills in the evaluation and restoration of health" (Article 50.1). Article 50.2 states that in order to practice these techniques of folk medicine, a citizen of the Russian Federation must obtain a permit. However, permits' issue and revocation are left to the regional governments.

For its part, conventional usage in Russia's medical field differentiates between ethnically marked "folk" medicine—like, say, Bashkir herbalism or Buryat bonesetting—and "traditional" medicine, which usually refers to evidence-based procedures and pharmaceuticals derived from different traditions of folk medicine but registered as isolated techniques incorporated into the system of medical accreditation and training. Thus, different types of ethnic herbalism are lumped together into clinical phytotherapy, all forms of manual therapy are reclassified as therapeutic massage, and so forth. In practice, this means that any given doctor can employ any given traditional medical technique for which they are accredited, even though, since 2012, the category of "traditional medicine" as such was struck out of Article 50, leaving only "folk medicine" as the sole legal signifier of medical alternatives to biomedical treatment. There are thus a number of officially recognized therapeutic approaches loosely marked as "traditional" in Russia—from homeopathy and bioresonance therapy to phytotherapy and acupuncture—with different degrees of legal incorporation and legitimacy. The histories of these practices, as well as their theoretical premises and therapeutic techniques, are frequently radically distinct, if not outright mutually contradictory.

The term "folk" (*narodnyi*) itself is somewhat ambiguous and can be taken to refer to popular practices that pertain to people (humans) as a whole—a generic category that presumably transcends national, historical, and cultural differences. Alternatively, it might be understood to reference discrete cultural groups, hearkening back to Soviet ideas of a unity of "the people," despite their distinct cultural forms, under a single presumably ideologically uniform state. This is important in order to understand the ways in which the legitimacy and authority of different forms of therapeutic knowledge play out in Buryatia's medical field. There is no simple ideological map for interpreting the power relations and hierarchies that organize different ways of knowing and treating the body, and the valence of these relations is often a question of perspective. More importantly, navigating these uneven conceptual terrains is not only challenging for a researcher or an outsider, but is frequently not a self-evident task even for those who are firmly part of the local professional medical sphere. At the time of my fieldwork, a different law stated more explicitly what specific techniques might be counted as folk medicine. According to Article 8 of the Russian Ministry of Health Protection Order N 142 dated 29.04.98 "on the types of medical activity subject to licensing," seven distinct types of folk (traditional) medicine required a license to practice. These included leech therapy (*hyrudotherapy*), homeopathy, manual therapy, medical massage, reflexotherapy, traditional diagnostics, and "traditional convalescence systems" (*traditzionnye sistemy ozdorovlenia*). Although the purpose of this law was to regulate the accreditation of medical practitioners, it also served a rhetorical purpose by officially recognizing folk medicine as a domain of medical activity on par with other forms of mainstream biomedical expertise. At the same time, Order N 142 operated to exclude certain nonbiomedical practitioners, most prominently phytotherapists (naturopathics), from the category of folk medicine—leaving their practice in an ambiguous gray area that is neither explicitly recognized nor explicitly forbidden.

Since Russia's health protection law draws a categorical distinction between religious healing and medical practice, it leaves certain types of nonbiomedical therapies outside the medical field entirely. Thus, religious healing (*tselitel'stvo*) is in fact regulated by Russia's labor code. "Occult and religious services," religious rituals, and *tselitel'stvo* are reclassified as private entrepreneurship under the subheading 93.05.12.150 of the Russian Classification of Products by Economic Activities and defined as "other personal services." These services are featured alongside a broad range of miscellaneous activities, such as escort services, astrology, mediumship, matchmaking, pet-sitting, and the activities of organizations that carry out genealogical research. As a result, healing that is explicitly marked as religious falls into a miscellaneous catch-all category of small business ventures. By contrast, "folk" or "traditional" medicine can be licensed, but only on the condition that the practitioner already has biomedical certification. After the federal level administrative body that used to license folk healers was dismantled in the early 2000s, the task of licensing folk medicine was outsourced to regional governments, and no systematic licensing system existed. In other words, *religious* folk healing was officially recognized as labor, but not medicine, while "traditional medicine" was grandfathered into being recognized as medicine, but not necessarily a legitimate form of medical labor in itself. And while Ayurveda and Chinese Traditional Medicine are recognized as "traditional medicines," Tibetan medicine is not. To summarize the rather complicated legal framework that brackets Tibetan medicine in Russia, *emchi* can practice Tibetan medicine, but only as biomedical doctors, or they can relabel what they do as religious healing and practice it as a small business venture, in which case they cannot claim that their activities are a form of medical labor that intends to treat the sick.

In the ambiguous space between legal regulation and medical practice, the most readily invoked metaphor for authorization that I have heard from my informants over the years is the concept of *krysha*, or "roof"—a slang term for a kind of protection racket scheme that became widespread during the rapid neoliberal changes that swept Russia in the 1990s. The concept of *krysha* has persisted in everyday language where, in its most general sense, it refers to a symbiotic (or parasitic) relationship where the existence of one form of professional activity or structure enables the continued, but contingent, existence of another. Many of the *emchi* I have come to know in Russia state more or less explicitly that to practice, one needs a *krysha*—both a cover and a form of protection. This statement refers to a variety of differentially available strategies. An *emchi* might practice in a state hospital "under the cover" of a biomedical doctor's white coat. Alternatively, if they are male, *emchi* might practice in a Buddhist temple and therefore have the de facto protection of a religious organization that can deflect critics by accusing them of inciting interethnic strife or hate speech, which, in Russia, is a punishable offense. Or, for practitioners practicing privately outside either the state medical or religious spheres, a *krysha* might be a quite literal callback to its original meaning of having powerful advocates in government or law enforcement agencies, who might make the strategic and timely phone call if one gets into trouble. For many of the practitioners I have worked with, there is a strong (if risky) impetus to take on such social actors as patients.

The analogy of *krysha* used by *emchi* in Buryatia is provocative in another way: it calls into focus the particular moral conundrums and compromises that securing legitimacy on terms external to the epistemologies of one's therapeutic expertise might bring with it. The East-West Medical Center operated as one such purveyor of *krysha* for *emchi* who wanted to practice Tibetan medicine and still retain an explicit association with a medical domain. My interlocutors often grumbled about the practical necessities of this arrangement, but the risk of being left without institutional protection outweighed the freedom to practice Tibetan medicine in a way that did not become translated or transformed away from what these practitioners understood to be the core principles and approaches of their therapeutic craft. Thus, the alliance between East-West and practicing *emchi*, under the aegis of medical integration, was a deeply fraught one and brought into focus the limits of an integrative vision within a clinical space in Russia. *Emchi* were not alone in this—other experts expressed doubt about the ways in which the incorporation of Tibetan medicine unfolded in a legislative space that constantly demanded its legibility to multiple evaluating regimes that simultaneously enabled and imperiled it. The rest of this chapter ethnographically explores some of these frictions.

"LIKE CROSSBREEDING A HEDGEHOG WITH AN ADDER"

The office of Bayar Badmaevich was located on the second floor of the East-West polyclinic, one of the four offices where practitioners who identify their specialty with Tibetan Medicine resided.[1] He shared this space with several other doctors, since there was a shortage of available rooms for receiving patients. For all its lavish interior, the remodeled mansion that houses the center is not designed for clinical efficiency. The office is used for massage at times when none of the doctors need it—during lunch hours, for example. Inside, it would look like any biomedical space, with its large desk and patient couch, its white curtains and hygienic paraphernalia, if not for the large Buddhist *tankgha* reproduction of Yutogpa the Younger, an important spiritual figure of worship in the more esoteric aspects of Tibetan medical practice. Another reference to Buddhism was a papier maché replica, perched atop a cabinet, of the Ivolginsky Datsan, the main Buddhist temple in Buryatia and the seat of the Buryat Buddhist Sangha. Bayar Badmaevich himself wore the white frock typical of Russian biomedical doctors, as did all the other members of the medical personnel at the center. The obligatory white gown worn by practitioners and the blue plastic slippers that patients were asked to don over their shoes upon entering the vestibule signaled the center's clinical identity.

The plaque outside of Bayar Badmaevich's office described him as a "therapist, phytotherapist, and Buryatia's recognized medical professional"—an honorary title bestowed on those medical professionals who have been in the field for a long time and have actively pursued medical research. In many ways his self-presentation was fairly typical of what I had come to expect of Buryat medical professionals I had met over the years—mostly soft-spoken, at times brusquely direct, and uproariously funny with his patients. Yet, he was primarily known to his patients and his colleagues at the center as a "Tibetologist"—a somewhat misleading designation of a practitioner of Tibetan medicine, used in Buryatia interchangeably as a synonym for *emchi*.

Bayar Badmaevich's patients, frequently older Buryat women, waited for their turn. They came one after another, sometimes accompanied by a family member, sometimes asking for medical advice not just for themselves but for their neighbors and friends. He examined the pulse in silence, his gaze turned away from the patient and toward the window, feeling for the texture of pulsations first on the right, then on the left hand (and in reverse if the patient was male), then examined the patient's tongue. He asked no questions—the patient volunteered the information herself, painstakingly listing an array of diffuse symptoms, aches, pains, and wheezes, betraying an assiduous scrutiny of her interiority. He joked, diffusing the gravity of a patient's narrative, each manifestation of the body already a potential sign of life-threatening failure, and recast it in the terms so typical of Tibetan medicine, of a body in constant flux—"Your wind has gone up again, and it's making your phlegm come out of balance. I'll give you something to warm you up, to calm the wind, and the phlegm should settle."

Aside from the immediate clinical encounter with the patient happening behind closed doors, Tibetan medicine made few appearances in Bayar Badmaevich's practice, despite the fact that this was indeed the specialty for which he was best known. For most "Tibetologists" who worked at East-West, this was one of the difficulties of practicing Tibetan medicine in a state-sanctioned integrative clinical setting. Since there was no official recognition for Tibetan medicine, and since the East-West Medical Center operated under the administrative supervision of Buryatia's Ministry of Health, all diagnoses had to be recorded in an administratively legible language. In the center's reports to the regional Ministry of Health Protection, patients' conditions were formulated in the generic repertoire of biomedicine, and available treatments were almost exclusively reported in accordance with the legislative categories mentioned in the first section of this chapter. As a result, Tibetan medicine was reclassified as "phytotherapy." Meanwhile, the specificity of Tibetan medicine, with its particular approach to illness and the making of medicines, was curiously invisible, despite the fact that, by reading between the lines of the center's official reports, it became clear that practitioners of Tibetan medicine taken together were responsible for the biggest part of the center's revenue and treated the highest number of patients. For doctors like Bayar Badmaevich, the administrative invisibility of their specialty was a source of irritation: "We supposedly practice traditional medicine here, but the diagnosis has to be European," he bemoaned. Similarly, he often expressed annoyance at the necessity to identify himself as a phytotherapist, the closest official gloss for Tibetan medicine practices, based on the fact that he relied on the prescription of botanical remedies in his treatments. As he explained, "The theories are completely different. Phytotherapy is really *modern* medicine."

For his part, Bayar Badmaevich argued that the East-West Medical Center as a medical site ought to emphasize "traditional medicine" over "European medicine." The center's administration, on the other hand, had a different vision of the institution's role—for the center's head doctor, administrative legibility was crucial to the center's continued existence as, specifically, a state medical institution; therefore, East-West had to position itself primarily as a site of rehabilitative care (*vosstanovitel'naya meditzina*). As such, she saw it as a medical project where integrative approaches that offered a combination of "regular, and good quality, European medicine" and "techniques of traditional medicine" were put to the service of rehabilitative and restorative medical practice.

When I asked Bayar Badmaevich how he envisioned this fusion of traditional and European medicine, he laughed. *Kak pytat'sia skrestit' uzha I yezha, poluchaetsiq bezobrazie*: "It is like trying to crossbreed a hedgehog with an adder. You get something unseemly." The English translation does not do justice to the original pithiness of the comment—in Russian *uzh* (adder) and *yozh* (hedgehog) sound remarkably similar until they are forcibly combined. One may question, then, what species of new "unseemliness" are engendered by the blending of different forms of therapeutic knowledge and expertise co-present in a space like East-West. In practice, it may be difficult to define what makes the center a space of "integration"—other than the administration's claims that it is. During my fieldwork at the center's polyclinic, the public relations staff frequently asked me, partially in jest and partially genuinely baffled, "What is integration, anyway? You're from America, you should know." Their appeal to me as the Western "expert," who might be able to interpret the strange buzzword that many of them felt needed to be present in the center's description, destabilizes the concept much along the same lines as Bayar Badmaevich's comments on the possibility and seemliness of cross-species breeding

Another dimension complicates the distinctions between traditional and modern medicine and the possibility of bridging them. Doctors and staff use a shorthand to classify traditional therapeutic modalities practiced at the center in terms of their relative "Easternness" and "Westernness." In other words, although the official distinction remains along the lines of modern and traditional medicine, in practice, there are separate gradients of differentiation along which therapeutic approaches might be categorized. For example, both phytotherapy and homeopathy might be traditional, but they are posited explicitly as Western knowledge systems, informed by logics that, from the point of view of Tibetan medicine, share a fundamental kinship with "Western" biomedicine. Even acupuncture becomes divided into its "Western" and "Eastern" interpretations. Russian reflexotherapy, which includes but is not limited to acupuncture, is taught in the neurology departments of medical universities, and it has been regulated since the late 1970s. Reflexotherapy is officially recognized as an additional professional specialization for neurologists and traumatologists. "Eastern" acupuncture is viewed as a more direct import from China and Mongolia, and doctors I spoke with describe it as the less "Westernized" approach.

Similarly, the pharmacological principles of Tibetan medicine rely on the ability of plant-derived medicinal substances to affect the three constitutions, and practitioners combine the *materia medica* in such ways as to regulate the *nyes pa*; traditional "Russian" or "Western" phytotherapy is based on composing botanical mixtures in such a way that each ingredient is matched to a specific condition or physiological system (such as the digestive tract, the cardiovascular system, or the nervous system). This approach within Russian phytotherapy allowed practitioners of Tibetan medicine to identify it as quintessentially belonging to biomedical practices, despite its official classification as traditional, on the principle that biomedicine was based on a symptom-active ingredient pairing. According to a logic of root causes, focusing primarily on both symptoms and bodily systems elides the underlying working of the *nyes pa*, or culprits, and the ways in which different organs are made to relate and influence each other. The most typical example I heard of this apparent short-sightedness attributed to modern medicine is the treatment of ear disorders by acting only on the ear itself without checking on the kidneys, which in Tibetan medicine have a direct connection to hearing. In other words, while both Tibetan medicine experts and phytotherapists use botanical substances, practitioners of Tibetan medicine critique phytotherapy's focus on symptoms and its failure to address the root cause of the illness—much in the same way that they critique biomedicine. More pragmatically, for an *emchi*, a pairing between specific botanicals and anatomical disease categories in biomedical terms ignored the ways in which different ingredients combine and interact.

"70 PERCENT OF PEOPLE DIE FROM PILLS"

The work of maintaining these multiple, nonaligned distinctions between Eastern and Western, modern and traditional ways of knowing and treating the body required a formulation of what characterizes Western (or modern) therapeutic approaches. I turn again to Bayar Badmaevich and his vehement critiques of integration in order to delineate the ways in which biomedicine is imagined and experienced in a place like East-West. In a sense, Bayar Badmaevich was an extreme case—of all the doctors at the center, he was the most vocal about the impossibility of combining Eastern medicine with European medicine. Trained in clinical medicine at a medical university in the Russian Far East and subsequently expanding his specialization through courses in phytotherapy and, finally, Tibetan medicine, Bayar Badmaevich identified himself strongly as a practitioner of traditional medicine who was trapped in a clinical space that, institutionally, privileged European medicine as the default medical modality.

Bayar Badmaevich articulated his discomfort with biomedicine based on the unique motivations that he felt drove medical progress. His commitment to traditional medicine—and his original interest in phytotherapy and, subsequently, Tibetan medicine—centered on the ethics of medical practice and pharmaceutical prescription. "You know, American statisticians have established that about 70 percent of people die from pills," he offered one day during a conversation we had about his choice of specialization. "One of those days, calculate how much money all your medicines in your medicine kit (*aptechka*) come out to cost. You won't believe it!" he challenged. In Bayar Badmaevich's explanation, the widespread iatrogenic harm of artificial substances was largely ignored or taken to be a necessary price to pay for efficacy, as the interests of pharmaceutical companies drove the population to ever increased medicalization and chemical dependency. Although, in his opinion, Russia up until recently had avoided the overmedicalized fate of its more Western neighbors, the process was well underway.

Reducing patients' dependence on pills was an explicit goal for doctors at East-West; the point of traditional medical procedures is formulated in terms of decreasing or replacing patients' reliance on chemical interventions so that one might be able to understand what they suffer from, as opposed to diagnosing and responding to ever-proliferating symptoms. Alternatively, by introducing nonbiomedical techniques, practitioners hoped to reduce or mediate the side effects or toxicity of chemical interventions. Certainly, among patients, attitudes toward pills (*tabletki*), understood as synthetic pharmacological compounds, vary greatly—from acceptance as a necessary evil to explicit and vehement avoidance. However, performances around the excesses of pharmacologization were a fairly common element of patients' lives at the center. As I shadowed Zhamso Sayanovich, the clinic's chief neurologist and acupuncturist, on his daily rounds at the East-West's in-patient clinic, he sometimes demonstratively went through the patient's *aptechka*—a bag of both prescription and over-the-counter pharmaceuticals patients brought with them to take during their treatment. After questioning the patient and familiarizing himself with her medical record, he would sit at the foot of the patient's bed and demonstratively sift through the bag of medicines, tossing the superfluous packages of pills into a haphazard pile on the blanket: "This you don't need, this you don't need, this we can keep" (*Eto ne nuzhno, eto ne nuzhno, eto mozhno ostavit'*). In the view of doctors practicing at the clinic, patients were often taking "too much"—some medicines were redundant, others were simply not suited to their specific conditions, and all of them could ideally be avoided through the integrative approaches of restorative medicine.

East-West's personnel attempted to discipline the unruly pharmaceutical mixtures materially manifested in patients' habits of indiscriminately acquiring and consuming a variety of chemical medicines and therapies. They also shared the suspicion that patients were already engaged, on their own, in troubling practices of therapeutic integration, mixing therapies, medicines, and procedures in a maximizing logic that lacked systematicity and was ignorant of the ways in which different therapeutic interventions interacted. This sense of overmedicalization has concrete repercussions for practitioners of Tibetan medicine at East-West. I was frequently told that because patients' bodies are a site of constant therapeutic interventions, it becomes remarkably difficult to get to the root cause of their illness because their symptoms are muddled, shifting, and uncertain.

In view of these efforts to restrain patients' medical omnivorousness, it is ironic that the therapeutic practices of the center rely on increasing and multiplying nonbiomedical interventions. Both practitioners and the center's administration tend to encourage patients to undergo as many traditional treatments as possible, and although they pay attention to certain kinds of dangerous combinations, such as combining medicinal leeches with balneological procedures (mostly constituted of herbal-infused baths), there is a general sense that the more procedures the patient undergoes, the more efficacious and productive their stay at the clinic will be. Certainly, there are financial benefits from such maximization: because most traditional procedures are not covered by the obligatory medical insurance system (OMS) and are paid for out of pocket, there is a pragmatic interest on the part of the institution in increasing their number. However, this maximization of therapies had another goal—to reset the baseline of a patient's overmedicalized and overtreated embodiment to something that might be closer to normal functioning. Practitioners at East-West and other integrative medical facilities where I did fieldwork tend to think of nonbiomedical treatments as good replacements for most chemical interventions, especially in cases of systemic disorders like polyarthritis, diabetes, and neurological and cardiovascular dysfunctions.

Alternatively, such procedures are understood to increase the efficacy of synthetic pharmaceuticals, and therefore their dosages can be reduced. Once the pharmaceutical excesses have been contained, practitioners of Tibetan medicine at the clinic say that they can begin treatment "proper"—rebalancing the body's constitutions.

"I DON'T EVEN KNOW WHAT THESE MEDICINES MIGHT DO"

In explicit conversation with this framing of reducing pharmacological dependence, East-West promoted its own pharmaceutical line of Tibetan medicinal teas, which are prescribed to its patients through the pharmacy. Patients can also buy medicines from the pharmacy independently of a prescription, and many do just that, since it is regionally one of the only state-affiliated pharmacies that specializes exclusively in botanical medicines. In their public presentation, these herbal formulas simultaneously claim the authenticity of traditional *emchi* medicine, the legitimacy conferred by laboratory and clinical testing, and an added intangible appeal derived from their alleged naturalness and locality.

Mariana, one of the pharmacists, was in charge of preparing the plant-based formulas the center produced and prescribed—which ranged from single-component remedies, sold in bulk, such as willow bark, to the much more complex, multicomponent formulas typical of Tibetan medicine. In 2017, when I returned to the field, she explained that one of the central problems that people faced in present-day Russia—and, indeed, everywhere—is that medicines, by and large, no longer worked. When I asked her to explain, she rephrased. "The only thing that works now is the herbs." What I first took for an ideological statement about the superiority of natural medicines over chemicals—a salient category among much of Russia's therapeutic publics—was in fact a practical one for her. People who come to East-West and who specifically purchased the herbal formulas had, in many cases, already tried everything else. I asked her what had changed. "The bodies," she answered, without hesitation. "We are no longer the same people as when these medicines were developed."

For Mariana and her colleagues at the pharmacy, the contingency of therapeutic action is intimately connected with an ontologically open-ended, uncertain world. Because plants are themselves subject to environmental pressures—in other words, because they are dynamic organisms—their therapeutic properties change alongside the human bodies with which they cohabit. Moreover, she argued, plants themselves have deeply localized entanglements, both with concrete ecological conditions and with the particular Buddhist (or other) deities and place spirits that populate Buryatia's local landscapes.

Mariana's colleague Lyudmila, a pharmacist in her mid-fifties, paid attention to the constraints of incorporating Tibetan medicine formulas in a different way: much of her work consisted in coordinating across an ad hoc and unregulated network of growers, suppliers, and wildcrafters, often offering their products from different regions of Russia, in the absence of any system of oversight or centralized regulation for evaluating the safety and efficacy of the plants the pharmacy used for medicine-making. The pharmacy had access to some basic testing equipment—for example, to test for heavy metal poisoning—but they also conducted pharmacological studies of each new batch of plants they obtained, which tended to demonstrate fairly divergent chemical content. The problem with plants is that they are not fungible. Thus, a plant wildcrafted in Buryatia, with its shortened reproductive cycle caused by the region's protracted cold season, would be pharmacologically quite distinct from one grown in a more moderate climate with a longer summer. Lyudmila's professional difficulties had to do with the fact that the lifecycles of plants and their suppliers have different kinds of temporalities, in particular under the uncertain conditions of doing business in present-day Russia. Reliable suppliers, whose plants can be predicted pharmacologically, go out of business on a regular basis, and the work of finding new sources translates into pharmaceutical contingency: the labor of analyzing each batch of plants and estimating their usability—including how much of a particular botanical ingredient should go into a formula as a corollary of its phytochemical content—has to be constantly repeated. Ironically, this led Lyudmila to conclude that the sort of work the pharmacy does cannot be done effectively without top-down coordination: in other words, the particular brand of plant work that Lyudmila does would ideally require a centralized, planned economy. "It was all much easier in the Soviet Union," she explained.

There are other epistemological instabilities in play for Lyudmila's pharmaceutical practice. The Tibetan medicine lines produced by this pharmacy trace their descent from canonical formulas found in Tibetan pharmaceutical compendia, adapted through scientific research carried out at the local sciences center. However, the hospital's pharmacy finds itself in a uniquely complicated position in its effort to approximate the classic pharmacopeia of Tibetan medicine for clinical purposes. Because these medicines are distributed through a medical institution directly operating under the purview of the Ministry of Health, the pharmacy's formulas must comply with Russia's official State Registry of Medicinal Substances, a document that recognizes only a fraction of the ingredients that might be found in Tibetan medicine's pharmacopeia and confines them solely to a list of some 120 plants, excluding most mineral and animal compounds or anything that might be toxic. Complicating matters further are the cascading substitutions that have transformed canonical formulas over the course of Tibetan medicine's history in the region. During the nineteenth and the turn of the twentieth centuries, Mongol and Buryat lamas composed medical compendia that sought to adapt Tibetan medicine pharmacology to local ecologies. And while pharmaceuticals flowed—and still flow—across variably porous borders between Russia, China, and Mongolia, the majority of the ingredients that make up Buryatia's Tibetan medicine pharmacon are local substitutes.

The second bout of formula translations took place when these compendia were interpreted by the laboratory of experimental biology at the local research center between the 1980s and the present, with an eye to the existing regulatory frameworks within which these medicines would have to be distributed. Thus, researchers and clinicians also face legislative pressures from *outside* the medical field that often move apace independently (and somewhat faster) than translational work, biological research, or clinical trials. An illustrative case might be ephedra, or *mtshe ldum*, which I discuss in Chapter 6. It is a key ingredient in one of the locally famous formulas called Taban Arshan (or "five nectars" in Buryat)—a five-component mixture used externally for medicinal bathing and incorporated into clinical balneology. While ephedra was, until recently, authorized for medical use, in 2012 it was reclassified as a narcotic precursor for ephedrine and its use and collection made illegal. As the pharmacists working at East-West explained to me, there are several ironies to such efforts at regulation—the biggest one perhaps that one cannot turn ephedra into a drug, since commercial ephedrine is a synthetic molecule. The regulation is also blind to use—for example, to the fact that in the clinic, the ephedra-containing formula was used topically, not internally. The new legislation excluded what the pharmacists and clinicians felt had been a useful and effective compound for a range of conditions that could be managed without more invasive pharmaceutical interventions, ironically on the grounds of its excessive potency.

The tensions that arise between the interpretations of Tibetan medicines at work in the local clinical context become clear at moments when they are made to explicitly intersect during treatment. One such incident occurred when Aleksandra, whose *emchi* training and practice were often in tension with the demands of the clinic, was asked by a member of the senior medical staff to administer "her own" medicines to a newly admitted patient. Like most classically trained practitioners of Tibetan medicine in Buryatia, Aleksandra devotes much of her free time to collecting botanical ingredients and preparing formulas she subsequently deployed in her practice at the outpatient clinic where she worked as a (biomedically trained) pediatrician. On the other hand, during her shifts at the inpatient hospital of East-West, she also had to prescribe the Tibetan medicine pharmaceuticals produced by the hospital's pharmacy, most of the time in consultation with senior doctors who were not specialists in Tibetan medicine, and therefore matched the formulas to the patient's biomedical symptoms. When Aleksandra was asked to supplement these prescriptions with her own, she was irate: "They are already getting Tibetan medicines," she tried to argue, to no avail in convincing her senior colleague.

Beyond an example of foiled hierarchical defiance, the incident is remarkable for the underlying, yet usually unacknowledged tensions around the questions of labor that shape the efforts at pharmaceutical translation this medical institution undertakes. One source of Aleksandra's annoyance at being asked to add "her own" formulas to the clinic's official in-house prescriptions stemmed from the way the clinic simultaneously claimed equivalence between its pharmaceutical production and the medicines individually prepared by its *emchi* employees while making additional demands on these practitioners' medicinal supplies and labor time, which is practically entirely taken up by plant work.

When I suggested to Tsyrenma, another *emchi* who had practiced at East-West but eventually left to practice at a Buddhist temple, that she try to get a better sense of how much labor goes into the production of a single formula, she offered an analysis of a fairly common compound medicine, *srolo 6*, which is used to treat upper respiratory infections. A year's supply of the medicine for the number of patients that Tsyrenma treats requires the coordination of complex disjointed networks across multiple social and ecological landscapes. It mixes the manual labor of wildcrafting plants and minerals with the emotional and social labor that takes shape through an economy of favors and personal relationships.

The medicine itself is already a kind of contingent, uncertain assemblage, in part because it involves multiple cycles of substitutions. Take *sro-lo*, the ingredient that gives its name to the formula, according to the standard nomenclative principles of Tibetan medicine. In original Tibetan medicine compendia, three types of *sro-lo* are identified and classified by color—namely, white, red, and brown. All three have, by and large, similar pharmaceutical properties, but plants that fall under the category of *sro-lo* belong to different species according to standard scientific botanical classification. In Buryat Tibetan medicine pharmacology, only *sro-lo smug po* is used, and involves double substitutions: *Rhodiola crenulata* is substituted for *Rhodiola rosea*, in turn substituted with *Stellaria dichotoma*, because *Rhodiola*, despite being a Siberian endemic, has in recent years become rare, mostly overharvested by the cosmetic industry, and is technically under protection of the Russian state as an endangered species. A classically trained *emchi* would not tweak a formula—the prescriptions are canonical. But the legislative armature that brackets different plants and their collections changes over time because plant populations are not stable entities. There is some redundancy built into the system, such that one might prescribe a different formula with similar effects, but Tibetan medicine formulas are subtle in their pharmacological action and therefore do not substitute easily. In practice, what this results in is a kind of ethical conundrum for practicing *emchi*—balancing how many patients one is able to treat and which patients might be considered more deserving of the more powerful formulas—which are often the ones that are more personally dangerous to produce.

Conversely, if a plant must be ordered from elsewhere, one must maintain cordial relationships with a reliable supplier, and this frequently exceeds a relationship of commodity exchange—because, once the crossing of borders is concerned, importing large quantities of botanical products is technically illegal. Similarly, for the treatment of some ingredients that require calcination, one must avail oneself of a friendly chemist or geologist who might have access to a high-heat furnace and be willing to let the *emchi* use it in the off hours. In total *srolo 6* takes Tsyrenma about a week of full working days to make—except that this time can never be entirely dedicated to the formula. The labor of plant work is done at the edges of other, more recognizable forms of working obligations—such as seeing patients and the care work of running a household. And yet, ironically, it is the single most important part of *emchi* practice in Buryatia—and the only object of a financial transaction: the only thing *emchi* charge for is the medicines. Tsyrenma makes about thirty formulas on a yearly basis, with anywhere from four to twenty-five ingredients—all of it done outside of what she conceptualizes as her working day. "It's all I ever do," she laughs when we calculate some of these numbers. Other *emchi* with larger practices make as many as 500 formulas a year and have come to rely on both paid and unpaid labor to be able to maintain their supply.

With this in mind, if we return to Aleksandra's frustration with the hospital's demands, in the calculus of individual medicine-making, where the work of wildcrafting plants, taming toxic ingredients, and assembling formulas are all forms of invisible and often personally perilous labor carved out of whatever time outside of professional work one is doing as a cover or *krysha* for one's Tibetan medicine practice, this was not just a matter of a medicine being used inappropriately. Rather, for Aleksandra, this was a preventable waste of the *emchi*'s limited labor power that potentially affected the careful scaffolding of her entire practice—not to mention that the hospital was rather cynically outsourcing the potential peril of illegality in exchange for a contingent *krysha*. Medicines made by *emchi* are the direct materialization of a kind of scarce labor time and limited ecological resources in a zero-sum game where literally every particle of medicinal dust matters. Yet, this form of labor is not visible or recognizable through Russia's juridical framework, which regulates the labor of traditional medicine, nor is it explicitly acknowledgeable by state institutions of integrative medicine where *emchi* sometimes find employment.

But there is also a deeper epistemological conflict at stake in this ethnographic example. After Aleksandra visited the patient in question to establish a diagnosis, she noted a "deep cold in the kidneys" that could easily account for the patient's symptoms of chronic urinary tract pain. In the meantime, while the hospital formula prescribed to the patient aimed at improving kidney function, Aleksandra noted that most of its ingredients, although compliant with the state's official medicinal registry of medicinal substances and indeed used in Russian phytotherapy to address kidney disorders, were cooling in nature.

Other practitioners of Tibetan medicine had in fact noted to me that the clinic's adapted pharmacopeia had mostly retained only cooling ingredients. From the logic of primary elements that accounts for disease etiology in Tibetan medicine, the medicines acted as a poison for this particular patient: "She has massive cold in the kidneys, we need to warm her, not cool her even further," Aleksandra explained. As I asked her what she thought of the efficacy of the clinic's own pharmacological line more generally, she stated that their assemblage, forced to conform to the rules of clinical phytotherapy and amalgamating substitutions of other substitutions, no longer reflected the epistemological principles of Tibetan medicine formulas. "I don't even know what these medicines might do," she added, frustrated.

"WHAT IS SO UNCONVENTIONAL ABOUT US?"

I sat in the public relations office, helping the three other active members of the organization committee with the rushed preparations. Alla, the center's lawyer; Liza, the PR representative; and Ayuna, a pediatrician by profession who, as a junior doctor, shouldered many of the organizational and logistical tasks associated with the conference, sat at their desks, furiously composing programs and pamphlets, responding to emails and phone calls as they tried to balance the influx of contradictory directives coming from the administration with the demands and queries of the potential guests. The atmosphere was rushed and tense, the anxieties and frustrations elicited by the approaching deadline defused by an unceasing stream of teasing, wisecracks, and Alla's seemingly inexhaustible supply of ribald humor, which would vanish without a trace in her flawlessly professional telephone voice, only to resume as soon as the phone call was over. The phone rang incessantly, and the other office dwellers largely ignored Alla's conversations until the habitual routine was broken by Alla's unusual tone—a thin veneer of officiousness over barely contained amusement. Between the long pauses, she proceeded to patiently explain to her invisible interlocutor what medical services the East-West Center provided. When she finally hung up, she turned to us and recounted the conversation, chuckling at its apparent linguistic absurdity. Someone had called to inquire whether the services

East-West offered under the label of "traditional" (*traditzionnaya*) medicine were really "nontraditional" or unconventional (*netraditzionnaya*) medicine. "What's so unconventional about us, I wonder?" (*Chto, interesno, v nas takogo netraditzionnogo?*) she queried with a flirtatious head bob, to the laughter of her colleagues. "Where had they called from?" Ayuna inquired. Still chuckling and repeating the offending term to herself in puzzlement, Alla explained that her interlocutor had called from Moscow—a statement met with silent nods of understandings from the others.

The humor of Alla's quip draws attention to the ways in which "tradition" becomes an especially laden term in Siberia—and in Buryatia in particular—a region already culturally marked as a kind of internal "other" in national imaginaries that take the Western part of Russia to be the unmarked equivalent of the nation as a whole. Alla's joke highlighted not simply that the term "nontraditional," when mobilized to designate therapeutic practices at East-West, is confusing because it brings into focus, by association, the other use of the term *netraditzionnyi* in Russia—specifically in the pairing of *netradiztionnaia orientaziia* to designated LGBTQ identities. More importantly, for this PR team of Buryat women, it pointed to the ways in which being an "outsider" simultaneously means an ignorance of Russia's cultural and religious ties to a transnational Buddhist world, and, more specifically, to Buryatia's connections to the realm of global Tibetan medicine, with a failure to recognize the commitment to the development of this local cultural heritage as such and not as an alternative to a norm. Indeed, East-West finds itself at the unexpected vanguard of federal-level efforts at medical integration, buttressed by its ability to garner federal financial support for development and expansion. The center's administration imagines the institution as perfectly reflecting the future of Russia's national policy toward traditional medicine. Yet, in Alla's comment, "tradition" scales up to articulate claims and discourses that are not just about therapeutic strategies, but equally about the relationship to local histories, the place of cultural alterity in Soviet (and post-socialist) ideologies of progress, and the present-day meaning of "recuperating" a local past to the benefit of both regional and national bodies. The silent consensus among Alla and her colleagues stemmed from the supposition that all of us understood traditional medicine to stand in implicit contrast with European medicine, where the latter was potentially as culturally and historically situated as the former, if not more so. In other words, while European medicine held an important place in the activities of the center, biomedical care was not perceived as unproblematically universal or divorced from its political and historical origins.

There are other stakes to rejecting a terminological usage that equates tradition to mainstream normalcy, beyond its positioning of biomedicine as the default system, to which all other therapeutic engagements are peripheral or alternative. First, "alternativeness" is doubly undesirable in the context of present-day Russia as a variety of identities and subject-positions, most powerfully ethnic and gendered ones, have recently become the target of vehemently normalizing biopolitical discourses. In a certain sense, then, Alla's playful comment was doubly efficacious because it drew on Russian publics' anxieties over nonheteronormative gender relations to reject the "unconventional" label wholesale: there was nothing any more unconventional about the center and its relationship to traditional medicine than there was about Alla and her relationship to her female colleagues.

Second, claims to autochthonous therapeutic practices that preceded and have persevered throughout the history of Soviet modernization highlight the absence of a pure medical tradition that might be easily associated with an ethnically Russian state, or Russian culture more generally. This indeterminacy is in fact at the center of how some experts define what is unique about Russia's case. For example, Russia's Professional Phytotherapy Association claims a longstanding (ethnically) Russian practice of natural herbal medicine, developed into present-day clinical applications. However, these medical practices are described as unique because they were established at the intersection and through the mutual influences between Western and Eastern medical traditions (Karpeev et al. 2006, 11). Such claims appear to recuperate and cite a historically recurrent discourse frequently scaled up to the level of state ideologies and perpetuated by Russian (and Soviet) intellectuals that identifies Russian culture as a middle way between the Asian East and the European West.

However, such claims to national exceptionalism via a celebration of hybridity open up a space of critique. *Emchi* in Buryatia frequently emphasized the stark differences between traditional and modern medicine, articulated through an opposition between East and West. One of the implications of these oppositions and refusals is that a "traditional" Tibetan medicine, native to Buryatia, can be mobilized in a politics of patrimony the Russian state might have access to only by virtue of its relationship and serious engagement with Buryatia's cultural, religious, and ethnic specificity. This unique regional configuration is formulated as inherently more syncretic and more global by virtue of Buryatia's culturally equidistant ties to the East and the West. Conversely, biomedicine itself, insofar as it is linked to European medicine, becomes open to critical localization and a challenge to its universalist claims.

"THAT'S WHY INTEGRATION FAILS"

In this final section, I shift to an external critique of the institutionalization of *emchi* medicine in Buryatia, formulated by those practitioners who find themselves at the peripheries of the official medical establishment. In my first conversation with Erden Lama, an *emchi* working in one of the local Buddhist temples, I asked him how ideas about illness and health in European medicine differed from those in *emchi* medicine. He replied, as many of my *emchi* interlocutors did, that Western medicine lacked a theory because it was simply incapable of getting to the root cause of illness. Unlike European medicine, he explained, Buddhist medicine understood that all illnesses had, if reduced to their phenomenological foundations, a single root cause—namely, ignorance (or *nevedenie* in Russian). Confused by whether he meant ignorance in a more secular sense or whether he was offering a felicitously homophonic Russian gloss of the Sanskrit *Avidya*, or "delusion," an important Buddhist concept, I asked him to explain. After a period of mildly irritated reflection at my apparent obtuseness, Erden Lama finally volunteered the following example:

> If a person doesn't know how to live, they get sick. Which is why we have to begin with enlightening our consciousness, and only then move on to the body. Think about it, conventional medicine claims that one must "temper" (*zakalivat'*) the body, "dress according to the weather," "take contrasting showers"—it's all wrong, erroneous, mistaken! This is why it's always a failure when they try to study [our medicine] from the scientific point of view. We always present European medicine as anti-scientific. Why? Because how did they even think this up, that you should "temper" the body? We're not made of iron [sic] that we need tempering. And its take on chronic illness—it's wrong too. There are no chronic illnesses, only doctors who don't know how to cure. That's why

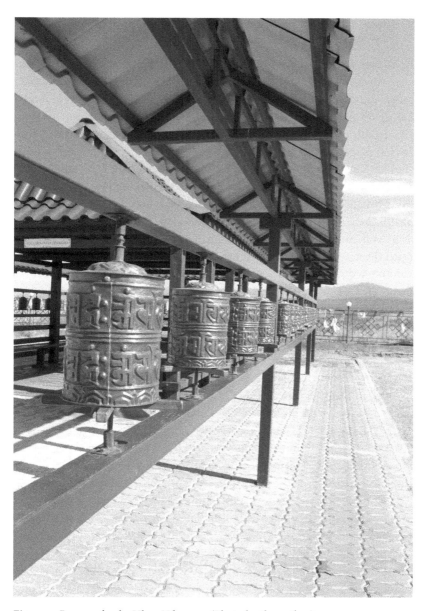

Figure 5. Prayer wheels, Ulan-Ude, 2017 (Photo by the author)

integration fails. In order to incorporate *emchi* medicine, you have to throw away your preconceptions.

In his response, Erden Lama cleverly combined a Buddhist critique of European forms of medical knowledge, invoking the failures to cure illness in those recalcitrant, chronic cases that frequently result in patients in Russia falling through the cracks of official health care—with a rejection of a specific health practice and ideology particular to both official Russian (and Soviet) medicine—namely, *zakalivanie* or "tempering." In order to understand this strange equation—by all accounts, *zakalivanie* is certainly not at the center of the practices of mainstream biomedicine in Russia—it is useful to briefly consider its history and position in present-day discourses on health. According to the Great Soviet Encyclopedia, *zakalivanie* is defined as a "system of procedures that contribute to the organism's capacity to resist the nefarious effects of the external milieu through the production of conditioned reflexes of thermal regulation with the purpose of its improvement" (Kondakova-Varlamova 1978).

A surface reading of tempering suggests a model of the human body as a relatively malleable substance that can be strengthened and qualitatively transformed through a specific set of bodily techniques—namely, "exposures" to the environment. "Tempering" was a widespread form of bodily self-management that gained popularity in the Soviet Union and is still invoked by many people to this day as part and parcel of quotidian practices associated with healthy living or, at least, is formulated as an ideal of healthy living toward which one must strive. In discourses on tempering, it is especially the child's body that becomes the focal point of regulatory interventions as advocates of the practice emphasize the need to activate the latent capacity of the infant, and of the human as a life-form more broadly, to withstand a harsh environment, a capacity progressively lost over time through excessive efforts to maximally optimize external conditions (such as temperature, movements of air, and hygiene). The logic of *zakalivanie* has a long and complex history in Russia and is not unproblematically tethered to exclusively Soviet bodily ideologies, although it does resonate with other Soviet scientific practices that strove to develop a philosophy of human health. As a concept, tempering also moves beyond the manipulation of strictly human bodies to encompass other living organisms. Despite its current accepted position within the Russian healthy lifestyle mainstream, some of the famous practitioners and advocates of *zakalivanie* had an ambiguous status, and none more than Porfiry Korneevich Ivanov. Born in 1889, Ivanov had a turbulent biography and relationship to the Soviet authorities, having spent about twelve years in prisons and psychiatric wards for his teachings on health, *zakalvianie*, and asceticism and for his charismatic healing activities. Most famous for his ability to walk year-round in nothing but a pair of long shorts, regardless of the weather, and for his long, waterless fasts, Ivanov accrued a semireligious following in the early 1980s, and a movement called *ivanovtsy* appears to be active to this day. While contemporary rereadings of Ivanov's works and ideas trace parallels between his teachings and Eastern Orthodox mysticism and neopaganism, based on Ivanov's own writings it is important to note that he positioned himself as a staunch supporter of communism and the revolution and that his teachings on tempering were very much articulated toward the good of the Soviet state. Following several failed attempts to communicate his ideas to the Communist Party and Stalin, he was repeatedly arrested and forcibly committed to an asylum with a diagnosis of schizophrenia. In his 1951 notebook, republished in 1993, Ivanov explains his broader philosophical position as follows:

> I became an innovator because from my early childhood I felt the strength and desire to accomplish something exceptional, useful for the people, even though at first I didn't know what exactly. I just knew something from the start: that one needs to help all the poor and suffering people, and that help must be found in something new, and not in the old and the ordinary. All my life, I strove from the old toward the new and unprecedented. I am an innovator because Nature created me this way and because life made me so. I am an innovator because I was born to the old life, surrounded by the need and ill health of the toiling people, because I read Karl Marx's "Capital" and learned that the toiling people should become the masters of the World and of all of Nature. This is why I participated in the revolution with everyone else, and that is why I then separated myself from everyone to try to distance myself from the people of the past, from the lazy and weak—toward the future, I began to sacrifice myself to work for the future, to enter it even if I were alone, to possess its riches, and to bring this pile of riches to the poor suffering people and show them the Way to these riches. . . . From early

childhood, I was very impressionable and curious toward Nature, toward all surrounding life and terribly, to the point of tears, felt pity toward people, especially the poor. I saw around me how people get sick, suffer, and die before their time because they have no means of resisting Nature, Her terrible forces—cold and illnesses. (Ivanov [1951] 1993, 2)

In 1934, following two emotionally significant dreams—one where he beheld the image of a beautiful man walking naked through the snow, seemingly impervious to the cold, and another where Ivanov was being buried by a cascade of wheat grains and yet remained unharmed and, in fact, found himself on top of the growing mountain of grain—he began to articulate his teachings:

In 1933 in the winter I saw a person who walked around without a hat, and didn't fear the cold and sickness. I suddenly was struck by the thought that a tempered person doesn't have to fear Nature. . . . From all this, in 1934 the idea and courageous decision matured in me to find and develop in myself the strength to not fear Nature, but to go into Nature, to possess her riches, her conditions and forces, so that they do not cause harm and horror, but benefit the people, so that a person wouldn't fear Nature, wouldn't depend and suffer from Nature because of his body, but become the master of his body and the whole of Nature. I decided to temper myself and transform [process] my body in such a way, that it would not be harmed, but benefited by Nature, to lay the way toward the riches of Nature for our people and for every person. (Ivanov [1951] 1993, 4)

Based on Ivanov's autobiographic accounts, what ensued was a series of movements back and forth between the need to adequately function in society, hold a job, and provide for his family and the drive to further experiment with *zakalivanie*. Ivanov writes that he was fired several times from different workplaces, the first time over an accusation of being an Orthodox priest, the second time for his folk healing activities. The relationship between *zakalivanie* and his ability to heal also took the form of a negotiation with himself: after being asked to heal an acquaintance's mother who had not walked for over seventeen years, Ivanov wrote that he made a deal with himself that if he managed to get her to walk, he would return full-time to his tempering practices, seeing them as directly related to his ability to heal others. At the next stage of his "experimentation," as he refers to his activities, he would thus attempt to walk barefoot in the winter. After about a week of treatment, the woman was able to move around independently, and Ivanov shed his footwear.

Ivanov commented on the way his training had enabled him to withstand the harsh conditions of incarceration: "Here, in Leningrad, I have prepared myself to meet the winter time. Every day, it comes and goes. I am not made of steel or bronze, I am a living person, and strongly feel every changeable thing, that my body hears it—[the changes] string it like a needle, they go through my body" (Ivanov [1951] 1993, 17). In other words, for Ivanov, the ability to withstand the harsh conditions of the environment did not necessarily equate to a form of imperviousness, of complete isolation from the living conditions of his body, but instead suggested a form of hyperattention to the minutest changes.

In 2008, Ivanov was rehabilitated as a "victim of Stalinist repressions," but his relative rise to acceptability happened much earlier, notably with the publication in 1982 of an article on his bodily practices, entitled, "An Experiment That Lasted Half a Century," in the journal *Ogonek*. The authors of the article had gone to live with Ivanov in his village for five days, following the rising popularity of Ivanov's teachings among the Moscow technical intelligentsia. They interviewed him about his life and experimented with dousing themselves in icy water, as per his recommendations. The article is stylistically ironic and flaunts the authors' own misconceptions about Ivanov's philosophy. "Can he really not feel the cold?" the reporters asked each other and their audience, only to be rebuked by Ivanov's own comment: "Of course I can feel the cold, probably better than you can." Ultimately citing the body's unexplored hidden potentials, the journalists went back to Marx's reading of the relationship between man and nature:

> It was Marx who said that the civilized man should be able to withstand nature in the same way that ancient people did. Porfiry Ivanov knows how to withstand nature. His system serves him as a foundation for this. He has moved toward it for almost half a century, and for almost half a century he follows it without deviation. (Vlasov 1982)

Despite Ivanov's ambiguous and marginalized position within the visions of Soviet medical practices, tempering was also advocated in more mainstream forms of health maintenance and, even in the 1960s, already had a semi-official status. Within methodological manuals on resort medicine and balneology produced since the 1960s and until the present day, tempering is described as one of the standard methods for increasing the body's resistance to the negative effects of the environment by using controlled and incrementally increased exposures to those very same potentially negative or pathogenic conditions—air, cold and hot water, and solar radiation (Marshak 1957; Parfenov 1960; Bogolyubov 1985).

Going back to Michurin's grafting techniques, later marshaled by Lysenko's attack on genetics, the possibilities and frustrations associated with extracting lifeforms from their original environments and transplanting them elsewhere—in an ultimate vision of human dominion over nature—runs through the history of Soviet agricultural and population management, from forced relocations of populations to sparsely peopled regions of the Soviet Union to Khrushchev's enthusiasm for planting corn above the permafrost line. Further buttressed through a Pavlovian logic of nervous conditioning, tempering did indeed become a mode of disciplining all sorts of bodies.

By the 1980s, tempering became firmly entrenched in the Soviet wellness mainstream and proved unusually resistant to the cultural shifts of the 1990s, eventually coming to constitute an unquestioned, self-evident background for health maintenance. A surface reading of this health ideology suggests a model of biological life as a highly malleable phenomenon that can be qualitatively transformed through a specific set of techniques that build up resistance to a hostile environment. A variety of tempering methods and systems are presently available in Russia's popular self-healing literature, such as the works of the scandalous TV personality and folk healer Genady Malakhov, who draws a parallel between the tempering of the body and the tempering of metal: like metal, he writes, the "durability and hardness" of the human organism could be improved to "withstand unfavorable natural factors" (Malakhov 2003, 13).

For his part, Erden Lama grounded tempering in the history of the Soviet state's shifting health ideologies. In his own medical practice, he related Russia's much-discussed demographic crisis to what he described as an epidemic of infertility among young women, caused, in his opinion, by the logics and practices of environmental "independence." And while Russian biomedicine had a long and robust tradition of thinking about the environmental aspects of health, Erden Lama's critique runs deeper than the simple rejection of a somewhat clichéd Soviet medical utopia about impervious bodies operating at the margins of the possible. I take his equation between what he calls "European" (read "Soviet") medicine and "tempering" as an effort to articulate a theoretical-level abstraction about biomedical knowledge practices in general. Like many other traditional healers in Buryatia, Erden Lama was engaged in a politics of "weirding" biomedicine by localizing it. In "Sovietizing" what he called "European" medicine through an invocation of "tempering," Erden Lama's critique rejects claims to "universal" human bodies or a single, "universal" way of managing them.

Localizing bodies was a recurrent concern in many conversations I had with practitioners of *emchi* medicine, as well as scientists who did research on the topic. Tibetan medicine in Buryatia was thought to have adapted to the environmental and cultural conditions of its relocation in Siberia. Practitioners often suggested that the Buryat version of *emchi* medicine differed subtly from its other expressions in Nepal, China, India, and Mongolia. For example, Dr. Zhapovich, a well-known local practitioner, explained that a history of working with European bodies had left its mark. Because Russian bodies tended toward more phlegm, while Buryat bodies exhibited an excess of bile, its medicinal formulas were adapted accordingly. Articulating a similar attention to emplaced bodily becoming, Erden Lama explained that even though there used to be profound differences between indigenous Buryats and Russian settlers, with time ethnic distinction became skin-deep, progressively collapsing through processes of cohabitation, cultural hybridization, and the exercise of Soviet state power.

Despite their critiques, *emchi* in Buryatia do not actually reject biomedical knowledge wholesale. At his small clinic, Erden Lama's work desk sported Buddhist ritual paraphernalia alongside stacks of X-ray slides. When I asked him about what to me seemed like a contradiction, he patted the stack fondly. "X-rays, they're a great technology. Remarkable. Imagine, I give the patient medicines, they come back, and they show me that the kidney stones are gone!" But *emchi* mobilize biomedicine, in particular its imaging technologies, to give their patients material proof of the efficacy of *emchi* therapeutic orientations. Like other *emchi*, Erden Lama addresses biological life as always already an emplaced, local affair, one that cannot be abstracted from the environmental, cultural, and historical conditions that form it. The increased phlegminess of European bodies, the tendencies of local Buryat bodies to accumulate heat by way of bile, the infertility of modern young women become indices of the medical histories of Soviet and post-socialist life. Implicit in these claims is the sense that the failure of state medicine in Russia, from the *emchi*'s perspective, lies in its curious double blindness: state-backed ideologies of health simultaneously produce local forms of embodiment and subsequently mistake them for the universal abstract body of biomedical science, while obscuring the ideological imaginaries and pragmatic conditions that make these embodiments possible in particular.

"European medicine has no theory," Erden Lama declared during one of our conversations. "So it can't get to the root of the illness." While he was invoking the classical logic of root causes of Tibetan medical epistemology, Erden Lama's pronouncement also spoke back to Sergei's question. When *emchi* like Erden Lama reject projects of medical integration, it is precisely because a medicine that mistakes itself for a human universal is blind to its own rootedness and to its trajectories of travel and offers no adequate terrain on which integration, in any real sense, might be imagined as a desirable future.

6

"NOTHING IN THE WORLD THAT COULDN'T BE MEDICINAL"

The Limits of Extraction

LIVELY MIXTURES

This chapter interrogates the concept of *syrye* (Rus)—"raw materials"—used both in Buryat-Tibetan medicine and in wider discourses on the production and transformation of medicinal substances in Russia, a conceptual category that, in phytopharmacology, refers to natural substances that have not yet been transformed for medicinal purposes. Thinking of raw ingredients as *syrye*—in Russian meaning literally "wet" or "uncooked"—is certainly not limited to the practices of Tibetan medicine but is in fact a broader economic category. It characterizes those branches of industry that use natural materials as the basis for their products, phytopharmaceutical research and production being two of them. According to the economics dictionary, *syrye* refers to "useful minerals and other natural resources, as well as those products derived from them that require further processing."

Since the 1990s, economic and policy studies have tended to unproblematically classify Russia's post-socialist economic strategy as an extractive economy par excellence, one that, according to analysts promoting the values of private property, democratic political arrangements, and free markets, will ultimately reach the limits of its extraction potential and crony capitalism and fail as a nation (Acemoglu and Robinson 2012). Anthropology focusing on Siberian regions as a frontier of Soviet (qua Western)

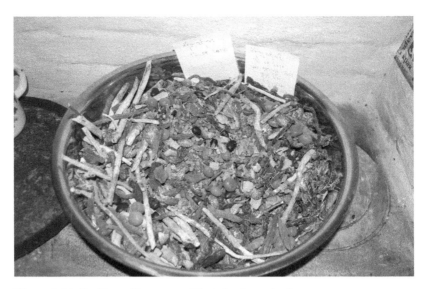

Figure 6. Medical ingredients, 2011 (Photo by the author)

resource extraction and colonial domination tends to focus on an opposition between projects of land and resource exploitation and indigenous rights activism.[1] The central question of this chapter is informed by a somewhat different set of concerns—namely, what sorts of ideologies of extraction emerge in the wake of post-socialist deindustrialization. Instead of focusing on received oppositions between a capitalist orientation to an inert nature defined primarily in terms of its resource potential, accessible and commodifiable through extractive practices, and accounts of sustainable indigenous engagements with the environment, I am interested in tracing the ways in which certain things become inextricable—too deeply rooted to bother, or too deeply entangled to travel.[2]

By focusing on the pharmacological practice of Tibetan medicine in Buryatia, I aim to illustrate the complex ethical, financial, spatial, and epistemological commitments to a particular form of labor required to produce a packet of Tibetan medical powders from raw materials. In tracking these practices, I am also interested in the ways in which botanicals complicate their own ideological genealogies as *syrye*. I show, through a series of ethnographic episodes, that in the pharmaceutical craft of Tibetan medicine in Buryatia medicinal plants are far from inanimate extractable matter, passive objects on which humans exercise their will to mold and shape them into desirable products. As Lyudmila's struggles with the unpredictability of medicinal plants illustrated in Chapter 5, the work of harnessing the efficacy and agency of plants in Tibetan medicine complicates extractive logics writ large, whether it is in the domain of gathering botanicals or in the pharmaceutical logic of isolating chemically active compounds. There is nothing inherently medicinal or self-evidently therapeutic about the *materia medica* used in Tibetan medicine in Buryatia when they are in their natural setting. But the raw materials of local therapeutic practices are naturally hyperactive, agentive, unpredictable, locking bodies with which they interact in a total and consuming relationship that requires and cultivates specific modes of attention to botanical lives, as well as to local ecologies and histories. With the descriptions that follow, then, I argue that the therapeutic efficacies of Tibetan medical formulas are produced through densely layered relationships and rooted tangles.

This chapter is thus as concerned with unpacking Tibetan medicines to trace the implications of their physical and intellectual production as it is with shedding light on the complex imaginaries of inextricability in Buryatia. I focus here on the liveliness of botanical substances and the different relations they generate and demand from those who work with them. This allows me to track the means by which Tibetan medicine (*tibetskaya meditzina*) as a form of practice and Tibetan medicines (*tibetskie lekarstva*) as material assemblages are productively held in place.

BAGS OF BONES

Not unlike other patients at the Blue Beryl Medicine Center located on the outskirts of Lukovo, a small Siberian village in the vicinity of Ulan-Ude, Irina, a former architect in her mid-seventies, has been a regular user of Tibetan medicine for over ten years. Diagnosed with benign kidney tumors and obstructive lung disease over a decade ago and faced with the prospect of extensive surgery, she followed the advice of Aleksandr, her *emchi* and the owner of Blue Beryl. As a result, she forwent the kidney removal surgery and subsequent permanent reliance on dialysis that her biomedical doctors were recommending. Since then, she had been taking the powders and decoctions Aleksandr makes and prescribes, and she felt that her health had stabilized, although she no longer bothered with regular bio-medical check-ups. Instead, she assiduously monitored her well-being, her attention turned inward for minute changes and processes, and consulted with Aleksandr whenever possible so that he could adjust her medication to compensate for these changes. Irina's migration patterns coincide with those of her *emchi*. Aleksandr runs Blue Beryl in the summers, from May to mid-October, and practices out of Moscow the rest of the year. As one of the regular workers at Blue Beryl explained to me, the seasonal variations are a necessary part of how the operation is run, but they also cater to the ways in which patients' bodies are themselves unstable and cyclical. In line with the *Gyüshi* and other canonical texts, practitioners expect seasonal changes to influence the changes in patients' *nyes pa*—fall and spring might bring an escalation of symptoms, as *rlung* (wind) becomes more active, while winter might overstimulate *badgan* (phlegm) and summer exacerbate *mhris* or *shara* (bile). The summer months are both the ideal time to undergo intensive therapy and rife with their own dangers of squandering health through an inappropriate life-style, such as overcooling.

Blue Beryl also reflects a model of how the more successful independent practitioners of Tibetan medicine in Buryatia organize their work life. For those practitioners who have the financial means, social connections, and real estate opportunity to split their work between Buryatia and Moscow, or other metropolitan centers in Russia, Ulan-Ude and its environs become, first and foremost, a source of botanicals, but also a therapeutic site in their own right. The diverse ecology of the region supplies them with some of the necessary ingredients for making medicines, provided they have access to a four-wheel-drive vehicle that allows them to navigate the unevenly maintained and, in places, downright decaying Soviet-era trans-portation infrastructure. In addition, they mobilize Buryatia's emergent status as a destination for ecological tourism in which ecological and geo-logical features, such as Lake Baikal, the many natural water springs, the solar radiation, and the "air itself" are formulated as therapeutic agents, especially for those urban bodies whose vitality has been sapped by the stresses of urban life.

Most of the year Irina lives in Moscow, although she is an avid traveler and vacations in the seaside town in southern Russia where she was born. Part of her summer is spent in Siberia for intense Tibetan medical treatment, which supplements the medicines she regularly takes through-out the year with infused baths, massage, diet, and a kind of minute behav-ioral regimentation that characterizes the everyday pace of Blue Beryl. She is not a Buddhist and often smiles indulgently at the Buddhist sensibilities of Blue Beryl, its owner, and its workers. Although religion is not usually at the forefront of Irina's medical concerns, a story she likes to narrate about her own complicated relationship vis-à-vis the powders, decoctions, and procedures that she constantly uses to maintain her health illustrates some of the complicated ways in which patients in Russia engage with the ther-apeutic substances that get commonly generalized as *tibetskie lekarstva* (Tibetan medicines).

When Irina was just beginning her use of Tibetan medicine, she went to an Eastern Orthodox church to converse with a priest. The conversation took the shape of a confession, and as the priest encouraged Irina to share things that weighed on her conscience, she spontaneously informed him that she had been using Tibetan medicines to cope with her flagging health. She was not much concerned with the repercussions of this information, she explained, simply bringing the subject up because her lengthy struggle with her aging physiology and the recent death of her husband following an unsuccessful surgical procedure were closest to the surface. The priest expressed concern about her choice, but, contrary to what may be expected, he did not object to the relationship between Tibetan medicine and Bud-dhism and hence Irina's potential "defection" to a different faith. Instead, he focused his concern on the content of the medicines themselves: "You don't know what goes into these powders. What if they include human remains?" he asked Irina.

She recalled the incident to me during an informal conversation as we sat around a cast-iron *kazan* full of a slowly simmering mixture of milk and "burning-bush" root (*Dictamnus albus*). Irina shrugged, smiling slyly, and noted that at the time, her answer surprised even her: with a regal wave of her hand, which she replicated for my benefit, she had announced to the priest that, to her, it made no difference: "*A mne vse ravno.*" The priest, she recalled, was understandably disgruntled by her statement, but, for Irina herself, the final morality of using Tibetan medicines was that they alleviated human suffering, improved health, and allowed her to avoid a dangerous operation, potentially extending her longevity past what it would have been had she gone to a biomedical facility.

In justifying her therapeutic choices, Irina invoked a criticism I heard time and time again from patients in Russia who distrust the state's official medical system and its workers, especially when it comes to surgery. They also distrust surgery itself—this is a point of emphatic agreement between both traditional medicine practitioners and patients: at its wits' end, contemporary "Western" medicine can do nothing more than prescribe the knife and "cut off pieces," people frequently informed me. Even within the logic of Eastern Orthodoxy, Irina felt validated. At the peak of her illness, she went to see an Eastern Orthodox mystic, who, after one look at her, pronounced, "You are ill. You need a good doctor." Shortly after that, she recalled, she met Aleksandr.

Irina maintained her position even after some of the workers at Blue Beryl, also gathered around the makeshift rusty barrel that served as a stove for the bubbling *kazan*, had brought to her attention the bag of human skulls stashed away in one of several wooden cabins that served as storage for ingredients. When I asked her if this bothered her, she shrugged. "Do we ever know what goes into our [regular] medicines, anyway?" she asked me. I later quizzed Aleksandr about the skulls—where did they come from? What are they used for? He explained that it was something a patient had brought one year, as a form of payment for treatment. As far as he knew, they came from a marshy area of Belarus, where a multitude of wars—dating to even before the two world wars, Aleksandr added—have strewn the ground with the remains of soldiers, bandits, and who knew what else. The bones come and go, absorbed into the unstable soil of the marshland, only to reappear on the surface later as water levels shift and erosion exposes the underlying layers. As I laughed, profoundly uncomfortable at the mental image of human remains acting much like mushrooms that appear after the rain and disappear for no discernible reason, as enterprising locals walk around with woven baskets to collect the grim harvest, Aleksandr remained solemn. They are unclaimed, he reminded me, discarded and forgotten, nothing remaining of their lives or biographies, to the point that even archaeologists don't have an interest in them—nothing significantly different from any other kind of raw material required for the making of medicines. Meanwhile, there is an excellent recipe to treat intracranial hypertension in infants, especially when there is no underlying structural cause, that uses ground-up skull bone as one of its many ingredients. "You know what our natal wards are like," he reminded me. "If something is wrong, the baby is mostly ignored and simply dies." Aleksandr hadn't used the skulls yet, but he kept them around. The *Gyüshi*, after all, reminds its readers that there is nothing in the world that couldn't be a medicine.

The skulls on Aleksandr's compound were also a source of horrified pleasure for the workers and patients, highlighting the apparent "otherness" of Tibetan medicine. Unlike other ingredients, however, which have to be replenished each season, the skulls remained untouched, a permanent fixture that functioned as a sort of didactic *memento mori*. The use of human remains is certainly a controversial question for local practitioners, and, as far as I was able to gather, no one actually uses them in practice—Aleksandr included—arguing that, in the end, there are perfectly efficacious and long-established substitutions for most problematic ingredients in the Tibetan and Buryat *materia medica*. For example, bear flesh and bear bile are considered an effective replacement for what the *Gyüshi* euphemistically calls "great meat." Derivatives from bear bile are also widespread in Russia's official pharmacopeia, and products based on ursodeoxycholic acid are quite common for treating gallbladder disorders.

Medical anthropologists have long paid attention to the ways in which substances derived from dead bodies—both human and animal—have figured in cutting-edge biomedical intervention and have troubled the ways in which seemingly irrevocable divisions between life and nonlife are understood and imagined (Lock 2001b; Sharp 2006). In this sense, Himalayan medicine is certainly not alone in the harvesting of dead matter—whether animal, botanical, or mineral. That plants do not evoke the same ethical dilemmas as animal and human materialities merits closer examination. Troubling the conceptual boundary from the other side of the divide, works in science studies and political ecology are beginning to complicate assumptions that life is qualitatively distinct and segregated from nonlife. In doing so they rethink notions of agency and draw attention to the unboundedness and permeability of organic formations to their inorganic counterparts (Bennett 2010). The ways in which Buddhist medical logics and the everyday practices of assembling botanical medicines parse the relations among living and nonliving entities or conceptualize the liveliness of things and the possibilities and stages of transforming them into therapeutically efficacious substances do not easily align with mechanistic imaginaries of producing therapeutic substances from inert, standardizable, and interchangeable raw materials whose chemically active essence is their only relevant component. The division into active element and inert ballast is profoundly unsettled by the logic of therapeutic efficacy in *emchi* medicine in Buryatia. These differences in apprehending and parsing out the inert from the lively is not simply a question of conceptual incommensurability. The very process of working with botanicals necessary for assembling therapeutically efficacious mixtures upsets visions that would confine both organic and inorganic bodies to the status of things from which active components might be extracted.

This chapter follows ethnographically how the liveliness of bodies—human and botanical—is attended to and managed by different groups of experts. This focus follows from a series of contextual observations—first, that in the botanical practices of Tibetan medicine in Russia the vitality of plants is an unruly, messy affair and the transformation of plants into medicinal ingredients demands labor that would control, manipulate, and discipline this excessive activeness, albeit with no guarantee of success. Here, I argue that much conceptual and practical work goes into making medicinal plants into recognizably therapeutic objects. Raw materials do not simply exist "out there," waiting to be gathered, but require a particular form of attention that anticipates and traces their liveliness across distinct temporal and material scales and does not limit itself to their actual biological life.

Second, ideas about the ways plants and human bodies mutually implicate each other inform the therapeutic imaginaries of natural medicine as something that stands in contradistinction to and potentially remedies or complements the epistemic and practical lacunae of biomedical and scientific visions of bodily health. Here I draw on the insights of anthropologists who have suggested that the consumption of substances understood to have medicinal properties, be they foods or medicines—or often both—encourages us to attend to the ways in which everyday forms of bodily practice and their associated forms of reason and reasoning come to bear on broader political formations and processes (Farquhar 2002; Landecker 2011; Etkin 2008).

Finally, this chapter follows the production of a distinct pure ecology in Buryatia. Here, claims about the region's peripheral qualities are destabilized by practicing *emchi* who make their own medicines from both local and imported flora and fauna. Looking at pharmaceutical craft and the alignments and forms of expertise Tibetan medicine necessitates brings into focus the social and practical implications of what a post-socialist pure ecology might resemble.

IN THE WEEDS: THE MANY LIVES OF *"MTSHE LDUM"*

Aleksandr is both an anomaly in the field of Tibetan medical practice in Buryatia and its archetypical representative. An ethnically Russian, Siberian-born man in his mid-sixties, he started off his career as a promising geologist, gaining acceptance to a doctorate program in the prestigious Moscow State University, at a time when access to MSU, especially for someone from "the provinces" with no connections and political caché, was considered a rare feat. After receiving his education, he returned to his native Buryatia and began to work for the Buryat Research Institute, where he came into contact with lamas working on the translations of Buryatia's Buddhist textual archive. Like a number of his colleagues who came in contact with this project, he became fascinated with Buddhism and Tibetan medicine. However, the original drive to shift careers and devote himself to learning Tibetan medicine came from his own experience of illness. Crippled with slowly degenerative ankylosing spondylitis in his youth, Aleksandr faced the choice of becoming an invalid or seeking out alternatives. During an interview in 2010, he recalled that Tibetan medicine "put him back on his feet" in six months, at which point he decided to seek out a mentor.

Like many narratives that *emchi* told me to account for their choice of profession, Aleksandr explained that his request was predictably and repeatedly met with a categorical refusal until the prospective student wore down the potential teacher's resistance through systematic pestering. In Aleksandr's case, his prospective mentor gave him a woman's stocking filled with sand and fractured pieces of bone, in imitation of a broken limb. He was told not to return until he managed to reassemble the bone inside the stocking without removing it from the sand, a task that had taken him a week to master. When I asked him if anyone ever tried to cheat, with the lama being none-the-wiser, Aleksandr laughed, saying that it would entirely defeat the point of the exercise. These sorts of tests, he explained, were as much for the student as they were for the teacher—it is a chance for students to gain enough self-awareness to realize that they would not have sufficient dedication for the practice.

As we drove around the countryside in search of medicinal herbs, Abba blaring at full volume inside Aleksandr's new Toyota SUV, he occasionally veered off the main track in unmarked places, shifted the truck into four-wheel drive, and directed the vehicle toward sites where he knew from previous experiences one could find the plants necessary for this year's medicine production. His improvised collection team—two patients, one paid worker, a friend of the family, and one anthropologist—exited the vehicle, collected the burlap sacks stashed in the trunk, and followed Aleksandr in his search for ingredients. On this particular occasion, Aleksandr pointed out *mtshe ldum*—a short creeping plant with leaves resembling pine needles and small crimson spherical berries reminiscent of poorly formed raspberries. Our task that particular day was to collect the small berries in a container as well as amass entire *mtshe ldum* plants, roots included, in a separate bag. Someone asked what the Russian name for it was. "*Efedra*," Aleksandr responded.

In the time I had spent helping with the gathering and preparations of medicines, *emchi* practitioners almost never used the Russian plant name unless I or one of the other workers asked. Among those who had worked with Aleksandr for a long time, using Tibetan botanical terms in reference to ingredients, even those common and familiar in everyday life, appeared to be second nature, and recalling the Russian folk name for the plant or the Linnaean designation required effort. In part, this is at once a performance of craft and a matter of convenience. Practitioners who learned Tibetan medicine in the traditional way, through an apprenticeship with an older mentor, often commented about the difficulty of translating the pictures and names of plants found in Tibetan and Buryat sources to match the actual material they were meant to collect. Commenting on the way he had learned from his teacher, an *emchi* practicing at one of the city's Buddhist temples laughingly narrated his failures:

> It's difficult, you have this drawing of the plant, but it doesn't look like anything. You have to follow your teacher, so he can go and show you, and he's old, a grandpa, he doesn't want to go, his daughter protests— where are you taking my dad again? So he says, "Quiet, woman," just to be contrary, and goes anyway, you follow him, he shows you the plants. Or then, sometimes, he sends you off alone—"go get this plant"

all the way over there on that mountain, so you go, it's a long way, you go on horseback, half a day there, half a day back. You find the plant, you bring it back, and he says, "That's the wrong plant. Go again." It's hard.

Deciphering the botanical referents of Tibetan medicine is not only a challenge for practitioners learning to identify the correct botanicals based on highly stylized drawings or trying to find substitutions for those plants that are not easily available locally. For botanists and scientists in Russia, translating the terms of the original Tibetan text is also rife with potential pitfalls. The drawings of plants, or the metaphorical language that describes their different parts—their leaves, flowers, roots, fruits—do not always map onto Russian botanical terminology, nor do they easily align with a Linnaean taxonomy. Moreover, the two forms of epistemological commensuration—finding substitutions for rare plants to use in recipes and translating the Tibetan text into the language of modern botany—are not independent endeavors but are, instead, intimately interlinked. The same Tibetan name is frequently used for both the original component and its substitutes, even when the two are not in fact in the same botanical family. Batorova and Antzupova (1989) list two distinct methods that scholars working on establishing equivalencies between the Tibetan and Latin or Russian terms have used: the comparative survey method and the pharmaco-linguistic method. The first approach relies on interviewing local practitioners and was widely used in Soviet research on Tibetan medicine in the 1970s, while the second method performs a complex calibration between the plant's Tibetan name and its pictorial representation with other sources, including the data collected from the survey method, Russian, Chinese, and Ayurvedic reference manuals, and herbarium data (Batorova and Antzupova 1989, 16). The uneven translational opacities in the *emchi*'s commentary cited previously and the methodological discussions in the literature on Buryat *materia medica* suggest that the use of medicinal plants is not a matter of simple one-to-one correspondences between what is formally known as a plant's depiction and the form in which it is actually encountered. Nor is it based on drawing equivalencies between its chemical components and its therapeutic efficacies or between its status in an officially recognized pharmacopeia and its therapeutic usage.

Even when one focuses on a single plant—in the case of this example, ephedra—its singularity and coherence as a specific object is tentative at best. *Mtshe ldum* is the Tibetan term taken in the Russian scientific literature on the terminological equivalencies of plants to refer to a number of species of Ephedra L. Depending on the source, *mtshe ldum* might refer to Ephedra monosperma C.A. Mey, or, alternatively, to Ephedra sinica, Ephedra distachya, or Ephedra saxatilis (Aseeva 2008; Dudin 1993). Conversely, ephedra might be referred to by other terms, such as *brag-mtshe*, translated as Ephedra equisetina Bunge, *lug-mtshe*, as Ephedra gerardiana Wall. ex Stapf, *ra-mtshe*—as Ephedra minuta Florin, or *chkhu-mtshe*, which stands for Equisetum diffusum D. Don—in other words, not a species of ephedra at all (Kosoburov 2006). According to the *mDzes mtshar mig rgyan*, a medical reference book and commentary by the Mongolian author Jam dpal rdo rje (or, in the Buryat equivalent pronunciation, Jambaldorje) first translated in 1986 into Russian and subsequently republished in 2011 in Buryatia's *Republican Typography*, ephedra is referred to by *mtshe*, and the source lists only two types of ephedra—those with fruit, called *lug mtshe*, and fruitless ephedra, referred to as *ra-mtshe*.

In addition to the terminological ambiguity, the therapeutic efficacies of *mtshe ldum* proliferate and multiply. According to Aseeva (2008), *mtshe ldum* differs in its uses in traditional Tibetan and Buryat medical practices. Thus, for example, in the *Gyüshi*, *mtshe ldum* stops bleeding and treats both new and old liver heat (Aseeva 2008, 137). By contrast, in Buryat practice, *mtshe ldum* is used to treat "cholecystitis" (gall bladder inflammation), stomachaches, and women's reproductive disorders. It is also used in cases of uterine tumors (Aseeva 2008, 137). Its qualities are listed as "dry and cool," and it is used to heal the vessels, blood, and liver heat, both internally and externally as part of the "five amrita" bath infusion (Jambaldorje and Zhabon 2011, 78). One way to account for these differences is to look at the other ingredients with which the plant will be combined—in other words, *mtshe ldum* is meaningless outside a contextual assemblage. Alternatively, ingredients that are differently processed might acquire new qualities. The same plant or mineral might be boiled in milk, water, or vodka and would as a result acquire entirely different properties—become hot, cold, neutral, or be transformed into *amrita* (healing nectar). Processing plants in water, milk, and other ingredients such as cow urine might also be used to tame the plant if it contains toxic compounds. In traditional Russian phyto-therapy and naturopathy, species of Ephedra are also known as *Khvoynik* and *Kuzmich* grass and are widely used to treat bronchial spasms, arthritic joint pain, and allergy.

Recall that *mtshe ldum* was one of the plants that posed a particularly difficult problem for the pharmacists working at the East-West Center, since it is, from the perspective of the Russian state, illegal to use. Despite its long history of use and wide popularity in Russian phytotherapy, Chinese medicine, and some uses in official medicine, all species of ephedra are included in Russia's legislation on narcotic substances, and their mass cultivation, defined as ten or more single plants, is forbidden along with other narcotic precursors such as the opium poppy, the cocaine plant, and the peyote cactus.[3] Russia has some of the strictest legislation in the world regarding ephedra regulation, despite the fact that its use for the production of ephedrine within Russia itself is considered negligible. As of January 2013, possession and propagation (commercial or otherwise) of "large or exceptionally large" quantities of dried ephedra, respectively equaling 500 grams and 5 kilograms, is prosecutable by law.[4] From the perspective of the legislation, the ephedra plant stands in a synechdocal relationship to one of its active ingredients, ephedrine. The fifty different species of the plant are undifferentiated, despite the differences in alkaloid content. Neither is there a distinction between the different elements of a single plant, the stage of maturation, the specifics of its natural habitat, and ephedrine and the other substances it might contain, such as tannins. Thus, for example, the sweet red berries that have a very low alkaloid content and that are traditionally used in Siberia to make jams and preserves fall in the same category as the rest of the plant.

My point here is that the ingredients of the Tibetan-Buryat pharmaco-poeia are always already a kind of unruly assemblage with many different claims made on their natures, their therapeutic efficacies being only one of the ways in which they can be narrated and seen, and even those take on a relational quality as they are extracted into distillates or combined with other ingredients. This is not unique to botanicals that are hypervisible to the institutional structures whose goal is to regulate the traffic of illegal substances. Russia's Registry of Medicinal Substances (2008) numbers some 700 plant-based products, with about 300 different plants in official use, which is to say available for sale and prescription in licensed pharmacies and medical establishments. These different products include composite teas, tinctures, and balms produced both in Russia and abroad. Although some of these 300 plants are used in Tibetan medicine, the majority of the botanical components necessary for producing Tibetan powders are not in fact officially recognized by the Russian legislature as medicinal—either because their properties have not gone through the process of scientific study and licensing or because they belong to a conceptually different category of product, such as food or nutritional supplements. While there are certainly a number of botanicals that are both food and medicine, many of the common ingredients used in preparing Tibetan medicines, such as red pepper and cardamom, are not, from the perspective of Russian legislature, recognizably medicinal. Conversely, an entire category of plants labeled strong-acting (*silnodeystvuyushie*) or toxic, some of which figure in Tibetan prescriptions, are excluded from the production of nutritional supplements, and their use and preparation require a special license.[5]

I highlight the example of ephedra in order to draw attention to the ways in which botanical ingredients—and plants more broadly—become a kind of boundary object (Star and Griesmer 1989; Star 2010) that mediates the relationship between different communities and groups of experts, but also stipulates the nature and efficacies of other lively substances such as other plant and human bodies. Plants are incorporated into different kinds of efficacious assemblages: illegal drugs, whether therapeutic or recreational; biologically active extracts distributed through official channels like pharmacies and medical institutions; remedies in one's medicine cabinet; canned preserves stored in kitchen pantries; and life-forms allowed to only exist "in the wild," and whose cultivated bodies are subject to elimination and destruction, but whose "wild" equivalents might be collected and processed into any of the aforementioned alternatives. Whether the efficacy of a plant is measured through its ability to forestall soil erosion in arid desert or steppe ecosystems, to provide berries that make a tasty jam, to stimulate the nervous system or cause weight loss, to be commercially exchanged as a narcotic substance, to form the basis of legislature, to destabilize linguistic categories of botanical translation, to decrease allergic reactions, or to "cool and dry" the body's constitutions is as much a question of unequally distributed power relations, forms of knowledge, and ensuing priorities as anything intrinsic to a specific botanical life-form or to a concrete plant that might or might not have been *mthse ldum*, ephedra, or *Kuzmich* grass.

TAKING "LITTLE HERBS"

In this section, I move from the conceptual instabilities of plants to their lively agencies in the preparation of medicines. I work to situate the place of botanicals in the Russian therapeutic imaginary and pharmaceutical market and trace the ways in which *emchi* who produce their own medicines attend to raw materials and their subsequent processed afterlives, which relativize perceptions of an over-abundant local environment.

In September 2010 a Muscovite acquaintance had asked me to recommend to her a Tibetan medicine doctor who practiced in the capital. She wanted to pass on the recommendation to a couple she knew who suffered from infertility and had gone through all kinds of biomedical infertility treatments with no success. After providing her with a list of names of those practitioners I knew would be in Moscow in the winter, I left the field. The next time we spoke, I inquired about her friends and asked whether they had decided to consult with one of the Tibetan medicine practitioners I had suggested. My acquaintance explained that they had, but, once again, without success. She extrapolated: "Well, all he did was give them some little herbs (*travki*). They said that this is just not serious." She added that, in the end, they decided to forgo taking them altogether.

The seriousness of herbal-based medicines in Russia is certainly a question of perspective. During field research I frequently asked patients whether they used herbal medicines at home and almost inevitably was given an exposition of their "green pharmacy"—the plants they grew in their gardens, on balconies, and windowsills for culinary, therapeutic, and decorative purposes (with any of these functions potentially overlapping). From common parsley, garlic, or chamomile to various flowering species classically used in Russian folk medicine—*Inula* for the digestive system, St. John's wort (*Hypericum*) for colds and sore throats, *Chelidonium majus* to treat warts, skin tags, and calluses. Patients frequently described the common vegetables that could be used to treat burns, headaches, rashes, and other everyday ailments, narrating their success stories of healing themselves using a recipe they found in the popular media or press or through their friends' recommendations. When I asked patients where they found out about the properties of any given herb or why they decided to employ a specific method of preparation (for example, making a tincture instead of a tea infusion), they listed a variety of eclectic sources—"common knowledge," reference books, aging relatives, neighbors, television programs, popular print media were all providers of recipes or prescriptions in a kind of equal-opportunity space where any source was potentially effective and reliable, but whether the plant would work for the sufferer herself was to be tested empirically.

Folk pharmabotanical knowledge in Russia—by which I mean the knowledge about the therapeutic properties of various plants—circulates through various media and is consistently marked as "folk" in the process. This quality of folkness both invokes its timelessness and indexes a kind of grassroots populist groundedness—a knowledge by and for the people, unfettered by the exigencies of official institutional recognition or scientific legitimacy. While research institutions such as the Buryat Research Center's Institute of Biologically Active Substances conducts pharmaceutical experiments on the curative properties of the components included in the pharmacopeia of Tibetan medicine, the use of phytopharmaceuticals is not necessarily mediated by these scientific discoveries or resultant products.

The market for herbal-based nutritional supplements in Russia is a lucrative industry, estimated to generate about 1.5 billion U.S. dollars a year, of which only 350–400 million dollars are accounted for by official pharmacy sales, the rest being attributed to network marketing. According to Russian legislation, it is illegal for doctors to recommend or prescribe nutritional supplements to their patients. In Buryatia, a thriving black market of plant- and animal-based nutritional supplements (called *biologicheski aktivnye dobavki*, or "*BAD*") and natural cosmetics, usually imported from China and distributed through network marketing schemes, capitalized on the "sundress-radio effect" (*effekt sarofannogo radio*), loosely translatable as "rumor mill," and so was frequently invoked by both patients and doctors to account for how people learned about new therapies or drugs.

About ten Russian corporations are listed as the biggest producers of herbal pharmaceuticals, although an estimated 80 percent of plant medicines sold in Russia are in fact imported from China and Europe to supplement a demand allegedly not met by the domestic producers (Vasylyev and Poloz 2000). While the market share of medicinal botanicals is estimated to constitute only 0.5–1.5 percent of the entirety of pharmaceutical sales, financial analysts have been drawing attention to the yearly growth in the demand for herbal medicines, and most pharmacies stock a large selection of plant-based remedies, from loose-leaf and individually packed herbal mono- or multicomponent compositions (*sbor*) to tisanes, syrups, alcohol tinctures, oils, and "phytoteas." In part, the small portion of total revenue has to do with the fact that herbal-based medicines are significantly cheaper than synthetic medicines. For example, a packet of medicinal tea might cost around 30 to 50 rubles (1–2 dollars). Most of these products fall into two categories: the "monocomponent" botanicals may have a variety of effects and uses, from ingestion to topical application, while the multicomponent ones usually aim at improving the functioning of specific bodily systems. Almost every bookstore features a thriving section on herbal therapy that provides everything from substantial reference manuals that offer do-it-yourself recipes to treat a wide array of illnesses to small pamphlets on the miraculous benefits of a single garden herb. Herbal therapy, or the use of plants for therapeutic purposes, is currently referred to in Russian with two different terms. The term "phytotherapy" (*fitoterapiya*), derived from the Greek "plant" (*phyto*), is usually assigned to the scientific study and deployment of plant-derived medicines from within the medical sphere. The term "*travnik*," on the other hand, usually refers to a person outside the biomedical profession who is knowledgeable about herbal medicines and prepares botanical remedies. From a legal standpoint, a phytotherapist is a licensed medical professional who has completed both medical school and a specialization in one of the possible medical fields and then completed a course in herbal therapy (Egorov 2010). The legitimacy of the *travnik* is a lot more tenuous.

To some extent, the appeal of Tibetan medicine for patients is mediated through the familiarity of taking "little herbs," and in practice, their efficacies as therapeutic substances are understood through patients' assumptions about the "softer," innocuous agencies of botanicals. Unlike these more familiar, homely preparations, however, Tibetan medicines are almost entirely opaque to their consumers. At the end of a typical *emchi*-patient encounter, the patient is sent home with a packet of medicines, usually to be taken over twenty-eight days—a lunar month. A course is usually begun on an auspicious day on the Buddhist calendar, and the *emchi* will inform the patient when to begin taking the medicines. At the end of the first course, the patient is encouraged to come back for a follow-up, where another batch of medicines is prescribed if necessary. In part, this practice is a reflection of the way in which illness is conceptualized in Tibetan medicine—since the treatment aims to remove the root cause of the disease, understood as a disorder of one or more of the three bodily constitutions, the first step is to force the cause to manifest itself more clearly. As such, the first batch of medicines can exacerbate the symptoms. The second batch targets the cause itself, once the root of the problem has been made apparent. A third course of medication may be given to "fixate" the therapeutic effects of the second part of the treatment, making them more permanent. For patients who are "drinking powders" (*pit' poroshki*), as the local expression often describes the process, these effects might mean that their first experience with Tibetan medical treatment might involve a temporary worsening of their condition.

Mostly referred to as "*tibetskiye poroshki*" (Tibetan powders) or "*tibetskoye lekarstvo*" (Tibetan cure) by patients who take them, the medicinal substances themselves can only be known by their effects. In fact, this ascription of "Tibetanness" is itself problematic and is complicated by the ways in which ingredients are acquired and combined. While some practitioners who have emigrated from Tibet to Buryatia use local Buddhist networks to import already prepared medicines from China and India, most local practitioners either make their own or import them from Mongolia, where ready-made Tibetan medicines are more easily available. Even among those practitioners who do assemble their own medicines, obtaining certain rare ingredients locally is not always the chosen course of action. While arguments about the autochthonous nature of Buryat-Tibetan medicine emphasize its tradition of finding substitution for the original ingredients that fail to grow in the harsh Siberian climate, for practitioners making their own medicines it has become easier in recent years to practice a kind of "reverse substitution," replacing the local Buryat ingredients with the originals, imported in bulk from East Asia. At the same time, importing ingredients, especially ones that have not been pulverized, is not taken to be the same thing—and is not as vehemently critiqued—as importing ready-made medicines.

Unlike imported Tibetan medicines, the majority of locally produced medicines in Buryatia take the form of finely ground, often volatile pungent powders that come either in individually wrapped, pre-dosed paper packets or in small sealable plastic bags combined with a plastic dosing spoon, depending on the training and personal preferences of the *emchi* who prescribes them. The powders might be taken with hot water, honey, or sometimes vodka, depending on the kind of "horse" (*kon'*) or conduit the prescription requires. Alternatively, powders can be boiled into decoctions, on occasion requiring a long reduction time to either concentrate or extract the medicinal components, or as a kind of final step in the "taming" process if the medicine contains toxic substances. Typically, a packet of powder may not include a name, or, if it does, it may be written in Tibetan, which the majority of patients would be unable to read. It also does not include a list of contents, and as Tibetan medical components are finely ground, sifted, and homogenized, the only distinguishing features of the powders would be their smell, taste, color, and the thinness of the powder itself. Medicines do, however, include detailed instructions about how they are to be ingested, at what time of day, and for what length of time. These instructions are usually supplemented with the *emchi*'s verbal recommendations on the changes of diet and behavior that the patient ought to undertake for the treatment to be maximally effective. For example, medicines that aim to reduce *rlung* or wind might require the patient to increase the amount of "warm" meats (notably, mutton and beef) and meat-based meals, such as soups and broths, in their diet, while reducing their coffee and tea intake and the consumption of "rough" foods, like uncooked fruits and vegetables. While a person familiar with Tibetan medicine might be able to reverse-engineer what someone is being treated for based on these recommendations—an activity that my *emchi* informants liked to indulge in when they asked me what medicines I had been given and by whom—for the majority of patients the Tibetan medical prescription is known only experientially as its efficacies within their bodies. While it might be possible to argue that all medicines, biochemical pharmaceuticals included, are characterized by a certain "unknowability," I would like to suggest that there is something fundamentally unique in the logic of the Tibetan medical prescription as it is given in Buryatia. One simply cannot look up what one is ingesting—or, if a name is provided, comprehend the information—without prior expertise in a variety of fields and an access to specialized kinds of resources—Tibetan medical disease etiology, medical *chzhor* (formula books) or their translated versions, the Tibetan or Mongolian language, and a familiarity with botany, geology, and zoology. In this sense, unlike folk phytotherapy, Tibetan medicine and Tibetan medicine powders in Russia are, in daily practice, familiar but intensely opaque.

While plant-based medicines are commonly construed in Russia as a more natural, safer, and cheaper alternative to taking biochemical pills, plant-based medicines have come to occupy a somewhat contradictory position in the Russian therapeutic imaginary. On the one hand, reports by WHO on the prevalence of traditional medicine and growing demand for plant-derived natural medicines are invoked as a cause for concern because of the increasing scarcity of resources and depletion of biodiversity (Smirnov 2009). On the other hand, regional media often present the production of botanical medicines as a potentially unexplored gold mine for the depressed postindustrial regions of Russia, ideal because of the relatively low start-up capital necessary to begin a lucrative business (Klyuchevskaya 2010). At the same time, the safety and quality of botanical medicines produced in Russia are a frequent area of skepticism and concern in professional journals and popular media: because, the argument goes, most Russian-based herbal medicine production is undertaken by small private businesses or individual entrepreneurs with little to no accountability, and since medicinal herbs are usually not collected by professionals, the quality and safety of the final product may be severely compromised.

This, of course, is something Russian botanists and practicing phytotherapists writing about the collection of medicinal raw materials talk about extensively. Methodological treaties on phytotherapy prescribe both how, when, and under what circumstances plants ought to be collected and how to properly process them, from drying and storing to grinding and packaging. Most medicines are prepared during the summer season. In the practices of Tibetan medicine and in Russian phytotherapy, the collection of plants is strictly regimented, depending on which part of the plant is to be harnessed. Thus, the flowering part of a plant is ideally collected in early summer; the stems, leaves, and fruit in mid-summer to early fall; and the underground parts—roots and tubers—in late fall, but before the ground freezes. These different collection times speak to the efficacies of plants— in Russian scientific accounts, the plant's "BAS" (biologically active substances) content depends on the maturity, the stage of the life cycle, the immediate weather conditions, and the climate and soil where the plant grew more broadly (Dzuba et al. 2004).

Working with ingredients used in Tibetan medicine, whether botanical, animal, or mineral, requires the management of their unpredictability, as the very material aspects of the craft become a source of both anxiety and pleasure, stretched over weeks, months, and years, where single actions—one's own and those of others—have both immediate and far-reaching consequences, extending into future possibilities of sustained practice. I first became alerted to the unruly materiality of the *materia medica* my *emchi* interlocutors were constantly negotiating through a conversation with Aleksandra. During a period of inactivity between patients' procedures, we sat in the doctors' lounge, and Aleksandra launched into a story about taming calcite—a procedure necessary for the incorporation of calcite into medical recipes. She recounted the way in which her mentor had left out some important details about the technique, something that he did frequently, seemingly to test his students' ability to extrapolate from his instructions and figure out their own approach to the procedure. "Taming" calcite requires heating the mineral at a high temperature, but unlike lime, the mineral does not pulverize when burned, but requires extra treatment—it is dunked in milk or vodka while the stones are still red-hot. This detail was something that Aleksandra's mentor omitted, and she complained, half-jokingly, that she almost caused the geology lab where she was performing her experiments to explode. Eventually, through trial and error, she worked out a way to transform the mineral into the necessary substance—something akin to thick sour cream, she recalled—navigating around the blanks in the literature and her teacher's instructions, calibrating her experience to that of other practicing *emchi*. Yet, she said, it doesn't always work, even when one does everything right. She mentioned a Buryat acquaintance whose grandfather was a practicing *emchi* and who had refused to let his female grandchildren anywhere near the preparation of medicines. The acquaintance suggested that Aleksandra's failures were linked to her being a woman—unpredictable and fickle bodies and materials mixing poorly together. After that, Aleksandra explained that she was out to prove that she could do it, unreliable female physiologies notwithstanding.

Most of the unruliness of ingredients is far less dramatic, but no less harrowing thàn Aleksandra's calcite narrative, as raw materials bring together a number of different (fickle and unreliable) agents responsible for their eventual conversion into medicinal components. Even after a plant has been collected, it must undergo a drying process before its remaining liveliness derails attempts to capture its therapeutic properties. Tree buds might bloom into leaves even after they have been cut from the tree when placed in a warm environment. Certain compactly packed plants not scattered on a drying rack in time are susceptible to fast oxidation, not only risking the degradation of their chemical components, but potentially starting a fire. Others, treated in milk, like the burning bush root that introduced this chapter, when not properly rinsed or not dried fast enough might succumb to mold forming on the surface, where remnants of curdled milk are caught in the cracks of the root bark. These transformations—smoldering grass, molding roots and stems, overripe berries and fruits whose collection one missed by a few days—become constant sources of anxiety and sustained and continuous labor.

Beyond the process of drying and storing plants, both the collection of botanicals and the final preparation of powders are rife with their own unpredictabilities. Processing dry ingredients involves mixing them in the correct proportions and grinding the resulting mixtures into fine powders; depending on the kind of preparation used to ingest them, powders have different stages of granulation. Boiled or reduced tinctures necessitate larger particles, while those that will be swallowed as is are ground and sifted into a thin dust. Although some of my interlocutors preferred the traditional method of grinding that involves a narrow boat-shaped metal container and a heavy metal wheel that one passes back and forth over the mixture until the desired consistency is acquired, others use mechanized machinery, from coffee grinders to more industrial-sized professional mills imported from China. In his own practice, Aleksandr used a mix of these, because each method is rife with its own difficulties, depending on the nature of the particular recipe. The process of making a single recipe—about three to five kilograms worth of powders—often took two or three full days of work, from dawn to well into the evening. Most of the labor involved incremental degrees of pulverization and sifting, although different components of a single recipe have a variety of properties that do not lend themselves easily to forming homogenous mixtures. Ground into smaller pieces, plants acquire new lively efficacies, resisting the bodies and mechanisms that try to organize and discipline them. Tiny trichomes accumulate into small balls of yellow fluff as one tries to filter them through a thinner sieve and refuse to fall through the mesh; pomegranate seeds' sticky resinous mass clogs and jams the cogs of the mechanized grinder until its metal body heats and the air becomes saturated with the smell of burned sugar; finely ground pepper or nutmeg coats and burns the mucous membranes of the nose and throat, settles in eyes, and provokes a constant flow of tears.

Making Tibetan medicines also involves a different kind of balancing act: working with resources whose apparent abundance and availability in the surrounding landscape decrease under one's eyes as herbs that filled several large burlap sacks desiccate and deflate to fill smaller and smaller containers. In an effort to alert his heterogeneous crew of workers, some new and some more experienced, to this radical reduction, Aleksandr asked his helping crew to literally gather dust. Equipped with a small soft-haired brush, he proceeded to demonstrate that the thin layer of powder coating the edges of the grinding wheel, stuck in the crevices of sieves, on the surface of nylon bags through which ingredients pass on their way out of the mechanized mill, and at the bottoms of aluminum basins where the final mixtures are collected before being transferred into specialized storage containers, is enough for dozens of doses as measured by a tiny white plastic spoon, no bigger than a fingernail, provided to patients along with their packet of powders. Aleksandr's didactic trick of scale was to draw attention away from the macroscopic quantities of dried ingredients crammed into burlap sacks and later left out to dehydrate on drying racks, toward the microscopic preciousness of what one might mistake for an irrelevant byproduct.

As I understand it, its purpose was not only to maximize the quantity of the final product, but to cultivate a gaze that could apprehend the saturation and inevitable waste of medicinal substance, as one suddenly became hyperaware of the fine dust that coats one's clothing and hair, of the multitude of specks twirling in the sunlight, of the little mounds of ground-up material that have accumulated on surfaces and in spaces from which they are no longer recoverable, each one potentially amounting to 1/28th of a medicinal regimen—an entire day in a patient's therapeutic month.

The ability to hold in focus the uneven scalar shifts of raw botanicals on their way to becoming medicinal powders is something that informs emchis' practices of plant collection but also scales up to a particular orientation to regional ecologies. Tibetan medicine practitioners in Buryatia do not simply work in conditions of scarcity, as the very experience of the scarcity of botanicals is certainly not intuitive. It emerges in concrete, embodied practices like gathering dust and is in fact in tension with the narratives of Buryatia's ecological abundance I have highlighted in Chapter 3. It is specifically plants' vitality or liveliness that troubles visions of their status as extricable raw materials in an untouched and abundant space. In the following section, I argue that extractability (the transformation of raw materials into medicinal substances) and extricability (the possibilities of recontextualizing these therapeutic substances as part of other assemblages) are not necessarily part of an unquestioned hegemonic imaginary of a modernist relationship with nature. In the next section, I trace the ways in which plant collection is informed by conflicting visions of (post-socialist) ecologies.

EXTRACTABILITY AND BIOTIC COMMUNITIES

In the scientific and methodological literature on phytotherapy, plants are understood to be polyvalent agents, which is to say that their effects in the body are never one-directional, entirely predictable, or singularly focused or targeted. Never simply the sum of their biologically active parts, it is the patterned interactions and interferences between several components of a botanical recipe that enable their therapeutic effects, as noted by both phytotherapists and practitioners of Tibetan medicine. In Russian phytotherapeutic theory, each botanical ingredient is taken to have one primary and a host of secondary uses, frequently expressed differently depending on the other accompanying components. The main principle according to which botanical compositions are then assembled takes into account that different parts of a plant contain different substances such as alkaloids, bioflavonoids, oils, phenylpropanoids, and so on—and that these different substances might simultaneously act upon several bodily process or systems. Classifying the effects of each element becomes a complicated task, as a single component—for example, the phenylpropanoids contained in Melissa officinalis L.—might act as a sedative; a spasmolytic (muscle relaxant); an immunomodulator (a substance that either boosts or diminishes immune responses); an antimicrobial; an antihistamine; or an antiviral, depending on context (Alekseeva, Mazur, and Kurkin 2011). The practical implication of this is that the same plant might be used in remedies that have diverse properties and are prescribed for different conditions and that different plants might be used interchangeably to achieve the same effect in a single recipe.

It is precisely plants' ambiguous, polyvalent liveliness, which borders on capriciousness and extends far past the specific plant's biological life (or death), that makes them therapeutic but also consistently threatens their efficacies as medicinal. The same vitality also challenges efforts to extract and standardize their efficacies in the form of predictable pharmacological assemblages. That there is something about the efficacy of botanicals that cannot be reduced to their active components or, alternatively, that is lost in the very processes of extraction seems to trouble scientific research on phytotherapy in Russia, motivating some scholars to look for more abstract theoretical explanations for why a whole plant or a combination of plants is more effective than an extract. For example, writing on the use of botanicals to treat infertility and sexual dysfunction, Barnaulov and Poslepova (2010) note that certain plants seem to have a nonspecific effect on the reproductive capacities of different organisms, both human and animal, and appear to be efficacious for both genders—in other words, there is no one-to-one correspondence between the presence of a plant hormone and the effects of the plant on reproductive systems. In order to make sense of these findings, Barnaulov and Poslepova choose to view plants as self-interested, symbiotically agentive living organisms:

> Treatment with synthetic and naturally derived substances, extracted from denatured natural compounds, is characteristic of scientific European medicine and is based on an initial logical error: that humans can be cured through the use of substances. Substance has no biologically determined motivation for the reproduction of humans and animals. The unity of the biogeocenosis suggests that many plants have a positive effect on animal reproduction. (Barnaulov and Poslepova 2010)

Drawing on V. N. Sukachev's coinage of biogeocenosis in an elaboration of Karl Mobius's work, the authors propose to view medicinal plants as living in a single biotic community with local humans and animals and to therefore have evolved to support the reproductive capacity and vitality of these other life-forms to enable their own reproduction and propagation (see Sukachev 1964).[6] The formulation is also remarkably similar to Nikolai Badmaev's rejection of the extractive logic of studying the active substances of plants in European pharmacology, cited in Chapter 1.

Such visions of local symbiotically aligned life-forms certainly have the potential to challenge assumptions about the extractability—both chemical and geographical—of therapeutic substances from specific organisms and ecosystems. In my conversation with both Tibetan medicine practitioners and institutionally trained phytotherapists, I was frequently reminded that the most effective remedies would originate from the very area where one lives—those local plants would be both genetically and environmentally more compatible with specific, local, acclimatized bodies, and their therapeutic effectiveness would thus be maximized. Of course, locality in these claims becomes a supple category, defined through different parameters like climate, urban landscape, regional geography, national identity, the prevalence of certain foods, and even distinctly racially and culturally embedded physiologies.

PURE ECOLOGIES

These valuations of locality are, however, challenged by two recurrent topics on the quality of medicinal plant substances, two foci present in both the methodological literature on plant collection, and in everyday conversation by experts and laymen alike: whether the plant is "ecologically clean," and whether it is cultivated or wild. The relative ecological purity of Buryatia and its subsequent suitability for the collection of *syrye* or raw (botanical) materials are certainly topics of conversation among the region's administrators, practitioners of traditional medicine, and the broader public.

In one particular conversation with Tsyrenma, whose work at one of Ulan-Ude's Buddhist temples had earned her the head lama's joking moniker "*emchi*-ma" as a shortening and feminization of the standard "*emchi* lama" honorific, I asked about Russia's legislation for collection botanicals. What happens, I wanted to know, if the state forbids the collection of certain plants? In theory, she explained, you need a license if you plan to collect for commercial use. But who is going to check? I asked her if she had ever encountered problems with the forestry service. "No, of course not. Don't you have *dremuchyi les* in America?" she asked. While the literal translation of this expression is "thick forest," it fails to capture the connotation in Russian. Closer to "wild" or "impenetrable," *dremuchyi les* evokes the kind of forest one might find in fairy tales or in the imaginaries of the nineteenth-century Klondike romantic literature (or, certainly, in the Russian narratives of the Far East *taiga*)—hostile, entirely devoid of humans, uncharted, and dangerous—and of course, overabundant.

Tsyrenma's question points to a particular set of assumptions, quite prevalent in Buryatia, that certain natural features, even when incorporated into the legislative purview of the state, still sit largely outside of it and have powers of their own that are entirely beside efforts to control or dominate them. However, an *emchi*'s relation to this vision of wilderness is not one that assumes a kind of inexhaustible plenty or openness to unscrupulous exploitation that an imagery of the natural frontier might evoke. In practicing their craft, *emchi* are usually acutely aware of the complex relations to the surrounding ecology that their activities sustain.

However, what allows local administrators to make claims about Buryatia's "pure ecology" and for traditional practitioners to practice their craft is precisely the progressive decline of Buryatia's countryside into a new kind of impure, yet, paradoxically ecologically clean nature, one that is visibly and palpably reclaimed from the Soviet past as vegetation overtakes the sparsely interspersed ruins of former collective farms and occasional factories and infrastructure, which are little developed and unevenly maintained, around Russian and Buryat villages outside of Ulan-Ude. While I draw on recent discussions in environmental anthropology and political ecology that might pit capitalist natures against indigenous or local ways of knowing the natural world (Escobar 1999; Tsing 2005), I would like to focus on the fact that these models have a slightly different valence in Buryatia and in Russia more broadly.

There is a deep tension to the ways in which ecological purity is articulated in Russia's broader environmental context and in Buryatia and other rural regions in particular. In order to elucidate this point, it is worthwhile to discuss the kinds of metrics used in Russia to measure ecological cleanliness. According to "Green Patrol," a Russian NGO focused on monitoring the ecological status of the nation, Buryatia occupies seventeenth place out of the eighty-three subjects of the Russian Federation. In other words, it is the seventeenth ecologically cleanest region out of eighty-three. "Green Patrol" uses three parameters to rate ecological quality: the level of environmental protection taken up by local authorities, the ecological consciousness of the population, and the degree of pollution generated by industry. Classified solely along the latter index (industry pollution), Buryatia finds itself at number seventy-one, close to the bottom of the list. There is, of course, nothing surprising about this discrepancy—a region with only moderate investment potential, Buryatia's industrial infrastructure, where it is still functioning, dates back to as early as the 1930s and functions accordingly. In other words, those regions of Russia that are considered to be the most ecologically untouched and that are actively attempting to develop an ecotourist economy also house aging and outdated industries inherited from the Soviet state. These industries, in turn, still provide employment and a modicum of social security, which makes their dismantling a controversial issue.

My point here is not to suggest that Buryatia's ecological status is hopelessly tainted by its sub-regulated industrial production, but to draw attention to a kind of selective, strategic vision that allows local administrators, tourists, entrepreneurs, and, to some extent, experts interested in the raw resources of local botanicals to carve out a wilderness landscape that reinforces a sense of purity, emptiness, and timelessness, largely outside human activity and effort. Local claims about the therapeutic capacities of Buryatia's natural factors—about its therapeutic nature—are operating in a space of postindustrial renaturalization, where visions of a postmodern, socially fabricated nature do not mesh easily with the experiential reality of a visibly decaying bright future of Soviet modernity.

Tibetan medicine practitioners' intricate and fragile relationships to the environment rely on a different kind of selective seeing that renarrates the relationship between a Soviet history and a present post-socialist nature, flattening out the layers of the therapeutic nature fantasy such that all of the different actants and claimants that operate in relation to place and space are aligned and mutually implicated. One set of these emplaced agents is plants themselves. In the fall of 2010, I followed Tsyrenma, Aleksandra, and Ayuna—three practicing *emchi* with whom I worked extensively during my fieldwork—in their search for ingredients. The women easily identified sites where they had previously collected plants. Despite their confidence in navigating a largely unmarked and, to me, botanically opaque landscape, we had to change sites twice before we were able to find one with sufficient biomass. The first site had already been picked over by some other collectors, and they had left barely enough for the plants to be able to reproduce themselves next year, to the profound irritation of my companions. Being able to anticipate and mediate the effects of one's collection practices is an important part of *emchi* ethics. To illustrate this point, Ayuna explained to me that this kind of depletion is always a risk and is not necessarily or always the result of draconian or careless extraction—once, they had collected a plant on the prescribed date, but it hadn't seeded yet, and the next year the area was barren. Relocating to a hill with a view of the city, Ayuna moved swiftly through the waist-tall desiccated grass, pointing out a thistle plant we had come to collect. While large brown prickly thistles dotted the entire width of the hill, their territory was also bracketed by the telltale signs of encroaching development—a sandy road with some construction materials deposited alongside the beginning of a chain-link fence. The concrete multistoried high-rises whose roofs we saw below were slowly spreading up the hill. "They will be building here soon," Ayuna concluded. "We should collect everything there is, it'll be gone anyway next year."

Knowing how to identify sites for plant collection but also to pay attention to the human ecologies that bracket botanical life is a kind of embodied knowledge that is necessarily cumulative, compounded over time through relationships with specific places that one revisits every year. There is both a practical and a spiritual ethics to cultivating the relationship with a site and its flora—asking permission from the local *savdak*, or place owner, especially if the area has a nearby *oboo* or sacred site, and leaving it tribute by scattering rice or millet grains or, for lack of that, some small coins, a common practice and an important part of the proper conduct for a practitioner gathering herbs. *Savdak* are responsible for both human and botanical well-being, and improper conduct is often understood to result in the illness, or in extreme cases the death, of the offender. Similarly, making sure that one's collection activities do not simply deplete the population of a particular plant but, whenever possible, contribute to its reproduction—for example, by scattering its seeds or leaving parts of its root intact—ensures that one's relationship to a place continues. Places where one goes to gather specific ingredients are often well-guarded secrets. Collaboration between different practitioners around the gathering of ingredients is uncommon outside specific patterned relations, such as transmission lineages, or within particular communities, although practitioners who were trained together, especially those of a younger generation, often make medicines as a team. Alternatively, certain practitioners are credited with being serious about the practice and its ethics and are therefore able to maintain collegial relations. Yet, stories about draconian use of flora circulate in the community, and *emchi* have to compete with both Tibetan medicine practitioners and other botanical experts for access to specific plants, and any sort of collaboration or exchange is a matter of tentative and frequently careful negotiation.

As I have attempted to show here, places where botanicals are gathered are not disembedded spaces of pure nature, defined solely by the presence (or absence) of a particular herb or plant, but have institutional and relational histories to which *emchi* must attend in order to maintain a relationship with them over the years. One way of looking at the landscape is to see in it particular post-socialist natures, by which I mean to relate a place's Soviet past to its current state and to its possible futures. As we walked or drove around Lukovo, Aleksandr pointed out abandoned buildings, some one-story log cabins whose owners left and never returned, some partially crumbling skeletons of institutional brick structures: a kindergarten begun in the 1980s but abandoned when the funds "spontaneously" ran out, a school that operated in Soviet times, but then was closed for repairs and never operated again. The house, he explained, was poorly positioned and had "terrible Feng Shui" in relation to the lay of the land. Of course, the village was slowly losing its population, in part to migration, in part to alcoholism, but the land was an agent in the process as well—those houses that were poorly situated were more likely to contribute to their owners' desertion or decline. The village itself, Aleksandr explained, was well-placed under a mountain whose *khoziaka*—a female place spirit—was only slightly moody, but generally fairly well-intentioned as long as one maintained good relations with her. This continuous narration of an animated landscape, laminated over with history, different forces, and various inhabitants who each make claims to it or reject it, was something that many of the *emchi* I spoke to or worked with had in common, although Aleksandr's ability to bring together and make visible all the claimants and complex relationships that defined a place was perhaps the most striking. In these narratives, the Soviet past blended with both ecological processes and current human agency. "These used to be farmlands, wheat fields from a collective farm"—he pointed out, blanketing a vast hilly area, thickly wooded with short craggy pines. The collective farm fell apart in the first decade of post-socialism, he explained, and since no one had cultivated the land for the last twenty years, the *taiga* was slowly reclaiming its due. The space had also become a potential source of medicinal ingredients.

Conversely, botanical collection sites are always already laminated with the future possibilities of their incorporation and reinvention. Despite his rejection of local administrators' and official medical institutions' efforts to co-opt Tibetan medicine into reinventing Buryatia's economy, Aleksandr largely shared their vision of a distinctly local therapeutic nature and took concrete steps toward its implementation as an extension of his own therapeutic practices. On collection trips, he frequently brought our attention to a rock formation on a hill, the curve of the river, or a grass meadow, describing his plans for expansion and development, articulating a hypothetical dreamscape of what a truly therapeutic nature in the region might resemble. He narrated the geological formations as beneficial from the point of view of the flow of local energies, a perfect place to build a five-star hotel or a yurt eco-complex, places where patients could benefit not only from taking Tibetan medicines but from a kind of embedded therapeutic efficacy—the flows of water and energy that made the places uniquely beneficial to cure certain illnesses. A local *arshan*—a sacred water spring with high silver content—would make a perfect place for treating intestinal troubles as well as poor eyesight. The decrepit wooden structures of a Soviet-era sanatorium slowly rot around the water spring, their glass-less windows betraying their abandoned contents—twisted metal cots, peeling wallpaper, broken bottles. Faced with this destitution, Aleksandr often got angry: whatever Soviet institutional structures had been built, they have long fallen apart. His efforts to purchase the land from the local authorities and redevelop it were consistently met with refusal, not for lack of money, but because "they wouldn't sell," perhaps in an understandable move to resist what might be seen as a kind of well-intentioned privatiza-tion. The *arshan* is still very much in use, a rusty metal pipe jutting from underneath the earth and channeling the icy-cold water into a small riv-erbed, dark mud perpetually speckled with small coins and sweets in glittering wrappers left for the local *savdak*. As we arrived to collect water for the center, a delegation of Buddhist lamas from a local *datsan* stood in line behind us, plastic canisters in hand, chatting with Aleksandr about the prospects of formalizing *kumyz* (fermented mare's drink) therapy as another service that the temple might offer to the community. Next to the water spring, a small sign lists the *arshan*'s name and its benefits, a sheet of yellowing printer paper shielded from the rain and the elements with a little wooden box. I had seen similar signs around water springs throughout Ulan-Ude's environs, but when I asked Aleksandr whether the local forestry or resource management representatives put it there, he laughed. It had been one of his projects a few years back—he and his helpers drove around the local water springs, putting up signs like this one. Otherwise, people would not know what the water is for, he explained—each *arshan* has a different mineral content and should be used wisely and as directed.

Those *emchi* whose ability to make medicines depends on the collection of local plants seem to have a very clear sense of the ways in which the local environment is saturated with a diverse and emplaced *materia medica*, one that has a life of its own and is also deeply embedded in a constantly shifting ecology, closely entangled with both *emchi* activities and those of others whose interests do not come to bear on producing medicinal components but whose everyday practices and lives impact them regardless. To return to the bag of skulls that Aleksandr kept in his storage hut, one might be able to productively reread the *Gyüshi* admonition that "there is nothing on earth that could not be a medicine" more broadly: there is nothing in the world that couldn't be (or isn't already potentially) efficacious—in the sense of constantly acting upon human bodies. I argue that practicing *emchi* in Buryatia operate with this broader reading and set of assumptions in mind. Of course, it should not be surprising that the popular and widely circulating quotation is decontextualized from its original occurrence in that it appears to focus one's attention on the natural therapeutic potential of substances and plants rather than, as in the original text, on *why* anything can be viewed as therapeutic. Recall that for the *Gyüshi*, efficacy is the direct result of the qualities and properties of different substances, their relation to the five primary elements (air, earth, water, fire, and space), and the body's own materiality as an expression of these elements. The point then, was not that skulls were unclaimed and therefore opportunistically available, like any other kind of *syrye*, but that in their practices, *emchi* in Buryatia operate with the assumption that all living (and inert) bodies are already relational and mutually implicated and are engaged in a constant process of mutual transformation. From the perspective of an anthropology that attends to how ideas about nature articulate with local medical practices and global processes of capitalist resource use and extraction, I have attempted to outline the emergence of a variously populated therapeutic geography defined by its resistance to visions of extractability and circulation and holding a diffusion of efficacies that is as indebted to Buddhist medical logics as it is to the visceral experiences of post-socialist renaturalization.

MAKING THINGS MEDICINAL

At the end of my stay at Blue Beryl, Maksim, one of the workers at the complex and a long-term acquaintance, asked me what I had learned now that I had "gotten my hands dirty" with preparing medicines, as he joked. Before I could formulate an adequate response, he challenged me: "You see now why this can't really be made into something large scale? It simply can't be for everyone—there's just not enough. You can't just massively produce these medicines without losing their efficacies." Maksim's comment highlights an important dilemma for practitioners of Tibetan medicine in Buryatia, engaged both with the rhetorics of developing Tibetan medicine on a large scale and in the minute everyday practices of assembling medicines. That there isn't "enough," to use Maksim's words, isn't simply a matter of insufficient biomass. Medicinal plants, in these practices, cannot be understood as self-evidently therapeutic—as simply raw materials. I find the ambiguity of the admonition in the *Gyüshi* provocative in this respect as well. That there is nothing in the world that *couldn't* (potentially) be a medicine highlights the fact that making things medicinal is a complex, arduous, and highly contingent process. The efficacies of plants emerge through an intense and all-absorbing labor of collecting, manipulating, disassembling, storing, processing, and reassembling them, through attentive care and management, both on the part of the practitioner and on the part of the patient. Their efficacies are contingent at every stage, from the possibility of the plant's renewed growth each year to the moment of preparation and ingestion to their activities in particular bodies.

I have suggested in this chapter that therapeutic natures in Buryatia— and, arguably, in other regions of Russia that are currently promoting their ecology as resource in itself (as opposed to an ecology as *resources for* extractive projects)—rely on a selective economy of attention, one that elides and strategically skirts local histories of modernization and industrialization. While local practitioners of Tibetan medicine also participate to some extent in the construction of these therapeutic ecologies, their daily practices trouble these omissions by reinscribing the landscape with plural agencies, actors, and multilayered histories that are never fully or happily aligned, but whose mutual implications ensure that they will still operate alongside each other.

CONCLUSION

Markets, Magic, and Post-Socialist Surreal

"Here, citizens, you and I have just beheld a case of so-called mass hypnosis. A purely scientific experiment, proving in the best way possible that there are no miracles in magic. Let us ask Maestro Woland to expose this experiment for us. Presently, citizens, you will see these supposed banknotes disappear as suddenly as they appeared."

Here he applauded, but quite alone, while a confident smile played on his face, yet in his eyes there was no such confidence, but rather an expression of entreaty.

The audience did not like Bengalsky's speech. Total silence fell, which was broken by the checkered Fagott.

"And this is a case of so-called lying," he announced in a loud, goatish tenor. "The notes, citizens, are genuine."

—MIKHAIL BULGAKOV, *THE MASTER AND MARGARITA*

By 2017, after a complete administrative restructuring, East-West had moved away from its integrative model, which had made room for Tibetan medicine, and many of the practitioners of Tibetan medicine who had worked there left to continue in private practice or moved away from Ulan-Ude to work in private clinics in bigger metropolitan centers. Some of the practitioners I had worked with, like Aleksandra and Bayar Badmaevich, had tried to agitate for official recognition by the state and talked about drafting a petition letter to the government to have Tibetan medicine recognized under Russia's health-care laws, but were rapidly giving up and heading into the private sector. The freedom to practice without the infra-structure of *krysha* might have been liberating, but it opened up new forms of precarity: those associated with not having one's labor visible or recog-nized while being vulnerable to legislative action should a patient feel dissatisfied.

In many ways, this shift was in the works in 2011, when I had been gone from Buryatia for some time. The 2011 fuller incorporation of East-West into the OMS/DMS system did, in fact, affect the institutional philosophy and approach of East-West. The anxieties around this financial reconfigu-ration focused especially on the professional prospects for different prac-titioners. For those practitioners who had claimed a specific skill and therapeutic niche associated with a traditional medical practice, the tran-sition was not expected to increase financial or professional precarious-ness. Other doctors and staff viewed these practitioners' patient base as stable and reliable, precisely because each of these specialists could claim a unique therapeutic skillset in addition to having the baseline of a biomed-ical education. By contrast, for the center itself and for those doctors who did not have an added specialization in traditional therapies, the shift would potentially equate to a decrease in financial security and profes-sional status unless they (and the center) were able to maintain and expand a faithful (and financially solvent) patient base.

Practitioners and administrators at East-West were thus under pressure to think of their institution—and their medical activities—in ways that brought the commercial aspect of their practice to the fore. However, the center's staff did not reconceptualize patients explicitly as customers choosing the best option from a variety of increasingly multiplying thera-peutic offerings. Instead, their focus remained on what the center could provide as a medical institution whose agenda aligned with that of the Ministry of Health. The administration's responses to these financing changes focused on taking the next step on the path to medical integration by developing a systematic philosophy for combining the different thera-peutic modalities available at the center, but what that philosophy was had shifted away from the problem of epistemology, ethics, and emphasizing Buryatia's unique medical histories. In my conversations with Valerie, the neurologist and acupuncturist who had recently been appointed as the center's polyclinic's head physician, the problem of integration came to define what she understood as East-West's central conundrum. Like several of her colleagues, Valerie explained that the center lacked a properly integrative vision, and different therapeutic approaches lacked theoretical coherence—a hodge-podge of techniques thrown together with no methodology to organize them. The task of combining the center's many offerings ran into an impasse because of the theoretical premises the different kinds of therapies involved, but also because of how individual doctors thought of their practice. In a sense, she implied that the center operated under the model "every doctor is an island." In other words, the various forms of nonbiomedical specialization present in the center were made institutionally commensurable, but they refrained from substantive collaboration, or from deciding on a single medical epistemology that might unite them. The only grounds for dialogue across specializations were the bodies of patients and the common biomedical training shared by the staff.

Valerie voiced this critique by pointing out that each doctor is isolated: "sits in his or her office" (*sidit v svoem kabinete*), she intoned, miming a bracketed view by forming a box with her hands around her eyes. "Each one tries to do a little bit of everything, without actually specializing or excelling in any given thing." This statement struck me as paradoxical, especially in light of other staff members' insistence that the most successful practitioners were those who had an identifiable professional profile and a specific set of traditional therapeutic techniques that allowed them to be easily recognizable to patients. It also ran counter to aspirations of systematicity that I had encountered in the work of most institutions interested in a systemic view of treatment. By contrast, Valerie's new top-down view at the polyclinic had left her dissatisfied with practitioners' simultaneous redundancy and isolation. Instead, her proposed focus was not on the particular knowledge and skills each practitioner brought to their practice, but on patients. Her plan was to find which of the practitioners—with their aggregated assemblages of therapeutic techniques—excelled at treating specific illnesses. Her idea was to organize therapeutic intervention around patients' conditions, which would then structure a therapeutic division of labor.

For Valerie, the primary goal of developing the center's integrative model was to circumvent the kind of circulation that patients practice: "Patients run from one doctor to another, asking each if they would treat them," she explained. Many patients do, indeed, consult with several practitioners, and not just within the walls of East-West, but they also recruit other healers and private clinics into their therapeutic pursuits (Chudakova 2017). Valerie explained that patients naturally look for something that works, but this isn't their only prerogative. Instead, they seek a kind of maximization, a collection of treatments. It was this practice that Valerie wanted to forestall by reconceptualizing what medical integration meant at East-West.

I understand Valerie's efforts to rethink medical integration as a reflection of a broader concern with the ways in which patients in Russia are engaged in the pursuit of health. Practitioners at East-West did not view patients as customers in a therapeutic market, shopping for the best treatment available. Instead, they perceive what they understand as an irrational circulation that hopes to maximize and multiply therapeutic interventions—an accumulation of treatments against the specter of medical failure. Such divisions of a practitioner's labor have a multiplying effect. As I have discussed in this book, translating Tibetan medicine to make it legible to the Russian state often made it distinctly illegible in clinical practice: when the resulting translations do work, it is on terms unknown, as a kind of uncertain, open-ended third—neither a reconstitution of Tibetan medicine excavated and extrapolated from its canon nor the staunch dedication to proper Buddhist ethics attributed, and often pursued, by its individual practitioners. *Emchi* practice in Buryatia dwells in conceptual and practical interstices—at the edges of the clinic, sometimes mimicking phytotherapy, sometimes making itself speak to biomedical concerns in the language of an aspirational modernity if it means that the patients would benefit. In this sense, the sense of invisibility that I explored in the introduction—that Tibetan medicine in Russia is "barely smoldering," that it is not quite authentically real, that it only exists by virtue of something having to occupy the end of the line (regardless of content)—is not so surprising. Along with my interlocutors in Buryatia, this book has tried to look at this uncertain flickering through a kind of peripheral vision—one that might help recenter these presences.

Valerie's concerns with patients' irrationality speak back to popular descriptions of the first two decades of post-socialism in Russia, and of Moscow in particular, that tend to oscillate between the sense of moral scandal at the rapidly rising inequality and ideological unmooring of the masses—embodied, in particular, in the figure of the kerchiefed babushka begging for alms by the metro stop (see Parsons 2014), and, on the other hand, in an orientalizing obsession with the surreal quality of the everyday. The uncanny as a defining feature of post-socialist life appears as a recurrent political and cultural commentary, for example in Peter Pomerantsev's popular account of his work in Russia's TV industry, tellingly titled, in a recuperation of Vladimir Bartol's fictionalization of the Persian medieval Assassins guild, as *Nothing Is True, Everything Is Possible*, or in the grimly sardonic magical realism of Viktor Pelevin's fiction. But it also figures as a local descriptive category. I ran into people expressing a sense of uncertain ontology long before I began formal anthropological fieldwork in Russia in 2006. It circulated in the colloquial expression of *moskovski sur*—the Moscow surreal—to capture anything from weird architectural projects suddenly mushrooming in the familiar urban landscape to Kafka-esque interactions with various bureaucracies that no longer knew their own rules or purpose, to, as in Pomerantsev's account, cataloging the hallmark characters of the post-socialist (dis)order of things—motorcycle gangs of ultranationalist religious fanatics; soulful professional thieves that spewed poetry; lawyers and businessmen that consulted witches and psychics. Within the genre of the Western journalistic exposé, Russia's "surreal" is frequently viewed through the optics of a distinctly postmodern, "post-truth" regime that nonetheless serves to tighten ideological ensnarement and reframes reality to the specification of an authoritarian governing elite. The sense of brainwashing qua ontological instability in these accounts becomes framed as generative of a collective uncanny, as a kind of mass dissociative disorder from reality facilitated by the canny media and people's predilection for self-delusion.

Long after the formal period of my fieldwork in Buryatia came to an end, Tibetan medicine kept reappearing in the public eye, refracted through the familiar phantasmagoria of the uncanny spectacle. On September 3, 2016, the major Russian federal TV channel TNT riveted its Saturday primetime audience of over four million viewers to a somewhat unusual sight: a man, in the telltale dress of a Sufi whirling Dervish, twirled through a full parking garage in search of a woman concealed in a car trunk. At the end of the dance, interspersed with, at turn, skeptical, amused, breathless, and mildly uncomfortable close-ups of this spectacle's audience—an assortment of some twenty people sitting in a back room of the parking lot and observing the proceedings—the man fell to his knees in front of an unremarkable dark sedan, fixed a piercing blue gaze on its trunk, and announced, "Here." The audience, primed in advance about the location of the trunk's occupant amidst two rows of forty cars, gasped: the whirling mystic had guessed correctly.

The scene was part of the popular Russian competitive reality TV show "Battle of the Psychics." Modeled on the British show "Britain's Psychic Challenge," "The Battle of the Psychics" (*Bitva Ekstrasensov*) premiered in Russia in 2007 and has been one of the longest-running and most-watched Russian television offerings in its category for over ten years. The show typically stages a competition between finalists who all claim "extrasensory" powers—from healing to X-ray vision to channeling spirits. Contestants must pass a series of standardized, incrementally more complex challenges. These include finding a person locked in the trunk of a car in a parking lot full of vehicles; determining remotely what object is concealed inside an opaque box; and, in the final test, assisting with an unresolved police case long gone cold, usually by communicating with the spirit of the victim in order to help family members get closure. A panel of judges would decide which candidates should be eliminated at each stage while soliciting votes from the show's viewership.

The whirling man from the garage scene went on to become the winner of the show's sixteenth season. A self-identified Sufi mystic going by the hybrid Sanskrit/Tibetan moniker of Svami Bodhi Dashi, he became, like most of the show's finalists, the object of a sizable following and media buzz. Svami Dashi's critics argued that after his victory, his seminars and workshops in St. Petersburg escalated in price and popularity, corroborating one of the standard injunctions leveled against the show in the Russian media—that the contest's function is that of an elaborate PR campaign for aspiring self-help gurus and other entrepreneurial types.

Like many participants in the show Svami Dashi was circumspect about the details of his private life, but loquacious about his mystical credentials. Born in Leningrad, and allegedly fifty-seven years old, he identified himself as a member of the Naqshbandi brotherhood, a Sufi order founded in fourteenth-century Bukhara in Uzbekistan and present throughout Russia, the Caucasus, Central Asia, North Africa, the Middle East, and Indonesia. He claimed to be practicing the silent *zikr*, associated with the Naqshbandi order often referred to in the Soviet literature as the "whisperers." In later interviews he explained that he had become interested in esoteric techniques in the 1980s and moved to Buryatia. After that, he relocated to Uzbekistan, where he studied with Sufi mystics and converted to Islam, only to finally end up in India in the 1990s, where he stayed anywhere between ten and twenty years (it varies) at an Osho ashram. There, he was possessed by the spirit of Osho and studied breathing techniques—and came by the name of Svami Bodhi Dashi.

Svami Dashi's public persona fit with a long-established post-socialist autobiographic genre, taken up by some charismatic healers, who carefully craft alternative chronotopic narrations of the Soviet past that allow them to stand both inside and outside of it. For Mikhail Bakhtin, the chronotope—literally, time-space, or the discursive processes through which time and space are linked into a single experiential texture and made artistically visible—is at the heart of what produces different literary genres (Bakhtin and Holquist 1981). Like other Soviet and post-socialist era public healers, such as Merzakarim Norbekov and Gennadyi Rutzko, who traced their uncanny abilities to contact with Eastern mysticism, Svami Dashi seemed to exist entirely outside of the concrete temporality and the territorial isolation of Soviet politics and very much in the midst of Russia's economic present. Embodying a form of medical integration quite distinct from the ones practiced in Buryatia, he advertised his services as a practitioner of Tibetan medicine, among a cornucopia of other nonbiomedical healing.

The recuperation of a utopic Soviet multinationalism as part of the standardized aesthetics adopted by "The Battle of the Psychics" is quite distinct from the social realities of present-day Russia, with its sometimes performative and sometimes pedestrian xenophobic nationalism. But what interests me here is the distinctly post-socialist structure of these healers' performance of identity. Many of the participants in "The Battle of the Psychics" share a recognizable narrative and technical grammar with other famous socialist and post-socialist healers and public personalities, a grammar that simultaneously reproduces and subverts Soviet cartographic imaginaries of the state's internal plurality and external connections. Svami Dashi's revelations about far-flung apprenticeships were in line with how his late Soviet-era predecessors, who claimed familiarity with Tibetan medicine, articulated themselves as cosmopolitan travelers able to escape and reenter the geopolitical enclosures of the Soviet state.

Over the years, "The Battle of the Psychics" has generated a volley of criticism—which has not made the show any less popular. A regular target of ire on the part of the Commission for the Fight against Pseudoscience and Scientific Falsification—a watchdog organization founded in 1998 as part of the Russian Academy of Sciences in response to the rapid proliferation of traditional healers and occult services—the show has entire YouTube channels dedicated exclusively to its debunking. The show accompanied my research in Russia in the mid- and late 2000s as amusing, unapologetically tawdry background noise—a sort of conversation-starting curio that I and my friends and interlocutors would sometimes invoke to fill up companionable chatter about what it meant to do research about the field of traditional healing in contemporary Russia. For the medical doctors and practitioners of Tibetan medicine I spent time with, "The Battle of the Psychics" was simply lowbrow entertainment for which they had little time. Patients I interviewed sometimes followed the show, but with much less zeal than other popular TV programs that dealt with nonbiomedical therapies and healing. The world conjured up by "The Battle of the Psychics" seemed to occupy a qualitatively different lived space from the everyday realities of traditional medicine. There were the actual energy healers, *emchi*, babushkas, bonesetters, herbalists, and clairvoyants that populated Ulan-Ude's often unmarked and unremarkable therapeutic urban geography, one made knowable through, almost exclusively, the discursive labors of the rumor mill and the occasional unobtrusive and cheaply produced paper advertisement. There were the glossy, for-profit clinics marked with the generic "Eastern Medicine" label in Moscow's wealthy districts. And then there were the visible, highly mediated, larger-than-life public figures who fixed the nation's gaze on them every Saturday night.

Scholars have focused on the continuity of forms of nonbiomedical healing across the period of late socialism, suggesting that a taste for the uncanny was there all along, not just among the popular masses, but in the scientific community as well—from Yetis to UFOs to the possibilities of telepathy (Lindquist 2005; Belyaev 2010). The Soviet state occasionally initiated projects of research into the nature of these "uncanny" phenomena that captured the mass imagination of citizens (see also Lemon 2018). Various nonbiomedical therapies had already been integrated into the mainstream of Soviet medicine (for example, reflexotherapy), and an efflorescence of literature on the hidden reserves of the human body brought together utopian visions of future scientific breakthroughs and an interest in religious mysticism and technologies of the self. What changed in the late 1980s were the rules of circulation for these discourses and practices, making them suddenly much more visible. These disparate phenomena appear to have two main things in common: the reference to esoteric knowledge, often buttressed with claims to scientific rigor and rationality, and a focus on the body as both a site of ad-hoc therapeutic intervention and, in the case of the healers, as the inalienable locus of authority and efficacy. Hinting at a kind of embodied expertise that qualitatively transforms the healer's physical and mental abilities was an important part of the discourses and performances that characterized this group of public figures in the early 1990s.

Attention to the interplay of pleasure and horror at the encounter with the surreal, especially in its mediated form, used to diagnose the successes or failures of projects of cultural and political modernization is at the heart of the quotation that introduced this section. The passage is taken from Mikhail Bulgakov's 1966 satirical novel *The Master and Margarita*. The plot pivots around the Devil and his retinue's visit to 1930s Moscow and follows the social fallouts of the motley crew's romp through Soviet society at the height of Stalinism. In the scene cited, the demonic trio puts on a magic show at the Variety Theater and, as part of the performance, conjures a rain of banknotes, to the delight and grasping efforts of the audience. When time comes for the obligatory debunking of the performers' trickery—in line with the principles of Soviet scientific materialism that actively sought to exorcise all forms of superstitious animist thinking from the habits of modern thought—events take a turn for the decidedly more unpleasant. The master of ceremonies Bengalsky, who insists on restoring the performance to the ideologically correct frame of sleight of hand, literally loses his head at the behest of an irate audience, though the head is eventually reinstated with no physical trace of its removal, but with lasting damage to Bengalsky's mind.

For Freud, the aesthetic experience of the uncanny, or the "un-homely" (*Unheimlich*) erupts into everyday life from two different, but interrelated sources: from what he calls "superannuated" modes of collective thought, in particular animism, which interprets coincidences as meaningful events, and from repressed childhood complexes (Freud, McLintock, and Haughton 2003, 155). In both cases, the return of the repressed (or the putatively surpassed) wobbles at the edge of horror and causes psychological strain.

Even when the uncanny takes on the shape of wish-fulfillment, it is unsettling (Freud, McLintock, and Haughton 2003, 152). Here, I find it helpful to draw on Bulgakov as an interlocutor to Freud. Unlike Freud's analysis, Bulgakov offers a slightly different reading—that the experience of the uncanny *as* uncanny is the exception and that ontological uncertainty is readily and quickly reabsorbed into the rhythms and logics of unremarkable everyday life. The performance of black magic depicted in the novel does indeed have a purpose—but not the kind of debunking Bengalsky had hoped for. Rather, it is one in a series of social experiments designed to satisfy Professor of Black Magic Woland's—whom the reader knows to be the Devil—curiosity about whether the Soviet project of birthing into being the "New Soviet Person," endowed with physical, intellectual, and moral features qualitatively different from those of its bourgeois forebears, had succeeded. Woland resolves this in the negative. Following his entourage's antics at the theater, he concludes, "Well. . . . They are like people anywhere. They love money, but that has always been true. . . . They are thoughtless, but then again, sometimes mercy enters their hearts. They are ordinary people, very much like their predecessors, only the housing shortage has had a bad effect on them" (Bulgakov 1995, 104). In Woland's estimation, and despite the disciplinary techniques applied to cultivating them toward new states of personhood and embodiment, Soviet citizens are as people have always been—still thoughtless, still greedy, still occasionally moved to kindness—at most, corrupted more than usual by the scarcity of housing, but certainly not occupying a "higher sociobiological type."

It is precisely Woland's unsurprised dismissiveness of the New Soviet Man's robustly entrenched pecuniary desires that I find especially helpful as an analytical provocation for thinking about the efflorescence of magic, markets, and healing in the first two decades of post-socialism and in locating Tibetan medicine in their midst. To be sure, Woland's affirmation of an ineradicable human nature is a refusal of the Soviet project's utopian visions of redesigning human instincts, consciousness, and body in accordance with the principles of communism. But what seems to capture the Devil's attention is not so much the Soviet citizens' stubbornly bourgeois aspirations, but their differential willingness to accept or refuse ontological uncertainty. This is at the center of the novel's theological dialogue, which puts Woland in conversation with Immanuel Kant and Thomas Aquinas and their reflections on the possibility of proving the existence of

God. Woland's introduction of the "seventh proof"—the indirect confirmation that God must exist if the Devil and his demonic entourage amble about Moscow in all-too-fleshy, palpable presence, causing all sorts of mischief—is rooted in an empiricism of the senses. It is in relation to the different characters' ability to resist the "seventh proof" that Woland's social experiments acquire traction: while the materiality of magic-conjured money and luxury goods is greeted with a quick willingness to suspend disbelief, other proofs of the uncanny, no matter how irrefutable, are met with vehement resistance on the part of the novel's many characters, often at the expense of their sanity.

There is a robust tradition within anthropological analyses of magic that links the sudden efflorescence of the occult across different cultural contexts with the uncertainties, occlusions, and dangers associated with capitalist modes of production and exchange (Taussig 2010; Ong 1987; Comaroff and Comaroff 1999; Farquhar 1996; Lindquist 2006; Buyandelgeriyn 2007; Wood 2010). Similarly, as I mention in the Introduction, both popular and scholarly analyses of post-socialist nonbiomedical healing and its enduring presence in the post-Soviet world suggest that the willingness of the population to accept it seriously arises from the reaction between the thwarted ambitions of a Soviet mandated rationalism and the upheavals of market liberalization. Here, it seems to me that an explanatory reaching for neoliberalism, and in particular for its project of disciplining self-governing subjects, simultaneously forecloses other possible analytical avenues. A popular interest in the uncanny was already present in late socialism, where it took on the contours of a countercultural political stance that sought to situate its adherents firmly outside of Soviet politics and cosmology (Lindquist 2005; Belyaev 2010; Lemon 2018). Typewritten translations of Carlos Castaneda's fictional account of his shamanic apprenticeship circulated on the same conceptual footing as the writings of political dissidents and theological texts, propelled by the legitimacy conferred by illicit or semi-licit Samizdat networks. This is important when we consider the politics of (illicit) reading, where no helpful marketing rubrics situate a text along a gradient of fiction or nonfiction.

Second, the two poles of late capitalist biopolitics—the systematic economic, social, and political abandonment of certain kinds of subjects on the one end and the cultivation of perfectible, economically and socially viable selves on the other—derive part of their critical valence from the

Marxist assumption that the subject is caught in a net of false ideology that obscures the underlying reality of the social and economic forces that produced her. If we are to take seriously the hauntings of the state socialist past and its rationalities in the present, then it is worth remembering that Soviet projects of social engineering—like those aimed at forging the New Soviet person and of instilling a materialist, naturalist worldview—worked the same self-reflexive Marxist ingredients into their critical interventions as does post-Marxist academic critique. They posited subjectivity not as the outcrop of either biology or national character (or culture), but as the product of one's social and economic condition and ways of life, and therefore open to modification through disciplinary techniques on the road to a "higher sociobiological type," to borrow from Leon Trotsky's utopian musings on the lived contours of human emancipation from capitalism and the rise of a new, "higher social biologic type" (Trotsky [1925] 2005: 207).

Third, a turn to neoliberalism in interpreting these social forms obscures the parallel histories of a globally circulating self-help spiritualism and the politics of translation, cultural appropriation, and reinterpretation that accompany this circulation. In other words, many of the ideas and psychosocial techniques promoted through this literary and performative genre are not new, and while they do sometimes articulate well with the logics of capital, they are not just neoliberal. My point is that by privileging a reading that focuses on the construction of entrepreneurial selves in a time of uncertainty and transition, one risks analytical tautology by reducing the appeal and social efficacy of alternative discourses, techniques, social arrangements, and personae to the pressures of a social milieu legible solely as universalizing neoliberal capitalism.

STATES OF CONTINGENCY

While stories of the nineties have never been far from the surface of everyday conversations during my fieldwork, they seemed omnipresent in 2017. In 2014, after the ruble-to-dollar ratio collapsed following the changes in oil prices, Russia's conflict in Ukraine, and subsequent economic sanctions, the country entered an economic recession (Dreger et al. 2016). Jobs were lost, commodity prices skyrocketed, and the state began to implement budget cuts—a strategy still associated with Prime Minister Medvedev's paraphrased and widely parodied utterance "There is no money, but you hang in there" made during his visit to Crimea in 2016 (Khmelnitskaya 2017). The U.S.-led sanctions imposed on Russia and countersanctions imposed by the Russian government against European and U.S. corporations in response reconfigured what food products were available to the everyday consumer. In Buryatia, the feeling of relative prosperity—where average middle-class citizens could afford family vacations abroad, a car, and to eat out at restaurants on a regular basis—turned for many into careful budgeting and for many more into forms of livelihood that began to depend heavily on a shadow subsistence economy, one that had been prevalent during state socialism in Russia and elsewhere and became particularly salient during the first decade of post-socialism (Ries 2009; Rogers 2005). Practices like berry and mushroom picking—and selling one's harvest out of the back of one's car—or growing potatoes in one's vegetable plot to get through the winter are never far from the everyday tactics of my interlocutors. Neither are other, more nefarious forms of subsistence foraging that enter and restructure local landscapes: in Buryatia, this was the case with the catastrophic forest fires of 2016–17 caused, primarily, by illegal logging. For my local interlocutors, especially for those working at the infrastructural and financial edges of the legally precarious field of traditional medicine, the sudden economic and social changes of the recession were not experienced as something new—rather, they enlivened memories of the Soviet-era economic embargos and summoned the chaotic survival techniques incorporated into biographic narratives, both personal and distant. Together, they led to claims that life under economic isolation and general duress, is, in Russia, the normal state of affairs.

Researchers working on the aftermath of post-socialist transformations have argued that the experience of everyday precarity generalized as a new global condition—and recently theorized by anthropologists like Anna Tsing, Kathleen Stewart, Anne Alison, and others (Allison 2012; Stewart 2012; Tsing 2015)—has been a state of the long everyday for many post-socialist subjects, for whom the rapid neoliberal reforms of the nineties, such as aggressive market deregulation, privatization, the retraction of social safety nets, and rising economic inequality, were afoot long before the global North began to think about the ontological uncertainties of late capitalism (Matza 2012; Graan 2013). In Russia, for the people who labor in the interstices of the official medical system—some only starting in the field, and others over several decades, in some cases under radically different political regimes that have at times propelled them into public visibility (both positive and negative) or relegated them to obscurity—specific forms of economic precarity, legal uncertainty, and epistemological suspension are the stuff of everyday experience. They dwell in complicated, underdetermined spaces, ones that frequently highlight what lies outside or beneath the flows of capitalist logics, national political narratives, and formal, accepted histories.

If we consider nonbiomedical healing economies in Russia as intrinsic to a specifically (post)socialist structure of feeling, in Raymond Williams's sense, their persuasiveness and appeal stem not simply from their audiences' presumed vertigo in the face of new capitalist reconfigurations of economic, social, and ideological worlds. Nor are they simply a matter of something needing to occupy "the end of the line." Rather, they bear witness to the ways in which one inhabits ontological uncertainty not solely through disorientation, but also through an active reimagining of what might be possible. Anthropologist Marisol de la Cadena's discussion of cosmopolitics (De la Cadena 2010), which elaborates on the work of Belgian philosopher of science Isabelle Stengers, frames this ontological suspension as a project of translation, one that takes it upon itself to articulate different experiential worlds into mutual proximity. In Stengers's words, cosmopolitics is a politics where "cosmos refers to the unknown constituted by these multiple, divergent worlds and to the articulation of which they would eventually be capable" (Stengers 2005). In this book, I have explored the contours of an experience of everyday life where therapeutic and epistemic uncertainty is left unabsorbed and where different actors are actively invested in maintaining a sense of cosmopolitical open-endedness. This stance, I suggest, is an engaged one—not one where social actors are just helplessly thrown at the mercy of economic and social upheavals, but rather one that produces an ethic of ontological experimentation. In turn, in Buryatia, practicing *emchi* and their patients do not easily fit with a model of therapeutic appropriation or cultural absorption: rather, I have suggested throughout this book that they are often actively bringing alternative pasts into the present and reimagined presents into the past.

In his 1966 lecture *Le Corps Utopique*, Michel Foucault articulates the body as a site of both utopian erasure and emergence—experiencing oneself as a body appears, at first, to negate hopeful visions of a subjectivity not encumbered with the messy business of physicality. Eventually, Foucault's discussion turns on itself:

> All those utopias by which I evaded my body—well they had, quite simply, their model and their first application, they had their place of origin, in my body itself. I really was wrong, before, to say that utopias are turned against the body and destined to erase it. They were born from the body itself, and perhaps afterwards they turned against it. (Foucault 2006, 231)

I find Foucault's musing helpful in considering the articulations of post-Soviet bodies: both those aspirational bodies of socialist utopia and those of ordinary citizens engaged in the pursuit of nonbiomedical care. Foucault hints at an uninterrupted continuity between utopic embodiment and the actual lived body—it is not that the body is simply the actor (in the sense of primary character) of all utopias, but that it is the terrain out of which utopic visions of embodiment unfold. Scholars have noted that bodies—in particular dead bodies, but also, as anthropologist Alexei Yurchak has argued, bodies that are in an ambivalent zone that resists simple categorization as "alive" or "dead"—are an important vehicle for articulating the biopolitical limits of state power in socialist and post-socialist spaces (Gal 1991; Verdery 1999; Quijada 2009; Bernstein 2012; Todorova 2009; Yurchak 2008). For Verdery, dead bodies are particularly well-suited to anchoring the present to a cosmological order as well as reformulating relationships to the past (Verdery 1999). I suggest that the case of the therapeutic modalities I have described offers a glimpse of an alternative post-socialist body politics—not at the troubled margins of death and beyond it but erring on the side of surplus liveliness. It is not the deadness but the excessive vitality of their bodies, mediated through access to esoteric expertise, that allows healers like Svami Dashi to articulate a revision of an accepted Soviet temporality and structure of power—and to remain convincing to their audience and to themselves. I do not mean this as skeptical dismissal but rather as an inversion of how medical efficacy is typically framed by outlining its constitutive outside—the exception that makes its articulation possible. Their living bodies are literally in excess of—both more than and standing outside of—an embodiment conditioned by Soviet time (and Soviet space). However, the public healer's utopian body is not, in fact, qualitatively different from the "ordinary" Soviet body, but a logical extension of it. It does not articulate a radical departure from Soviet logics of scientific rationality and materialism. Instead, it extends to its limit a recurrent discourse, found in Soviet and post-socialist popular and professional medical texts, that the body is always, at least potentially, in excess of itself—that it is, to use a Soviet cliché usually reserved to Lenin's (dead) body, "more alive than all the living."

Throughout this book, I have suggested that visions of medical integration in Russia operate at the site of the implicit gap between the human body as always potentially more than itself—exceeding the expectations of normal functioning—and an actually existing form of embodiment that falls short of the baseline taken to represent normal, let alone optimal health. Defining the "normal" body, and good health more broadly, entails claims about the state's responsibility toward individual and collective subjects, but it does not presuppose stasis: the body is always an asymptotic and symptomatic accumulation of histories, individual and collective, assembled together into disparate ontologies.

Medical translations between "traditional" and "modern," between "Western" and "Eastern," and between "official" and "unofficial" medicine populate Russia's post-socialist therapeutic landscape with multiplying therapeutic crossovers. While patients' search for treatment sometimes comes across to medical professionals as something driven by a collector's impulse—one that recognizes similarity, but values subtle incommensurability—this is not, I have suggested, what drives patients' trajectories. Patients are in fact quite sensitive to the ways in which practitioners invest their therapeutic practices, formulas, and procedures with potential uncertainties, with meanings that arise in the gaps between determined ontologies. No medicine works exactly the same. Many of the patients I spoke to draw subtle, but insistent distinctions between seemingly identically labeled formulas and seemingly equivalent practitioners, clinics, and sites of care. They do not necessarily shop around. Abstraction, extraction, and standardization in this mode become not only nonsensical, but impossible. If post-socialist bodies are experienced and understood as moving targets, always entangled and exposed, and always carrying both their own histories and those of the state, then no medicine is fungible. This does not just result in the chronic and multiplying pharmacologization of the population, as the doctors at East-West feared, but rather in the sense that patients in Buryatia—and perhaps more broadly in Russia—frequently articulate experiences of carrying the state's medical histories under their skin: often partial, sometimes unknowable and contested, but always deeply imprinted with the state's epistemic commitments and self-reinventions, its experiments, its shifting ideologies of health, its exclusions, as well as the negative spaces and medical afterimages of regulatory frameworks and their practical work-arounds. It is perhaps unsurprising, then, that the utopian body of Soviet and post-socialist imaginaries is so often an aspiration to deterritorialization. Conversely, Tibetan medicine in its many inflections—as the Buryat-Tibetan medicine of the republic's official narratives; as the practices incorporated into metropolitan markets; as the shadowy, interstitial work of *emchi* who find themselves laboring in biomedical or integrative spaces; and as the often orthogonal, slightly oppositional practices of *emchi* who work in the private sphere—become ways through which both medicines and bodies are rerooted and held together.

ACKNOWLEDGEMENTS

This project would not have been possible without the time, labor, and generosity of a great many people. I would like to extend my deep gratitude to my interlocutors in Buryatia who have made this book possible. While I cannot name specific people, I would like to thank all the practitioners of Tibetan medicine who generously shared the intricacies of their practice with me. I am indebted to their intellectual generosity, keen insight, unwavering ethical commitments, and to their quick wit as a continuous source of inspiration. If I got this wrong, I hope they will correct me at the first opportunity. I would especially like to thank a team of three women who have taught me just how complex their practice is and how skilled they are at coping with these complexities. I can only hope that the end result does justice to their stories and their practice.

I am also deeply indebted to the doctors, administrators, and patients at the institutions where I did fieldwork, both in Ulan-Ude and Moscow, and who took the time to explain their lives to me. I am forever grateful to the scientists and researchers at the Buryat Sciences Center for their ability to translate their intellectual worlds, their passions and commitments, and their long and complex careers: their scholarship, academic rigor, and intellectual span are inspirations—intellectual, professional, and personal. I would like to thank Tatiana Boyarkina and Tumen Darmayev for their kindness, generosity with their many contacts, incisive reflections, and above all for their friendship. They were a home away from home in Ulan-Ude, and never failed to make me feel welcome on my frequent returns to Buryatia over the years.

I have incurred many intellectual debts in the U.S. as well. Judith Farquhar has inspired and guided me through the long process of turning a fledgling project into a book, and I cannot thank her enough for her mentorship, insights, wisdom, and careful reading of drafts in various stages of disarray. I would like to extend my deep gratitude to the members of the University of Chicago faculty for their mentorship and insights. I would like to thank Susan Gal, Jean Comaroff, and Eugene Raikhel, as well as Victor Friedman, Joseph Masco, and Valentina Pichugin for their guidance.

Several centers and institutions provided their support at different phases of this project: the Wenner-Gren Foundation and the Social Science Research Council Eurasia Program made the ethnographic research and the early stages of muddling through it possible; the Davis Center for Russian and Eurasian Studies at Harvard offered an amazing intellectual community and forced me to engage more seriously with Soviet history. I am deeply grateful to the School for Advanced Research and to the UC Berkeley Department of Geography for providing a space to write and think. Tufts University supported subsequent returns to the field in the critical book writing stages, without which this project would not have the longitudinal view it strives for.

Tufts University's Department of Anthropology has been a wonderfully collegial and insightful place to write and teach. I am deeply grateful to Amahl Bishara, Alexander Blanchette, David Gus, Sarah Luna, Zarin Machanda, Sarah Pinto, Nick Seaver, Cathy Stanton, Lauren Sullivan, and Rosalind Shaw for providing such a supportive intellectual community and inspiring examples of scholarly engagement through their own work.

The members of the Translating Vitalities Collective have been a systematic source of inspiration, anchoring insight, and creativity. I am deeply grateful to Judith Farquhar and Carla Nappi for making this remarkable group of scholars possible and for sustaining it through the years. I am especially grateful to Stacey Langwick, Larisa Jasarevic, Volker Scheid, Angelika Messner, and Barry Saunders for pushing me past my blind spots in how I thought about bodies, medicine, and healing.

I want to extend my deep gratitude to Thomas Lay, Clara Han, Bhrigupati Singh, and the team at Fordham University Press for shepherding the manuscript into book form, and to the anonymous reviewers for their invaluable insights, suggestions, and guidance.

This book would not have seen the light without the support of many dear friends and colleagues. While they are too many to enumerate, I want to extend my deep appreciation to Mary Leighton, Xeniia Cherkaev, Magdalena Stawkowski, Marissa Smith, Maria Sidorkina, and Anya Bernstein for being intellectual co-conspirators at different times and places. The early forms of this manuscript would never have been completed without the support of "the Hive"—Caroline Schuster, Kathryn Goldfarb, Elayne Oliphant, and Alexander Blanchette—who kept me on track, pushed me beyond my comfort zone, asked difficult questions I frequently couldn't answer, and tirelessly provided editorial advice on innumerable drafts.

I would like to thank the members of my family and friends in Russia and elsewhere, who have supported me through this process. My grandmother, Klavdia Trofimova, welcomed me back for many years while I traveled back to Russia, and never tired of inquiring about the minutia of my work and about when I will have finished writing, already. Olga and Sasha Doroshenko opened their home to me and made me feel part of the family, whenever I returned. Finally, I would like to thank my parents for instilling an intellectual curiosity and a taste for critical thinking that brought me to anthropology, and for always supporting me in my various pursuits, with an open mind, quick wit, and advice at the ready.

Last but not least, Alex, Mira, and Begemot make it all worth it.

NOTES

INTRODUCTION

1. Lineage-based transmission of knowledge and expertise is an important element of the reproduction of Himalayan Medicine in other contexts, not just in Buryatia (see Hofer 2018).

2. I juxtapose these two claims—the religious leader's harsh pronouncement and the scientist's more cautious, wistful one—because this was a rare case of convergence between the representatives of two groups who are usually vehemently not in conversation. Practitioners in temples often dismiss the research undertaken by scientists as destined to fail a priori because of what they see as profound incompatibility between Buddhism and Western medical epistemology. For their part, scientists are unable (and sometimes unwilling) to initiate a dialogue with the former, occasionally suggesting that there might be nothing to talk about. Historically, this has not always been the case. Starting with the late 1960s, the Buryat Sciences Center had managed to recruit Buddhist lamas recently released from labor camps to assist with the work of translating the collection of Buddhist xylographs stored at the republic's archive and to help botanical expeditions identify the raw materials of Tibetan medicine pharmacology. However, in recent years, attempts at collaboration have run into frictions, and they mostly took place via the mediation of practicing *emchi* who attempted to navigate both worlds.

3. For example, Aseeva adopts the framework of adaptation of Tibetan medicine to its contemporary historical conditions and to its place in the Russian state's present-day therapeutic pantheon (Aseeva 2008).

4. For a discussion of the ways in which the centralization of political power in the Soviet Union enabled projects of urban infrastructural distribution, see Collier (2011) and Reeves (2014).

1. "MAY ALL LIVING BEINGS BENEFIT": PASSIONS OF TRANSLATION

1. While the origins of the *Gyüshi* are not entirely clear, it is generally recognized by Tibetan scholars as itself a translation of the Sanskrit medical text *Amṛtahṛdayāṣṭaṅgaguhyopadeśa*.

2. For example, Boris Gusev's biography of Pyotr Badmaev, often cited in this chapter, is written from that space of intimacy, since Gusev is Badmaev's grandson.

3. The term most commonly used in its Russian translation is *rLung*, or wind, translated as the Russian *veter* in everyday conversations with practitioners and patients. The other two constitutions tended to retain their original Mongolian and Tibetan terms, especially in the case of *badgan*. At the same time, when dealing with ethnically Russian (or primarily Russian-speaking) patients, practitioners would translate the terms into Russian and use them accordingly. Conversely, when speaking with other practitioners, code-switching between the Russian translation and the originals was common.

4. The distinction between "nomadic" (Rus. *kochevyie*) and "roaming" (Rus. *brodyachie*) largely maps onto a distinction between pastoralist and hunter-gatherer means of subsistence.

5. Geographer Mark Bassin (1991) has argued that the image of Siberia in Russia can be productively read against similar constructions of the Wild West by American settlers, accounting for the territorial contiguity of the metropole and the settler-colonial frontier. Bassin's argument outlines the nuances of the construction of Siberia in the imaginary of Western Russians: a drift in meaning from the imperial ambitions of Peter the Great in the eighteenth century to model Russia on Western European colonial empires and toward the nationalist ideologies of Russia's cultural distinction and unique historical mission of serving as a bridge between Europe and Asia emerging in the nineteenth century. Eager to participate in the geopolitical theater of Western European modernity, Bassin argues, Russia's mythologies of Siberia mimicked Western Europe's fashioning of itself against a constructed colonial Orient deployed as a foil (Said 1978). Bassin notes that this original image of Siberia as an "Asiatic" colony—as empty wilderness, inhospitable landscape, and as a mercantile annex for resource extraction—shifted over time, as other regimes of signification, including those of political opposition and social radicalism, reinfused and transformed this earlier, more explicitly colonial optics. Other scholars have drawn attention to the ways in which Buryats articulate competing politics of inclusion in relation to other symbolic geographies (Bernstein 2013; Buck-Quijada 2020). My argument reprises and expands this scholarship. Here, I draw on recent discussions in postcolonial and feminist science and technology studies (Harding 2013), which point out that the history of Western scientific development has often been told unilaterally, relegating the role of its non-Western interlocutors to the passive margins. By looking at the ways in which

imagined geographies refracted through the dialogical spaces of scholarly, religious, and scientific encounter, debates, and silencing, we can see how Buryats' participation in and refashioning of "Asiatic" encompassments were not solely metropolitan projections, but, rather, competing articulations of "centers" and "peripheries" in the theater of Russia's scientific modernization.

6. Dashiev, in his translation of the *Gyüshi*, remarks that the version of the treatise that circulated into Mongolia, then into the Transbaikal region, cannot be divorced from the circulation of its commentaries, the most prominent ones being the "Vaydurja-onbo" and "Lhantab" treatises undertaken by Desi Sangye Gyatso in the late 1600s—part of a broader process of consolidation and religious unification happening in seventeenth-century Tibet. Dashiev notes, however, that subsequent translations into Mongolian were multiple, somewhat reversing this process of consolidation and standardization (Dashiev 2009, 19).

7. Historians Vera Tolz (2005) and Sergei Glebov (2011) both argue that the Russian school of Orientology in the late nineteenth century was participating in constructing a vision of Russia as distinct from (and opposed to) Western European colonial relations and forms of representation and offered a nuanced reading of the ways in which scholarly knowledge produced about Russia's ethnic minorities was often quite vocal about the politics of representation, and in some ways prefigured (and, according to Tolz, informed) Eduard Said's arguments on Orientalism.

8. It should be noted that the first recorded translation of the first volume of the *Gyüshi* into Russian was undertaken by Dambo Ulyanov, a Kalmyk practitioner of Tibetan medicine and a member of the Don Kazaks, in 1901. This translation did not have the same level of circulation in Buryatia during my fieldwork.

9. A designation for ethnically non-Russian, non-Orthodox autochthonous subjects of the Russian Empire, formalized in the Speranski.

10. Pozdneev's own biography probably had something to do with the much less vitriolic reception of his work. Born in the city of Oryol in southern Russia in 1851 into a family of Russian Orthodox clergy, Aleksei Matveevich Pozdneev, whose reflections on his experience with translating the *Gyüshi* into Russian introduced this chapter, received his education at the Oryol Seminary and subsequently at the Lazarev Institute of Oriental Studies in St. Petersburg, with a specialization in Mongolian languages. He spent several years of fieldwork in Mongolia as part of his dissertation research, focusing both on collecting and translating Buddhist manuscripts and on observing the everyday life at Buddhist monasteries. Later, his ethnographic interests expanded to include the Kalmyk—a Buddhist ethnic minority settled in the Volga region—as well as the institutionalization of Buddhism in Buryatia (Shastina 2003).

11. As Susan Buck-Morss has argued (2002), the Marxist vision of dialectical historical unfolding classified different cultures along a teleological temporal continuum, and Bolshevik attitudes toward the nationality question were preoccupied

with accelerating the collective march toward a socialist modernity. Historians Terry Martin (2001) and Francine Hirsch (2014) both emphasized the ways in which Soviet nationality policy was not so much interested in promoting "national culture" in the sense of ideological, social, or religious distinction—it wasn't—but in developing standardized outward markers of national identity, such as territory, language, national elites, literature, museums, food, dress, and other folkloric elements. Meant to implement the fairly ambiguous slogan, formulated by Stalin, of "national in form, socialist in content," these efforts were not targeted at fostering organic cultural expression so much as they were meant to help translate socialist ideas across contexts, while combating what Lenin had called "Great Russian chauvinism."

12. After Lenin's death in his early fifties, some writers have argued that the aging Bolshevik elite became alarmed at its own mortality and supported various forms of medical experimentation with both biomedical and nonbiomedical forms of healing aimed at restoring their youth. Perhaps the most radical forms of experimentation had to do with research in endocrinology and early efforts at hormone replacement therapy conducted through research on apes and experimentations with blood transfusion (Krementsov 2011; Sergeeva 2015).

13. Writing about the purges against Tibetan medicine institutions in Lhasa Mentsikhang's during China's Cultural Revolution in 1966–67, Hoffer (2018) notes the ways in which China's communist activists were similarly concerned with expunging all traces of religious and cultural "superstitions," leading to the dismantling of the institutional centers of Tibetan medicine in Tibet. In Russia of the 1920s, the Soviet state's antireligious policy concerned itself first with separating church and state, paradoxically guaranteeing freedom of confession to Soviet citizens, but also working on establishing freedom *from* religion writ large. In practice, this meant bringing religious institutions, including Buddhist monasteries, under party control while removing juridical and property rights from religious organizations. By the 1930s, these socioeconomic measures were augmented by political repressions against lamas and practitioners, state-led confiscation of lands and Buddhist relics and artifacts, and the physical destruction (active and passive) of sites of worship. By 1940, no active Buddhist *datsan* were left in the republic (Mitypov 2011). By 1945, Buddhism was reestablished in Buryatia via top-down intervention and under party control, with the reopening of the Ivolginskii Datsan. Sablin (2019) observes that Buddhism posed an additional problem for the Soviet state in that it offered avenues for cosmopolitan connection and internationalist policy and consequently the potential spread of socialist ideas in postcolonial Asia—a mission the Soviet state-controlled reimplementation of Buddhism did not accomplish, he notes.

14. In Buryatia, there is a differentiation between an *emchi* lama (a proper, authorized practitioner who had mastered the philosophy of Tibetan medicine)

and an *emtey* lama. The latter term is derived from a Buryatization of *"emchi"* by adding the comitative case suffix—*tey*, literally meaning a lama with medicines (*em-*).

15. Such relegation to the status of "historical stage" or "museum piece" was not a neutral rhetorical move in the Soviet context, since it functioned to dismiss a cultural practice as a previous stage of historical development, and the Soviet Union was quite intent on battling all forms of anachronisms and "survivals."

16. "Tibetskaya Meditzina" [Tibetan Medicine], *Izvestiya* 81, April 10, 1936.

17. At the same time that the epistemology of Tibetan medicine had been relegated to religious superstition, some of its ingredients, openly labeled "products of Tibetan medicine," found a vibrant place in Soviet agriculture and foreign trade. Wild ginseng and deer horns were regularly exported to China, Korea, and Germany from the Russian Far East, and reports about expanding production were filed with the Soviet Ministry overseeing hunting and wildlife preserves.

18. A. Subbotin, *Kommersant*, 79 (4), June 5, 1998.

19. S. Zebelin, *Pravda Buryatii* 83 (21335), May 7, 1998.

20. A. Subbotin, *Pravda Buryatii*, May 7, 1998.

21. B. Bazaron, *Pravda Buryatii*, May 13, 1998.

22. E. Demin, *Pravda Buryatii*, March 31, 1998.

2. "TO SEARCH FOR THE SOLELY RATIONAL": ENGINEERING TIBETAN PULSE DIAGNOSIS

1. In Russian, the standard term for many research projects around Tibetan medicine is *"Ob'ektiviztzia"*—translatable as, literally, "making objective" (rather than making into an object).

2. Postcolonial studies have also documented the fraught encounters between Western technoscientific and biomedical regimes and local epistemologies and practice, especially in places with no prior tradition of Western scientific thought. As anthropologist Vincanne Adams and her collaborators have argued, encounters between biomedical science and its "others" are never unidirectional (Adams, Schrempf, and Craig 2011), and efforts to translate nonbiomedical approaches and cosmologies sometimes reshape the very scientific regimes, diagnostic categories, and healthcare rationales that work to incorporate them (Adams, Dhondup, and Phuoc 2010; Langwick 2011). The case of the pulsometer discussed here encourages us to also consider how such encounters play out when biomedicine itself is neither the primary nor the uniquely privileged interlocutor, and where separate disciplinary projects of making sense of bodies are made to align (see also Adams 2003; Craig 2011). In many ways, this space of encounter is equally influenced by the specific epistemological optics of Soviet medicine and by the lingering high prestige and social capital of physics and other "abstract" sciences in Russia.

3. The most frequently analyzed example of the impact of the Soviet regime in the scientific domain is the rise of Lysenkoism and the concurrent repression and dismantling of Soviet genetics (see Soaeifer 1994). See also Joravsky 2010; Graham 1993.

4. From what I have observed, it is not necessary for the practitioner to "match" the biomedical diagnosis perfectly, as most patients will accept the explanation that an illness that, according to biomedical wisdom, is confined to one organ may be seen in Tibetan medicine to have an entirely different etiology and location in the body. A simple confirmation of the diagnosis is not sufficient—pulse diagnosis must go beyond what the patient already knows about oneself to be convincing. This preoccupation with authenticity is not entirely dissimilar from the sort of post-socialist suspicions that Buyandelger (2013) has detailed in her study of Buryat shamanism and Pedersen (2011) described relative to the revival of shamanism in Northern Mongolia.

5. On the circulation of medical images, see Kevles 1997; Dumit 2012; and Saunders 2008.

3. "THE MEDICINE OF THE FUTURE, NOW AVAILABLE": GEOGRAPHIES OF MEDICAL INTEGRATION

1. Not the original name.

2. I heard the term *samochuvstvie* frequently used in clinical practice in Russia. Literally meaning "self-feeling" or "self-experience," the expression could be used as a synonym of *zdorovye* (health), although it more closely captures the fluctuation of day-to-day bodily experiences.

3. Alaina Lemon has traced the rise of this concept in both Soviet scientific projects and the way it captured the imaginaries of a late Soviet public (Lemon 2018).

4. *Gotov k Trudu I Oborone*—"Ready for labor and defense," a Soviet program of physical preparedness made mandatory in educational and professional organizations, and at the workplace.

5. This sort of logic is echoed in various forms of regional rankings, especially in the division into "dotational" (*dotatzionnyi*) and "donor" regions, depending on each administrative region's contribution to the state budget.

6. The political show "Open Studio" on Russia's Channel 5 introduced this debate on November 27, 2009, by citing a joke: "Will they still let you into Moscow from other parts of Russia without a visa?"

7. Two separate incidents might serve to illustrate the nature of these tensions. One involved a visit by the then-president Dmitry Medvedev to the Ivolginsky Datsan in 2009, where the local administration had allegedly ordered the mass poisoning of "stray" dogs who lived on the temple compound. The second, less

dramatic event involved the rapid "gentrification" of the "Sayany" neighborhood in the city for Vladimir Putin's visit in 2008.

8. Thus, for example, Aleksandr Khamchikhin, a Moscow-based political scientist from the Institute of Political and Military Analysis, suggested that Russia's image in neighboring China was of a "negative-disdainful character." Similarly, a report by Ruslan Muhametov cited the yearly report by BBC's GlobeScan about the international popularity of different states: as the conference report noted, rather sarcastically, "Russia finds itself as the fifth country from the bottom of the list, outperforming only Iran, Pakistan, Israel, and North Korea."

9. From a juridical point of view, a *region* in Russia refers to one of the subjects of the Russian Federation, which includes twenty-one republics, nine "*kray*," forty-six "*oblast*," two cities of federal significance, one autonomous "*oblast*," and four autonomous "*okrug*." Most of these terms could be translated into English as "region" or "area," but in fact designate distinct administrative categories.

10. Baikal Cellulose Paper Combine, founded in 1966, considered the leading source of pollution of Lake Baikal. The factory was privatized and purchased by Alpha Bank in 2008, and the management has been consistently critiqued in the media for refusing to pay any heed to protests from local administration, experts, or public opinion.

11. For example, the national anthem of Buryatia, written by Buryat poet and writer Damba Zhalsaraev, is an example of Buryat ecologically focused poetry, which extols the environmental beauty of the region.

12. A procedure that involves cooking the mineral after neutralizing it in either water or milk, depending on the particular chemical composition of the particular type of calcite, which is referred to in terms of the mineral's "gender."

13. An interesting reversal of the earlier conference on branding, where Buryatia was articulated as the "Heart of Russia in Asia."

14. Bergenia root is commonly used in Russian phytotherapy for multiple therapeutic purposes: for digestive disorders, as an anti-inflammatory and coagulative, as an antimicrobial, and as a diuretic.

4. "TREATING NOT THE ILLNESS, BUT THE PATIENT": INTEGRATIVE MEDICINE FOR DISLOCATED BODIES

1. Elected councils in charge of the social and economic development of their corresponding regions.

2. The most widespread citation that figures as evidence of these tenets is taken from *Obshie osnovy klinicheskoy meditziny*, a speech given by Botkin at the Imperial Military-Medical Academy on December 7, 1886: "The concept of disease is inextricably linked with its cause, which is always and exclusively conditioned by

the external environment, which either affects the diseased organism directly, or indirectly through its closest or remote progenitors" (Botkin [1886] 2012).

3. In the 1960s, Brekhman had a fairly direct connection with Tibetan medicine, not just conceptually, but economically: he was involved in the trade consortium "Medexport," which specialized in the foreign export of natural medicinal products, including those labeled "products of Tibetan medicine"—namely, deer horns and Siberian ginseng. (See "Results of the All-Union Meeting Seminar for Heads and Specialists of Hunting Enterprises, State Industrial Farms, Territories and Regions of the RSFSR on the Organization of the Procurement and Delivery of Goods of Tibetan Medicine for Export, in Vladivostok on April 13–18," 1964. GARF f. A358, op. 5, d. 304. l. 2).

5. "WE ARE NOT IRON THAT WE NEED TEMPERING": THE CONTINGENCIES OF MIXING MEDICINES

1. Bayar Badmaevich, and most other practitioners of Tibetan medicine at East-West, with the exception of Aleksandra, are ethnically Buryat.

6. "NOTHING IN THE WORLD THAT COULDN'T BE MEDICINAL": THE LIMITS OF EXTRACTION

1. Many of these accounts seem to focus on traditional peoples of the Russian Far North, with a certain penchant for viewing them in a kind of timeless context. These accounts focus on indigenous relations to the environment, notably modeling much of the anthropology coming from Amazonia (cf. Brightman et al. 2006).

2. Both Martix Saxer (2013) and Theresia Hofer (2018) have explored the ways in which Tibetan medicine in Tibet is located at the peripheries of different assemblages, and its history, industrialization, and revivals trouble both center-periphery logics and assumptions about the circulation and uptake of global forms. Examining the industrialization of Tibetan medicine pharmaceuticals, Saxer specifically has shown how global forms are recontextualized in multiple steps, in particular via national optics. Here, I simultaneously draw on and expand these insights by suggesting that Tibetan medicine in Buryatia calls on specific forms of practice that not only localize Tibetan pharmaceuticals, but also work against their subsequent circulatory potentials, making these medicines, and the practices on which they depend, rooted in place.

3. Postanovlenie Pravitel'stva Rossijskoy Federatzii ot 3 sentyabria 2004 g., no. 454.

4. Postanovlenie Pravitel'stva Rossijskoy Federatzii ot 8 oktyabria 2012 g., no. 1020.

5. Postanovlenie Glavnogo Gosudarstvennogo sanitarnogo vracha RF ot 5 marta 2008, no. 17, "Ob utverzhdenii SanPiN 2.3.2.2351-08."

6. The unity of different organisms and chemical elements in a single system. The concept of biogeocenosis is widely used in Russian (and Soviet) ecology studies, but is not well-known in Anglophone environmental studies literature, where "ecosystem" is the preferred term.

BIBLIOGRAPHY

Abaeva, L. L. 1998. *Buddhism in Buryatia*. Ulan-Ude: Buryat State University.

Acemoglu, D., and J. Robinson. 2012. *Why Nations Fail: The Origins of Power, Prosperity, and Poverty*. New York: Crown.

Adams, V. 2003. "Randomized Controlled Crime: Postcolonial Sciences in Alternative Medicine Research." *Social Studies of Science* 32 (5–6): 659–90.

Adams, V., R. Dhondup, and V. L. Phuoc. 2010. "A Tibetan Way of Science: Revisioning Biomedicine as Tibetan Practice." In *Medicine between Science and Religion: Exploration on Tibetan Grounds*. New York: Berghahn.

Adams, V., M. Murphy, and A. Clarke. 2009. "Anticipation: Technoscience, Life, Affect, Temporality." *Subjectivity* (28): 246–65.

Adams, V., M. Schrempf, and S. Craig. 2011. *Medicine between Science and Religion: Explorations on Tibetan Grounds*. New York: Berghahn.

Agadjamyan, N. A., R. M. Bayevsky, and A. P. Berseneva. 2004. "Funktsional'nyye Rezervy Organizma i Teoriya Adaptatsii" [Functional Reserves of the Body and the Theory of Adaptation]. *Vestnik Vosstanovitel'noy Meditsiny* (3): 19.

Agadjanyan, N.A., and A. Y. Katkov. 1990. *Rezervy Nashego Organizma* [The Reserves of our Organism]. Moscow: Znanie.

Agamben, G. 1998. *Homo Sacer: Sovereign Power and Bare Life*. Stanford, Calif.: Stanford University Press.

Alekseeva, A. V., L. I. Mazur, and V. A. Kurkin. 2011. "Melissa lekarstvennaya: Perspektivy ispol'zovaniya v pediatricheskoy praktike" [Melissa Oficinallis: Possibilities of Usage in Pediatric Care]. *Pediatriya* 90 (1).

Alexseev, M. 1999. *Center-Periphery Conflict in Post-Soviet Russia: A Federation Imperiled*. New York: St. Martin's.

Allison, A. 2012. "Ordinary Refugees: Social Precarity and Soul in 21st Century Japan." *Anthropological Quarterly* 85 (2): 345–70.

Alov, A. A., and N. G. Vladimirov. 1996. *Buddizm v Rossii* [Buddhism in Russia]. Moscow: Rossiyskiy NII kul'turnogo i prirodnogo naslediya.

Alter, J. 2005. *Asian Medicine and Globalization*. Philadelphia: University of Pennsylvania Press.

Amosov, N. M. 2002. *Entsiklopediya Amosova: Algoritm Zdorov'ya* [Amosov's Encyclopedia: Algorithm of Health]. Donetsk: AST.

Apanasenko, G. L. 2012. "U Istokov Valeologii: Formirovaniye kontseptsii individual'nogo zdorov'ya" [At the Origin of Valeology: The Formation of the Concept of Personal Health]. *Valeologiia* 2 (18).

Appadurai, A. 1996. *Modernity at Large: Cultural Dimensions of Globalization.* Vol. 1. Minneapolis: University of Minnesota Press.

Arkhangelsky, G. V. 1998. "Istoricheskiye Portrety: Pëtr Badmayev—Znakhar', Predprinimatel' i Politik" [Historical Portraits: Pyotr Badmaev—Healer, Entrepreneur, and Politician]. *Voprosy Istorii* 2:74–84.

Aronson, P. 2007. "Rejecting Professional Medicine in Contemporary Russia." http://www.sras.org/rejecting_professional_medicine_in_contemporary _russia.

Aseeva, T. A. 2008. *Tibetskaya Meditsina u Buryat* [Tibetan Medicine among the Buryats]. Ulan-Ude: Izdatel'stvo BNC So RAN.

Aseeva, T. A., and C. A. Naydakova. 1991. *Pishchevyye Rasteniya v Tibetskoy Meditsine* [Nutritional Plants in Tibetan Medicine]. Novosibirsk: Izdatel'stvo Nauka.

Ayusheeva, L. V. 2007. *Tibetskaya Meditsina v Rossii* [Tibetan Medicine in Russia]. Ulan-Ude: Izdatel'stvo Rinpoche Bagsha.

Badmaev, N. 1935. "Indo-Tibetskaya Meditsina" [Indo-Tibetan Medicine]. *Izvestiya* 72, March 24.

Badmaev, P. A. [1901] 1991. *Zhud-Shi: Glavnoye Rukovodstvo po Vrachebnoy Nauke Tibeta* [Gyüshi: Principal Guide on the Healing Science of Tibet]. Moscow: Izdatel'stvo Nauka.

Badmaev, P. A., B. S. Gusev, and T. I. Grekova. 1991. *Osnovy vrachebnoy nauki Tibeta. Zhud-shi* [Foundations of the Tibetan Science of Healing. Gyushi]. Moscow: Izdatel'stvo Nauka.

Baer, H. 2004. *Toward an Integrative Medicine: Merging Alternative Therapies with Biomedicine.* Walnut Creek, Calif.: AltaMira.

Baer, H. A., and I. Coulter. "Taking Stock of Integrative Medicine: Broadening Biomedicine or Co-option of Complementary and Alternative Medicine?" *Health Sociology Review* 17 (4): 331–41.

Bakhtin, M. M., and M. Holquist. 1981. *The Dialogic Imagination: Four Essays.* Austin: University of Texas Press.

Balzer, M. 1999. *The Tenacity of Ethnicity: A Siberian Saga in Global Perspective.* Princeton, N.J.: Princeton University Press.

Balzer, M., and U. Vinokurova. 1996. "Nationalism, Interethnic Relations and Federalism: The Case of the Sakha Republic (Yakutia)." *Europe-Asia Studies* 48 (1): 101–20.

Barnaulov, O. D. 2001. *Zhen'shen' i drugiye adaptogeny* [Ginseng and Other Adaptogens]. St. Petersburg: Elbi.

Barnaulov, O. D., and M. L. Poslepova. 2010. "Rasteniya, zainteresovannyye v reproduktsii cheloveka" [Plants Interested in Human Reproduction]. In *Materialy 2go Mezhdunarodnogo Syezda Fitoterapevtov i Travnikov: "Soveremennye problem fitoterapii I etnicheskogo travnichestva."* Moscow: Institut Fitoterapii.

Bashkuev, V. Yu. 2016. *Rossiyskaya meditsina i mongol'skiy mir: Istoricheskiy opyt vzaimodeystviya (konets XIX–pervaya polovina XX vv* [Russian Medicine and the Mongol World: Historical Experience of Interaction (End of the 19th–First Half of the 20th Centuries.)] Irkutsk: Izdatel'stvo Ottisk.

Bassin, M. 1991. "Russia between Europe and Asia: The Ideological Construction of Geographical Space." *Slavic Review* 50 (1): 1–17.

Bates, D. 1995. *Knowledge and the Scholarly Medical Traditions.* Cambridge and New York: Cambridge University Press.

Batomunkuev, S. D. 2004. "Znakovoye sobytiye i etnicheskaya obshchnost' (chto kampaniya protiv vyvoza Atlasa tibetskoy meditsiny rasskazala nam o sotsial'no-politicheskikh predpochteniyakh sovremennykh buryat" [Significant Event and Ethnic Commonality (What the Campaign against the Export of the Atlas of Tibetan Medicine Told Us about the Sociopolitical Preferences of Contemporary Buryats)]. *Vestnik Evrazii* 1:55–64.

Batorova, S. M., and T. Antzupova. 1989. *Rasteniya tibetskoy meditsiny: Opyt farmagnosticheskogo issledovaniya* [Plants in Tibetan Medicine: Experience of Pharmacological Research]. Novosibirsk: Izdatel'stvo Nauka.

Bauman, R. 2003. *Voices of Modernity: Language Ideologies and the Politics of Inequality.* Cambridge and New York: Cambridge University Press.

Bauman, R., and C. Briggs. 1990. "Poetics and Performance as Critical Perspectives on Language and Social Life." *Annual Review of Anthropology* 19:59–88.

Bazaron, E. G. 1989. *Ontsar gadon der dzod: Tibetskiy meditsinskiy traktat* [Ontsar gadon der dzod: Tibetan Medical Treatise]. Novosibirsk: Izdatel'stvo Nauka.

Bazaron, E. 1992. *Ocherki Tibetskoy Meditsiny* [Notes on Tibetan Medicine]. Ulan-Ude: Eko Art.

Bazaron, E. G., T. A. Aseeva, and V. È. Nazarov-Rygdylon. 1984. *"Vaydur'ya-onbo": traktat indo-tibetskoy meditsiny* [Vaudur'ya-onbo: A Treatise of Indo-Tibetan Medicine]. Novosibirsk: Izdatel'stvo Nauka.

Belyaev, D. 2010. "'Heterodox' Religiosity in Russia after the Fall of Communism: Does It Challenge 'Traditional' Religion?" *Religion, State & Society* 38 (2): 135–51.

Benjamin, W. 1997. "The Translator's Task." Translated by Steven Rendall. *TTR: Traduction, Terminologie, Rédaction: Etudes Sur Le Texte Et Ses Transformations.* 10:151–65.

Bennett, J. 2010. *Vibrant Matter: A Political Ecology of Things.* Durham, N.C.: Duke University Press.

Bennetts, M. 2010. "Faith Healer Anatoly Kashpirovsky: Russia's New Rasputin." *Observer*, June 5, 2010. https://www.theguardian.com/world/2010/jun/06/marc -bennetts-anatoly-kashpirovsky-russia-rasputin.

Bernstein, A. 2013. *Religious Bodies Politic: Rituals of Sovereignty in Buryat Buddhism.* Chicago: University of Chicago Press.

Biehl, J. 2005. *Vita: Life in a Zone of Social Abandonment.* Berkeley: University of California Press.

Biehl, J., B. Good, and A. Kleinman. 2007. *Subjectivity: Ethnographic Investigations.* Vol. 7. Berkeley: University of California Press.

Bobrovnitzky, I. P., A. M. Vasilenko, S. N. Nagornev, L. V. Tatarinova, and M. Yu. Yakovlev. 2012. "Personalizirovannaya vosstanovitel'naya meditsina: Fundamental'nyye i prikladnyye podkhody k meditsinskoy reabilitatsii i nelekarstvennoy profilaktike" [Perzonalized Restorative Medicine: Fundamental and Applied Approaches to Medical Rehabilitation and Nonpharmaceutical Prevention]. *Russian Journal of Rehabilitation Medicine,* 1:9–20.

Bocharov, V. V. 2011. *"Rossiyskaya vlast' v politiko-antropologicheskoy perspektive"* [Russian Power in a Political Anthropological Perspective]. *Polis (Politicheskiye Issledovaniya)* (6): 92–103.

Bogolyubov, V. M. 1985. "Kurortologiya i fizioterapiya" (Resort Medicine and Physiotherapy). Moscow: *Meditzina* 1:452.

Boronoev, V. V. 2010. "Opyt nauchnoy ob"yektivizatsii i avtomatizatsii metoda diagnostiki po pul'su" [Experience of Scientific Objectification and Automation of the Pulse Diagnosis Method]. In *Razvitiye traditsionnoy meditsiny v Rossii.* Ulan-Ud·e: GUZ RTsMP MZ RB.

Boronoev, V. V., V. D. Dashinimaev, and È. A. Trubacheez. 1988. "Datchiki pul'sa dlya prakticheskoy diagnostiki v tibetskoy meditsine" [Pulse Sensors for Practical Diagnosis in Tibetan Medicine]. In *Pul'sovaya diagnostika tibetskoy meditsiny.* Novosibirsk: Nauka.

Botkin, S. 1950. *Kurs Kliniki Vnutrennikh Bolezney i Klinicheskiye Lektsii* [Internal Medicine Course and Clinical Lectures]. Moscow: Medgiz.

Botkin, S. P. [1886] 2012. "Vvedeniye v Izucheniye Klinicheskoy Meditsiny (Rech' S. P. Botkina Na Torzhestvennom Akte Imperatorskoy Voyenno-Meditsinskoy Akademii 7 Dekabrya 1886 g.)" [Introduction to the Study of Clinical Medicine]. *Klinicheskaya Meditsina* 90 (9): 4–10.

Boykov, V. E., F. Fili, I. M. Sheyman, and S. Shishkin. 2000. "Uchastiye naselenia v finansirovanii zdravookhraneniya" [The Participation of the Population in the Financing of Healthcare]. *Zdravookhranenie* 2: 32–46.

Brainerd, E., and D. M. Cutler. 2005. "Autopsy on an Empire: Understanding Mortality in Russia and the Former Soviet Union." *Journal of Economic Perspectives* 19 (1): 107–30.

Brainerd, E., and E. Varavikova. 2001. *Death and the Market*. Prepared for the WHO Commission on Macroeconomics and Health.

Brekhman, I. 1980. *Chelovek i Biologicheski Aktivnyye Veshchestva* [The Human and Biologically Active Substances]. Moscow: Izdatel'stvo Nauka.

———. 1987. *Vvedeniye v Valeologiyu—Nauku o zdorov'ye* [Introduction to Valeology—The Science of Health]. Leningrad: Izdatel'stvo Nauka.

Briggs, C., and C. Mantini-Briggs. 2003. *Stories in the Time of Cholera: Racial Profiling during a Medical Nightmare*. Berkeley: University of California Press.

Brightman, M., V. Grotti, and O. Ulturgasheva. 2006. "Introduction: Rethinking the Frontier in Amazonia and Siberia: Extractive Economies, Indigenous Politics and Social Transformations." *Cambridge Anthropology* 26 (2): 1.

Broom, A., and P. Tovey. 2007. "Therapeutic Pluralism? Evidence, Power and Legitimacy in UK Cancer Services." *Sociology of Health & Illness* 29 (4): 551–69.

Brown, J., and N. Rusinova. 2002. "'Curing and Crippling': Biomedical and Alternative Healing in Post-Soviet Russia." *Annals of the American Academy of Political and Social Science* 583 (1): 160–72.

Brown, S. 2008. "Use of Complementary and Alternative Medicine by Physicians in St. Petersburg, Russia." *Journal of Alternative and Complementary Medicine* 14 (3): 315–19.

Buck-Quijada, J. B. 2020. "From Culture to Experience: Shamanism in the Pages of the Soviet Anti-Religious Press." *Contemporary European History* 29 (2): 187–201.

Buck-Morss, S. 2002. *Dreamworld and Catastrophe: The Passing of Mass Utopia in East and West*. Cambridge, Mass.: MIT Press.

Bulgakov, M. [1966] 1995. *The Master and Margarita*. New York: Vintage.

Burawoy, M., and K. Verdery. 1999. *Uncertain Transition: Ethnographies of Change in the Postsocialist World*. Lanham, Md.: Rowman & Littlefield.

Busygina, I., and E. Taukebaeva. 2015. "Federalism or a Unitary State as a Strategic Choice and Its Consequences (Comparative Analysis of Russia and Kazakhstan)." *Comparative Politics Russia* 6 (18): 101–10.

Buyandelger, M. 2013. *Tragic Spirits: Shamanism, Memory, and Gender in Contemporary Mongolia*. Chicago: University of Chicago Press.

Buyandelgeriyn, M. 2007. "Dealing with Uncertainty: Shamans, Marginal Capitalism, and the Remaking of History in Postsocialist Mongolia." *American Ethnologist* 34:127–47.

Caldwell, M. 2005. "A New Role for Religion in Russia's New Consumer Age: The Case of Moscow." *Religion, State & Society* 33 (1): 19–34.

Canguilhem, G. 1989. *The Normal and the Pathological*. New York: Zone.

Carr, E. S. 2010. "Enactments of Expertise." *Annual Review of Anthropology* 39: 17–32.

Cetina, K. K. 1999. *Epistemic Cultures: How the Sciences make Knowledge*. Cambridge, Mass.: Harvard University Press.

Chadha, A. 2010. "Cryptographic Imagination: Indus Script and the Project of Scientific Decipherment." *Indian Economic & Social History Review* 47 (2): 141–77.

Chari, S., and K. Verdery. 2009. "Thinking between the Posts: Postcolonialism, Postsocialism, and Ethnography after the Cold War." *Comparative Studies in Society and History* 51 (1): 6–34.

Charles, L. 1980. "Medical Pluralism in World Perspective." *Social Science & Medicine*. 14 (4): 191–95.

Chebankova, E. 2005. "The Limitations of Central Authority in the Regions and the Implications for the Evolution of Russia's Federal System." *Europe-Asia Studies* 57 (7): 933–49.

———. 2007. "Putin's Struggle for Federalism: Structures, Operation, and the Commitment Problem." *Europe-Asia Studies* 59 (2): 279–302.

Choyzhinimaeva, S. G. 2010a. *Kak Zhit' ne Boleya: Iz Praktiki Vracha Tibetskoy Meditsiny* [How to Live without Getting Sick: From the Practice of a Tibetan Medicine Doctor]. Moscow: Izdatel'stvo ZebraE.

———. 2010b. *Tayny tibetskoy meditsiny v praktike doktora S. G. Choyzhinimayevoy* [Secrets of Tibetan Medicine in the Practice of Doctor S. G. Choyzhinimaeva]. Moscow: Izdatel'stvo Redazktsiya Vestnik ZOZh.

Chrysanthou, M. 2002. "Transparency and Selfhood: Utopia and the Informed Body." *Social Science & Medicine* 54 (3): 469–79.

Chudakova, T. 2017. "Caring for Strangers: Aging, Traditional Medicine, and Collective Self-Care in Post-Socialist Russia." *Medical Anthropology Quarterly* 31 (1): 78–96.

Cohen, L. 1995. *The Epistemological Carnival: Meditations on Disciplinary Intentionality and Ayurveda*. Knowledge and the Scholarly Medical Traditions. Cambridge: Cambridge University Press.

Comaroff, J. and J. L. Comaroff. 1999. "Occult Economies and the Violence of Abstraction: Notes from the South African Postcolony." *American Ethnologist* 26 (2): 279–303.

Comaroff, J. L., and J. Comaroff. 2009. *Ethnicity, Inc*. Chicago: University of Chicago Press.

Connor, L., and G. Samuel. 2001. *Healing Powers and Modernity: Traditional Medicine, Shamanism, and Science in Asian Societies*. Westport, Conn.: Bergin & Garvey.

Conroy, M. 2006. *The Soviet Pharmaceutical Business during the First Two Decades (1917–1937)*. New York: Peter Lang.

Coulter, I., and E. Willis. 2004. "The Rise and Rise of Complementary and Alternative Medicine: A Sociological Perspective." *Medical Journal of Australia* 180 (11): 587–90.

Craig, S. 2011. "'Good' Manufacturing by Whose Standards? Remaking Concepts of Quality, Safety, and Value in the Production of Tibetan Medicines." *Anthropological Quarterly* 84 (2): 331–78.

Csordas, T. 1993. "Somatic Modes of Attention." *Cultural Anthropology* 8 (2): 135–56.

Dagbaev, E. D. 2010. "'Buryatskaya etnicheskaya identichnost': Mezhdu traditsiyey i modernizatsiyey." *Vestnik Buryatskogo gosudarstvennogo universiteta. Pedagogika. Filologiya. Filosofiya* 6:134–41.

Danishevski, K., D. Balabanova, M. Mckee, and S. Atkinson. 2006. "The Fragmentary Federation: Experiences with the Decentralized Health System in Russia." *Health Policy and Planning* 21 (3): 183–94.

Danishevskiy, G. M. 1934. *Problemy Massovogo Otdykha v SSSR* [The Problems of Mass Recreation in the USSR]. Moscow: Profizdat.

Dashiev, D. B. 2009. *Kunpan-dudzi: Poleznyy dlya vsekh ekstrakt amrity; Bol'shoy retsepturnyy spravochnik Aginskogo datsana* [Kunpan-dudzi: Beneficial to All Extract of Amrita: Great Formulary of the Aginsk Buddhist Temple]. Moscow: Izdatel'skaya Firma "Fostochnaya Literatura," RAN.

Daston, L., and P. Galison. 2007. *Objectivity*. Brooklyn, N.Y.: Zone.

Davydkin, N. F. 2002. "Fizioterapiya i kurortologiya dolzhna byt' otdel'noy i edinoy vrachebnoy i nauchnoy spetsial'nost'yu" [Physiotherapy and Resort Medicine Should Be a Single Medical and Scientific Specialization]. In *Trudy vserossiyskogo s"yezda fizioterapevtov i kurortologov i rossiyskogo nauchnogo foruma*. Moscow: Morag Ekspo.

De la Cadena, M. 2010. "Indigenous Cosmopolitics in the Andes: Conceptual Reflections Beyond 'Politics.'" *Cultural Anthropology* 25 (2): 334–70.

Dorzhiev, A. 1994. *Predanie o Krugosvetnom Puteshestvii, Ili, Povestvovanie o Zhizni Agvana Dorzhieva* [The Myth of the Travel around the World, or a Tale of the Life of Agvan Dorzhiev]. Ulan-Udė: Olzon, BNC SO-RAN.

Dreger, Christian, et al. "Between the Hammer and the Anvil: The Impact of Economic Sanctions and Oil Prices on Russia's Ruble." *Journal of Comparative Economics* 44, no. 2 (2016).

Dudin, S. A. 1993. *Lekarstvennoye syr'yë tibetskoy meditsiny* [The Medicinal Substances of Tibetan Medicine]. Ulan-Ude: Olzon.

Dukhovsky, S. 1896. Letter to I. L. Goremykin. ["The Case of the Police Department Proceedings Concerning the Buryat Doctor Petr Aleksandrovich Badmaev from 1899"]. GARF, f. 102, d. 1665.

Dulganov, K. P. 2009. *O khode istoricheskogo razvitiya tibetskoy meditsiny v Baykal'skom regione* [About the Historical Development of Tibetan Medicine in the Baikal Region]. Ulan-Ude: Izdatel'stvo Buryatskogo Universiteta.

Dumit, J. 2012. *Drugs for Life: How Pharmaceutical Companies Define Our Health.* Durham, N.C.: Duke University Press.

Dzuba, V. F., V. A. Nikolaevskyi, V. M. Sherbakov, and I. M. Korenskaya. 2004. *Lekarstvennyye rasteniya v fitoterapii: Prakticheskoye posobiye dlya studentov i provizorov-internov po spetsial'nosti 060108 (040500) – farmatsiya* [Medicinal Plants in Phytotherapy: Practical Manual for Students and Interns for the Specialty 060108 (040500)]. Voronezh: Izdatel'stvo VGU.

Egorov, V. V. 2010. "Pravovoye Regulirovaniye Deyatel'nosti Fizioterapevtov i Travnikov" [The Legal Regulation of the Activity of Phytotherapists and Herbalists]. In *Materialy 2go Mezhdunarodnogo S"ezda Fizioterapevtov i Travnikov: "Sovremennye problem fitoterapii i etnicheskogo travnichestva."* Moscow: Institut Fitoterapii.

E. P. 1933. "Tibetskaya Meditsina Imperialistkoy Pechati" [Tibetan Medicine of the Imperial Press]. *Izvestiia* 102, April 18, 1933.

Escobar, A. 1999. "After Nature: Steps to an Antiessentialist Political Ecology." *Current Anthropology* 40 (1): 1–30.

Esposito, R. 2008. *Bios: Biopolitics and Philosophy.* Vol. 4. Minneapolis: University of Minnesota Press.

Etkin, N. 2008. *Edible Medicines: An Ethnopharmacology of Food.* Tucson: University of Arizona Press.

"Eto kurs na investitsii v cheloveka, a znachit, i v budushcheye Rossii." *Rossiyskaya Gazeta,* September 7, 2005.

Fadlon, J. 2004. "Meridians, Chakras and Psycho-Neuro-Immunology: The Dematerializing Body and the Domestication of Alternative Medicine." *Body & Society* 10 (4): 69–86.

Farquhar, J. 1994. *Knowing Practice: The Clinical Encounter of Chinese Medicine.* Boulder, Colo.: Westview.

———. 1996. "Market Magic: Getting Rich and Getting Personal in Medicine after Mao." *American Ethnologist* 23 (2): 239–57.

———. 2002. *Appetites: Food and Sex in Postsocialist China.* Durham, N.C.: Duke University Press.

———. 2014. "Reading Hands: Pulse Qualities and the Specificity of the Clinical." *East Asian Science, Technology and Society: An International Journal* 8 (1): 9–24.

Fassin, D. 2009. "Another Politics of Life Is Possible." *Theory, Culture & Society* 26 (5): 44–60.

Field, M. 2000. "Soviet Medicine." In *Medicine in the Twentieth Century.* Amsterdam: Harwood Academic.

Foucault, M. 2006. "Utopian Body." In *Sensorium: Embodied Experience, Technology, and Contemporary Art.* Cambridge Mass.: MIT Press.

Freud, S., D. McLintock, and H. Haughton. 2003. *The Uncanny.* New York: Penguin.

Fries, C. 2008. "Governing the Health of the Hybrid Self: Integrative Medicine, Neoliberalism, and the Shifting Biopolitics of Subjectivity." *Health Sociology Review* 17 (4): 353–67.

Gal, S. 1991. "Bartok's Funeral: Representations of Europe in Hungarian Political Rhetoric." *American Ethnologist* 18 (3): 440–58.

———. 2003. "Movements of Feminism: The Circulation of Discourses about Women." In *Recognition, Struggles, and Social Movements: Contested Identity, Agency, and Power*. Cambridge: Cambridge University Press.

Galison, P. 1999. "Trading Zone: Coordinating Action and Belief." In *The Science Studies Reader*. New York: Routledge.

Gammerman, A. F. 1966. *Primeneniye solodki v meditsine narodov Vostko: Voprosy izucheniya I ispol'zovaniya solodki v SSSR* [The Use of Licorice in the Medicine among the Peoples of the East: Questions of Research and Usage of Licorice in the USSR]. Moscow and Leningrad: Izdatel'stvo Nauka.

Gammerman, A. F., and B. V. Semichov. 1963. *Slovar' tibetsko-latinsko-russkikh nazvaniy lekarstvennogo rastitel'nogo syr'ya, primenyayemogo v tibetskoy med-itsine* [Dictionary of Tibetan-Latin-Russian Names of Medicinal Botanicals used in Tibetan Medicine]. Ulan-Udė: Buryat. filial izd-va AN SSSR.

Gammerman, A. F., and M. D. Shupinskaja. 1937. "Predvaritel'noye khimich-eskoye issledovaniye lekarstvennogo syr'ya tibetskoy meditsiny, sobrannogo zabaykal'skoy ekspeditsiyey VIEM" [Initial Clinical Study of Tibetan Medi-cine Compounds Collected during VIEM's Trans-Baikal Expedition]. *Farmat-siya i farmakologiya*, 3–4:20–31.

Garcia, A. 2010. *The Pastoral Clinic: Addiction and Dispossession along the Rio Grande*. Berkeley: University of California Press.

Gerovitch, S. 2004. *From Newspeak to Cyberspeak: A History of Soviet Cybernet-ics*. Cambridge, Mass.: MIT Press.

Glebov, S. 2011. "Postcolonial Empire? Russian Orientologists and the Politics of Knowledge in Late Imperial Russia." *Ab Imperio* 1 (3): 385–92.

Godik, E. 2010. *Zagadka Ekstrasensov: Chto uvideli fiziki.* [The Riddle of the Extrasensy: What the Physicists Saw]. Moscow: Ast.

Gordeev, V., M. Pavlova, and W. Groot. 2011. "Two Decades of Reforms: Appraisal of the Financial Reforms in the Russian Public Healthcare Sector." *Health Policy* 102 (2): 270–77.

Gordeeva, O. B. 2013. "Tibetskaya meditsina u staroobryadtsev Baykal'skoy Sibiri v 30–50e gg. XX veka" [Tibetan Medicine among the Staroobryadsty of the Baikal Siberian Region in the 1930–50s of the 20th Century]. In *Izvestiia Irkutskogo gosudarstvennogo universiteta*, 2:1. Seriya: Politologiya. Religiovedenie.

Goremykin, I. L. 1897. Letter to Dukhovsky. March 26. GARF, F. 102, d. 1665.

Goryunov, A. V., and R. G. Kholpushin. 2005. "Rynok traditsionnoy meditsiny Sankt-Peterburga" [The Market of Traditional Medicine in St. Petersburg]. *Zhurnal Sotsiologii i Sotsial'noy Antropologii* 8 (1): 179–85.

Graan, Andrew. 2013. "Transitology Revisited, or How the Trials of Postsocialism Forecast the Precarity of Neoliberal Capitalism." *Anthropology News* 54 (10).

Graham, L. 1993. *Science in Russia and the Soviet Union: A Short History.* Cambridge and New York: Cambridge University Press.

Greenhalgh, T., and S. Wessely. 2004. "'Health for Me': A Sociocultural Analysis of Healthism in the Middle Classes." *British Medical Bulletin* 69 (1): 197–213.

Grekova, T. I. 1998. *Tibetskaya Meditsina v Rossii: Istoriya v Sud'bakh i Litsakh* [Tibetan Medicine in Russia: A History of Fates and People]. St. Petersburg: Aton.

———. 2002. *Tibetskiĭ Lekar' Kremlevskikh Vozhdeĭ* [Tibetan Doctor of Kremlin Leaders]. St. Petersburg and Moscow: Izdatel'skiĭ Dom "Neva" and Olma-Press.

Grekova, T. I., and K. A. Lange. 1994. "Tragicheskiye stranitsy istorii institutta eksperimental'no·y meditsiny (20–30 gody)" [Tragic Pages of the History of the Institute for Experimental Medicine (the 20–30s)]. *Repressirovannaya Nauka* 1:9–24.

Gross Solomon, S. 2004. "Social Hygiene in the Soviet Union." In *Health, Disease and Society in Europe, 1800–1930: A Sourcebook*, edited by Deborah Brunton. Manchester: Manchester University Press.

Grosz, E. 2005. *Time Travels: Feminism, Nature, Power.* Durham, N.C.: Duke University Press.

Hammer, O. 2001. *Claiming Knowledge: Strategies of Epistemology from Theosophy to the New Age.* Leiden and Boston: Brill.

Haraway, D. 1994. "A Manifesto for Cyborgs: Science, Technology, and Socialist Feminism in the 1980s." In *The Postmodern Turn: New Perspectives on Social Theory.* Cambridge: Cambridge University Press.

Hardiman, David, and Projit Bihari Mukharji. 2012. *Medical Marginality in South Asia: Situating Subaltern Therapeutics.* New York: Routledge.

Harding, S. 2013. "Beyond Postcolonial Theory: Two Undertheorized Perspectives on Science and Technology." In *Women, Science, and Technology.* New York: Routeledge.

Harrison, S. 2003. "Cultural Difference as Denied Resemblance: Reconsidering Nationalism and Ethnicity." *Comparative Studies in Society and History* 45 (2): 343–61.

Hart, R. 1999. "From Copula to Incommensurable Worlds." In *Tokens of Exchange: The Problem of Translation in Global Circulations.* Durham, N.C: Duke University Press.

Heelas, P. 1996. *The New Age Movement: The Celebration of the Self and the Sacral-ization of Modernity*. Cambridge, Mass.: Blackwell.

Hevia, J. L. 1995. *Cherishing Men from Afar: Qing Guest Ritual and the Macartney Embassy of 1793*. Durham, N.C.: Duke University Press.

Hirsch, F. 2005. *Empire of Nations*. Ithaca, N.Y.: Cornell University Press.

Hofer, T. 2018. *Medicine and Memory in Tibet: Amchi Physicians in an Age of Reform*. Seattle: University of Washington Press.

Hogle, L. F. 2005. "Enhancement Technologies and the Body." *Annual Review of Anthropology* 34 (1): 695–716.

Hrycak, A. 2006. "Foundation Feminism and the Articulation of Hybrid Femi-nisms in Post-Socialist Ukraine." *East European Politics and Societies* 20 (1): 69–100.

Irvine, J. T., and S. Gal. 2011. "Language Ideology and Linguistic Differentiation. In *Linguistic Anthropology: A Reader*. Chichester: Wiley-Blackwell.

Ivanov, P. K. [1951] 1993. *Istoriya i Metod Moyey Zakalki*. Dnepropetrovsk: Porogi.

Jain, S. L. 2010. "The Mortality Effect: Counting the Dead in the Cancer Trial." *Public Culture* 22 (1): 89–117.

Jambaldorje, and Y. Z. Zhabon. 2011. *Dzeytskhar-migchzhan: Mongolo-tibetskiy istochnik po istorii kul'tury i traditsionnoy meditsine XIX v* [Dzeytskhar-migchzhan: A Mongol-Tibetan Source on the Culture of Traditional Medicine of the 19th Century]. Translated from Tibetan by Y. Z. Zhabon. Ulan-Ude: OAO Respublikanskaya Tipografiya.

Janes, C. 2002. "Buddhism, Science, and Market: The Globalisation of Tibetan Medicine." *Anthropology & Medicine* 9 (3): 267–89.

Jašarević, L. 2017. *Health and Wealth on the Bosnian Market: Intimate Debt*. Bloomington: Indiana University Press.

Joravsky, D. 2010. *The Lysenko Affair*. Chicago: University of Chicago Press.

Kagarlitsky, B. 2002. *Russia under Yeltsin and Putin: Neo-Liberal Autocracy*. Lon-don and Sterling, Va.: Pluto.

Kagarlitsky, B., J. L. Twigg, and K. Schecter. 2003. "Ethnic Problems and National Issues in Contemporary Russian Society." In *Social Capital and Social Cohe-sion in Post-Soviet Russia*. Armonk, N.Y.: M. E. Sharpe.

Kaptchuk, T. J., and D. Eisenberg. 1998. "The Persuasive Appeal of Alternative Medicine." *Annals of Internal Medicine* 129 (12): 1061–65.

Karpeev, A. A., T. L. Kiseleva, Y. I. Korshikova, and E. I. Sakanyan. 2006. *Fitoter-apiya: Metodicheskiye Rekomendatsii MZ RF 2000/63* [Phytotherapy: Method-ological Recommendations for the Ministry of Health of the Russian Federation 2000/63]. Moscow: Izdatel'stvo FNKETS TMDL Roszdrava.

Kashkadamov, V. P. 1936. *Doklad predsedatelya initsiativnoy gruppy po izucheniyu tibestkoy meditsiny prof. V.P Kashkodamova ot 31ogo marta 1936 g* [Report by the Chairman of the Initiative Group for the Study of Tibetan Medicine, Prof. V.P. Kashkadamov]. GARF f. A 482, o. 25, d. 1146, l. 2–3.

Kayne, S. 2010. *Traditional Medicine: A Global Perspective*. London and Chicago: Pharmaceutical Press.

Keane, W. 2007. *Christian Moderns: Freedom and Fetish in the Mission Encounter*. Berkeley: University of California Press.

Keshet, Y., and A. Popper-Giveon. 2013. "Integrative Health Care in Israel and Traditional Arab Herbal Medicine: When Health Care Interfaces with Culture and Politics." *Medical Anthropology Quarterly* 27 (3): 368–84.

Kevles, B. 1997. *Naked to the Bone: Medical Imaging in the Twentieth Century*. New Brunswick, N.J.: Rutgers University Press.

Khmelnitskaya, M. 2017. "The Social Budget Policy Process in Russia at a Time of Crisis." *Post-Communist Economies* 29 (4): 457–75.

Khundanov, L. L., T. B. Batomunkueva, and L. L. Khundanova. 1993. *Tibetskaya Meditsina* [Tibetan Medicine]. Moscow: Izdatel'stvo Prometey.

Khundanov, L., L. Khundanova, and E. Bazaron. 1979. *Slovo o tibetskoy meditsine* [A Word on Tibetan Medicine]. Ulan-Ude: Buryatskoye Knizhnoye Izdatel'stvo.

Kichigina, G. 2009. *The Imperial Laboratory: Experimental Physiology and Clinical Medicine in Post-Crimean Russia*. Vol. 87. Amsterdam, N.Y.: Rodopi.

King, F. 2005. "Rural Healthcare in Russia, 1864–1914: A Northern Case-Study." In *Health and Medicine in Rural Europe: 1850–1945*, edited by Josep Lluís Barona and Steven Cherry. València: Seminari d'Estudis sobre la Ciència.

Kleinman, A. 1980. *Patients and Healers in the Context of Culture: An Exploration of the Borderland between Anthropology, Medicine, and Psychiatry*. Berkeley: University of California Press.

Kloos, S. 2010. "Tibetan Medicine in Exile: The Ethics, Politics and Science of Cultural Survival." Ph.D. diss. University of California Berkeley.

Kloos, S., H. Madhavan, T. Tidwell, C. Blaikie, and M. Cuomu. 2020. "The Transnational Sowa Rigpa Industry in Asia: New Perspectives on an Emerging Economy." *Social Science & Medicine* 245:1–12.

Klyuchevskaya, E. 2010. "'Zolotoy Koren': Vyrashchivaniye Lekarstvennykh Rasteniy Mozhet Stat' Pribyl'nym Biznesom" [Golden Root: The Cultivation of Medicinal Plants Might Become a Lucrative Business]. *Rossiyskaya Gazeta*. June 9, 2011.

Kuz'min, A. V., ed. 2010. *Imidzh strany/regiona kak strategiya integratsii Rossii i ATR v XXI veke* [The Image of the Country/Region as a Strategy for Integrating Russia and APAC]. Ulan-Ude: VSGTU.

Kogan, G. 1936. *Tezisy k dokladu prof. Gammerman* [Abstracts from the Report of Prof. Gammerman]. GARF f. A-482, o. 25, d. 1146.

Kondakova-Varlamova, L. P. 1978. "Zakalivanie." In *Bol'shaya Sovetskaya Entsiklopediya Tret'ye izdaniye ed.* Vol. 29. Moscow: Sovetskaya Entsiklopediya.

Korobeĭnikov, G. V. 1995. "Fiziologicheskiye mekhanizmy mobilizatsii funktsional'nykh rezervov organizma cheloveka pri napryazhennoy myshechnoy deyatel'nosti" [The Physiological Mechanisms of Mobilizing Functional Reserves of the Organisms during Intense Muscular Activity]. *Fiziologiya Cheloveka* 21 (3): 81–86.

Kosoburov, A. A. 2006. *Lekarstvennoye syr'ye tibetskoy meditsiny: Sovremennyy vzglyad* [Medicinal Compounds of Tibetan Medicine: A Contemporary View]. Ulan-Ude: Izdatel'stvo BNC So RAN.

———. 2011. *Samten: Uchebnik Tibetskoy Meditsiny; Novyy Rassvet ili Kratkaya Sut' Meditsiny* [Samten: Manual of Tibetan Medicine; New Dawn or the Brief Essence of Medicine]. Ulan-Ude: Izdatel'stvo BNC So RAN.

Kozhevnikov, V. et al. 2010. "Traditsionnaya Meditsina: Sostoyaniye i Perspektivy Integratsii s Sovremennym Zdravookhraneniye" [Traditional Medicine: Present State and Possibilities of Integration in Contemporary Healthcare]. In *Razvitie Tradictzionnoy Meditziny v Rossii*, edited by V. Kozhevnikov et al. Ulan-Ude: Izdatel'stvo Guz RTsMP MZ RB.

Krementsov, N. 2006. "Big Revolution, Little Revolution: Science and Politics in Bolshevik Russia." *Social Research: An International Quarterly* 73 (4): 1173–1204.

———. 2011. *A Martian Stranded on Earth: Alexander Bogdanov, Blood Transfusions, and Proletarian Science.* Chicago: University of Chicago Press.

Krippner, S. 1986. "Soviet and American Perspectives on Hidden Reserves and Human Potentials." *Journal of Humanistic Psychology* 26 (4): 84–97.

Kuriyama, S. 1999. *The Expressiveness of the Body and the Divergence of Greek and Chinese Medicine.* New York: Zone.

Kuzmin, A. 2010. "Buryatiya—Serdtse Rossii v Azii" [Buryatia—The Heart of Russia in Asia]. *Delovoy Mir Baykala* (6) 1.

Landecker, H. 2011. "Food as Exposure: Nutritional Epigenetics and the New Metabolism." *Biosocieties* 6 (2): 167–94.

Langwick, S. 2008. "Articulate(d) Bodies: Traditional Medicine in a Tanzanian Hospital." *American Ethnologist* 35 (3): 428–39.

Laruelle, M. 2004. "The Two Faces of Contemporary Eurasianism: An Imperial Version of Russian Nationalism." *Nationalities Papers* 32 (1): 115–36.

———. 2009. *In the Name of the Nation: Nationalism and Politics in Contemporary Russia.* Palgrave Macmillan.

Latour, B. 1987. *Science in Action: How to Follow Scientists and Engineers through Society.* Cambridge, Mass.: Harvard University Press.

———. 1993. *We have Never Been Modern.* Cambridge, Mass.: Harvard University Press.

Laughlin, C. 1997. "The Evolution of Cyborg Consciousness." *Anthropology of Consciousness* 8 (4): 144–59.

Ledeneva, A. 1998. *Russia's Economy of Favours: Blat, Networking and Informal Exchange*. Vol. 102. Cambridge: Cambridge University Press.

Ledneva, I. P. 2011. "O Teoreticheskikh osnovakh tibetskoy meditsiny" [On the Theoretical Foundations of Tibetan Medicine]. *Vestnik Buryatskogo Gosudarsvennogo universiteta* 12.

Lemon, A. 2009. "Sympathy for the Weary State?: Cold War Chronotopes and Moscow Others." *Comparative Studies in Society and History* 51 (4): 832–64.

———. 2018. *Technologies for Intuition: Cold War Circles and Telepathic Tays*. Oakland: University of California Press.

Leslie, C. 1980. "Medical Pluralism in World Perspective." *Social Science & Medicine* 14 (4): 191–95.

Leslie, C., M. Nichter, and M. Lock. 2002. *New Horizons in Medical Anthropology: Essays in Honour of Charles Leslie*. London and New York: Routledge.

Lindquist, G. 2005. "Healers, Leaders and Entrepreneurs: Shamanic Revival in Southern Siberia." *Culture & Religion* 6 (2): 263–85.

———. 2006. *Conjuring Hope: Magic and Healing in Contemporary Russia*. New York: Berghahn.

Lock, M. 1990. "Rationalization of Japanese Herbal Medication: The Hegemony of Orchestrated Pluralism." *Human Organization* 49 (1): 41–46.

———. 2001a. "The Tempering of Medical Anthropology: Troubling Natural Categories." *Medical Anthropology Quarterly* 15 (4): 478–92.

———. 2001b. *Twice Dead: Organ Transplants and the Reinvention of Death*. Berkeley: University of California Press.

———. 2002. "Symptom Reporting at Menopause: A Review of Cross-Cultural Findings." *Menopause International* 8 (4): 132–36.

Lock, M., and J. Farquhar. 2007. *Beyond the Body Proper: Reading the Anthropology of Material Life*. Durham, N.C.: Duke University Press.

Lock, M., and V. K. Nguyen. 2018. *An Anthropology of Biomedicine*. Chichester, West Sussex, and Malden, Mass.: Wiley-Blackwell.

Lock, M., W. Burke, J. Dupré, H. Landecker, J. Livingston, P. Martin, M. Meloni, G. Pálsson, R. Rapp, K. M. Weiss, and A. V. Buchanan. 2015. "Comprehending the Body in the Era of the Epigenome." *Current Anthropology* 56 (2): 163–64.

Logvinov, V. S. 1988. Predislovie [Introduction]. In *Pul'sovaya diagnostika tibetskoy meditsiny* [Pulse Diagnostics in Tibetan Medicine], edited by C. T. Tsydypov. Novosibirsk: Nauka.

Luehrmann, S. 2005. "Recycling Cultural Construction: Desecularisation in Postsoviet Mari El." *Religion, State and Society* 33 (1): 35–56.

Makarova, V. 2001. *V Budusheye s Optimizmom* [Into the Future with Optimism]. *Nauka v Sibiri* 36 (2322): 3.

Malakhov, G. P. 2003. *Zakalivaniye i vodolecheniye* [Tempering and Water Therapy]. Donetsk: Stalker.

Manning, N., and N. E. Tikhonova. 2016. *Health and Health Care in the New Russia*. London: Taylor and Francis.

Marishuk, V. L. 1983. "Pereraspredeleniye funktsional'nykh rezervov v organizme sportsmen kak pokazatel' stressa" [Redistribution of Functional Reserves of an Athlete's Organism as an Indicator of Stress]. In *Trevoga i stress v sporte*. Moscow: Fizkul'tura i Sport.

Marshak, M. E. 1957. *Fiziologicheskiye osnovy zakalivaniya organizma cheloveka* [Physiological Basis for the Tempering of the Human Organism]. Moscow: Medgiz.

Marsland, R., and R. Prince. 2012. "What Is Life Worth? Exploring Biomedical Interventions, Survival, and the Politics of Life." *Medical Anthropology Quarterly* 26 (4): 453–69.

Martin, T. 2001. *The Affirmative Action Empire: Nations and Nationalism in the Soviet Union, 1923–1939*. Ithaca, N.Y.: Cornell University Press.

Martínez, F. 2012. "The Erotic Biopower of Putinism: From Glamour to Pornography." *Laboratorium: Russian Review of Social Research* 4 (3).

Matza, T. 2009. "Moscow's Echo: Technologies of the Self, Publics, and Politics on the Russian Talk Show." *Cultural Anthropology* 24 (3): 489–522.

———. 2012. "'Good Individualism'? Psychology, Ethics, and Neoliberalism in Postsocialist Russia." *American Ethnologist* 39 (4): 804–18.

Michaels, P. 2000. "Medical Propaganda and Cultural Revolution in Soviet Kazakhstan, 1928–41." *Russian Review* 59 (2): 159–78.

Mikhel, D. 2004. "Meditsinskaya Antropologiya: Chto Eto Takoye?" [What Is Medical Anthropology?] *Kul'turologiya: Teoriya, Shkoly, Istoriya, Praktika*. http://www.countries.ru/library/antropology/medant.htm.

———. 2009. "Sotsial'naya istoriya meditsiny: Stanovleniye i problematika" [Social History of Medicine: Establishment and Problems]. *Zhurnal Issledovaniy Sotsial'noy Politiki* 7 (3): 3.

Mirskiy, M. 2005. *Meditsina Rossii X–XX Vekov: Ocherki Istorii* [Russian Medicine X–XX Centuries: Historical Outlines]. Moscow: Rosspèn Rossiyskaya Politicheskaya Entsiklopediya.

Mitypov, V. M. 2011. "Gosudarstvo i buddiyskaya tserkov' v SSSR/Rossii: osnovnyye aspekty zakonodatel'nykh otnosheniy" [State and the Buddhist Church in the USSR/Russia: Main Aspects of Legislative Relations]. *Vlast'* 5:13–17.

Mitypova, G. S. 2006. *K voprosu ob istoricheskom poselenii shkoly tibetskoy meditsiny na territorii Atsagatskogo Arshana* [About the Question of Historical Settlement of the School of Tibetan Medicine on the Territory of the Atsagat Arshan]. In *Buddiyskaya traditsiya: istoriya i sovremennost': Yubileynyye chteniya, posvyashchennyye 150-letiyu so dnya rozhdeniya Agvana Lobsana Dorzhiyeva. Materialy konferentsii 25—27noyabrya 2004 g*. St. Petersburg: IVR RAN.

Mol, A. 2002. *The Body Multiple: Ontology in Medical Practice*. Durham, N.C.: Duke University Press.

Mudrov, M. 2008. (1820) *Slovo o sposobe uchit' i uchit'sya meditsine prakticheskoy ili deyatel'nomu vrachebnomu iskusstvu pri postelyakh bol'nykh* [A Word on the Means to Teach and Learn Practical Medicine, or the Practice of Medical Art at the Bedside]. Moscow: Direkt Midia.

Muzalevsky, V. M. 2007. "Institualizatsiya Traditsionnoy Meditsiny v Sovremennoy Rossii" [Institutionalizing Traditional Medicine in Contemporary Russia]. Ph.D. diss. Volgograd: VGMU.

Myasnikov, A. 2007. "Myasnikov, A. L. o Botkine" [Myasnikov on Botkin]. *Kardiologicheskiy Vestnik* 2 (1) 57–60.

Nagornykh, O.S. 2017. "K biografii professora V.G. Vogralika: Metod igloreflekso- terapii i aspekty sovetsko-kitayskikh otnosheniy v 1950-e gody" [Toward a Biography of Professor V. G. Vogralik: Acupuncture Method and Aspects of Soviet-Chinese Relations in the 1950s]. *Istoriya Meditsiny* 4 (4): 437–46.

Nagornykh, O. S., and N. P. Shok. 2020. "Komandirovki Sovetskikh Vrachey v KNR v 1950-1960-e Gg.: Realizatsiya Planov Sotrudnichestva v Sfere Meditsiny i Zdravookhraneniya" [Business Trips of Soviet Doctors to the PRC in the 1950s–1960s: Implementation of the Plans for Cooperation in the Sphere of Medicine and Healthcare]. *Vestnik Tomskogo Gosudarstvennogo Universiteta. Istoriya* 65: 75–85.

Nichter, M., and J. Thompson. 2006. "For My Wellness, Not Just My Illness: North Americans' Use of Dietary Supplements." *Culture, Medicine and Psychiatry* 30 (2): 175–222.

Nikolaev, S. 1998. *Tibetskaya Meditsina: Voprosy i Otvety* [Tibetan Medicine: Questions and Answers]. Ulan-Ude: Buryatskiy Gosudarstvennyy Universitet.

Novas, C. 2006. "The Political Economy of Hope: Patients' Organizations, Science and Biovalue." *Biosocieties* 1 (3): 289.

Ochirova, G. N. 2001. "Svedeniya o lamakh i miryanakh, praktikovavshiye tibet- skuyu meditsinu v 1928 g." [Information on Lamas and Laymen Practicing Tibetan Medicine in 1928]. In *Ivolginskiy Datsan: Istoriya, Sovremennost', i Perspektivy*. Ivolga: "Dashi Choykhorlin."

Ol'khovskiĭ, A., and S. Tikhonov. 2010. *Zdravookhraneniye Rossii: Dvadtsat' Let Reform, Kotorykh Ne Bylo* [Healthcare in Russia: Twenty Years of Reforms That Weren't]. St. Petersburg: Nestor Istoriya.

Olson, V. 2010. "The Ecobiopolitics of Space Biomedicine." *Medical Anthropology* 29 (2): 170–93.

Ong, Aihwa. 1987. *Spirits of Resistance and Capitalist Discipline: Factory Women in Malaysia*. 2nd ed. Suny Series in the Anthropology of Work. Albany: State University of New York Press.

Osipova, N. 2003. "Etapy razvitiya refleksoterapii v strane" [Stages of Development of Reflexotherapy in the State]. *Perspektivy traditsionnoy meditsiny* 1:1–9.

Osnovy Zakonodatel'Stva Rossijskoy Federatzii Ob Okhrane Zdorovya Grazhdan [Russian Federation Legislative Foundations of Health Protection for Citizens]. 1993. 5487–1 (67).

Palmer, D. 2007. "Qigong Fever: Body, Science and Utopia in China." *China Quarterly* 193: 172–206.

Panchenko, A. 2004. "New Religious Movements and the Study of Folklore: The Russian Case." *Folklore (Tartu)* 28.

Parfenov, A. P. 1960. *Zakalivanie Cheloveka* [The Tempering of the Human]. Leningrad: Medgiz.

Parfitt, T. 2005. "Russian Politicians Fight to Legislate Against 'False Science.'" *Lancet* 36:1597–98.

Parsons, M. 2014. *Dying Unneeded: The Cultural Context of the Russian Mortality Crisis*. Nashville, Tenn.: Vanderbilt University Press.

Pedersen, M. A. 2011. *Not Quite Shamans: Spirit Worlds and Political Lives in Northern Mongolia*. Ithaca, N.Y.: Cornell University Press.

Perrow, C. 2011. *Normal Accidents: Living with High-Risk Technologies*. Princeton, N.J.: Princeton University Press.

Pertsov, I. A., ed. 1939. *The Health Resorts of the USSR: A Symposium of Articles Compiled from Data of the Central Institute of Balneology in Moscow*. Moscow: U.S.S.R. Society of Cultural Relations with Foreign Countries (V.O.K.S.).

Petryna, A. 2002. *Life Exposed: Biological Citizens after Chernobyl*. Princeton, N.J.: Princeton University Press.

Pordié, L. ed. 2008. *Tibetan Medicine in the Contemporary World: Global Politics of Medical Knowledge and Practice*. London: Routledge.

———. 2012. "Tibetan Medicine Today: Neo-Traditionalism as an Analytical Lens and a Political Tool." In *Tibetan Medicine in the Contemporary World: Global Politics of Medical Knowledge and Practice*. London: Routledge.

Pozdneev, A. M. [1908] 1991. *Uchebnik Tibetskoy Meditsiny* [Manual of Tibetan Medicine]. St. Petersburg: Tip. Imp. Akademii Nauk.

"Pridut Pod Imenim Moim" [They Will Come under My Name]. *Pravda Buryatii*, October 24, 1990.

Prozorov, S. 2009. *The Ethics of Postcommunism: History and Social Praxis in Russia*. New York: Palgrave Macmillan.

———. 2010. "Ethos without Nomos: The Russian-Georgian War and the Post-Soviet State of Exception." *Ethics & Global Politics* 3 (4): 255–75.

Pupyshev, V. N. 1989. *Na puti k tibetskoy meditsine (istoriya, metodologiya izucheniya, i perspektivy* [Toward Tibetan Medicine (History, Research Methodology, and Prospects)]. Ulan-Ude: BNC SO AN SSSR.

———. 1992 *Osnovy Tibetskoy Meditsiny* [Foundations of Tibetan Medicine]. Ulan-Ude: BNC SO AN SSSR.

Quijada, J. 2009. "Opening the Roads: History and Religion in Post-Soviet Buryatia." Ph.D. diss. University of Chicago.

Rabinow, P. 1992. "Artificiality and Enlightenment: From Sociobiology to Biosociality." In *Anthropologies of Modernity: Foucault, Governmentality, and Life Politics.* Malden, Mass.: Wiley-Blackwell.

Rabinow, P., and N. Rose. 2006. "Biopower Today." *Biosocieties* 1 (2): 195.

RAEX. 2019. Mezhdunarodnyy proyekt "Luchshiye praktiki privlecheniya investitsiy v region" [International Project "Best Practices of Attracting Investment into a Region"]. RAEX: International Group of Rating Agencies. Accessed February 22, 2021, https://raex-a.ru/ratings/regions/2019/att1.

Raffles, H. 1999. "44 Local Theory": Nature and the Making of an Amazonian Place. *Cultural Anthropology* 14 (3): 323–60.

Raikhel, E. 2010. "Post-Soviet Placebos: Epistemology and Authority in Russian Treatments for Alcoholism." *Culture, Medicine & Psychiatry* 34 (1): 132–68.

———. 2016. *Governing Habits: Treating Alcoholism in the Post-Soviet Clinic.* Ithaca, N.Y.: Cornell University Press.

Randolph, E. 1996. *Waking the Tempests: Ordinary Life in the New Russia.* New York: Simon & Schuster.

Rapp, R. 1999. *Testing Women, Testing the Fetus: The Social Impact of Amniocentesis in America.* New York: Routledge.

Razumov, A. N., and I. P. Bobrovnitsky. 2008. "Vosstanovitel'naya meditsina: 15 let noveyshey istorii—etapy i napravleniya razvitiya" [Restorative Medicine: 15 Years of the Most Recent History—Stages and Directions of Development]. *Vestnik vosstanovitel'noy meditsiny* 3:7–13.

Redfield, P. 1996. "Beneath a Modern Sky: Space Technology and Its Place on the Ground." *Science, Technology & Human Values* 21 (3): 251–74.

Rees, L., and W. Weil. 2001. "Integrated Medicine: Imbues Orthodox Medicine with the Values of Complementary Medicine." *BMJ: British Medical Journal* 322: 119–20.

"Results of the All-Union Meeting Seminar for Heads and Specialists of Hunting Enterprises, State Industrial Farms, Territories and Regions of the RSFSR on the Organization of the procurement and delivery of goods of Tibetan medicine for export, in Vladivostok on April 13-18." 1964. Gosudarstvennyy Arkhiv Rossiyskoy Federatsii (GARF) f (fond). A358, op. (opis') 5, d. (delo) 304, l. (list) 2.

Ries, N. 2009. "Potato Ontology: Surviving Postsocialism in Russia." *Cultural Anthropology* 24 (2): 181–212.

Rivkin-Fish, M. 2005a. "Bribes, Gifts and Unofficial Payments: Rethinking Corruption in Post-Soviet Russian Health Care." In *Corruption: Anthropological Perspectives.* London and Ann Arbor, Mich.: Pluto.

———. 2005b. *Women's Health in Post-Soviet Russia: The Politics of Intervention.* Bloomington: Indiana University Press.

———. 2013. "Conceptualizing Feminist Strategies for Russian Reproductive Politics: Abortion, Surrogate Motherhood, and Family Support after Socialism." *Signs: Journal of Women in Culture and Society* 38 (3): 569–93.

Rodriguez, A. April 13, 2006. "No Offense, Doctor, but You're Alternative Medicine in Russia." *Chicago Tribune.* http://articles.chicagotribune.com/2006-04-13/news/0604130134_1_folk-remedies-folk-medicine-russian-doctors.

Roerich, N. K. 1995. *Khimavat.* Moscow: TOO Agni.

Rogers, D. 2005. "Moonshine, Money, and the Politics of Liquidity in Rural Russia." *American Ethnologist* 32 (1): 63–81.

———. 2010. "Postsocialisms Unbound: Connections, Critiques, Comparisons." *Slavic Review*: 69 (1): 1–15.

Romanov, P., and E. Yarskaya-Smirnova. 2007. "Sotsial'noye Kak Irratsional'noye (Diagnozy 1990 Goda)" [The Social as Irrational (Diagnosing the 90s)]. *Novoe Literaturnoe Obozrenie* (83): 205–26.

Romanov, P. V., and E. R. Yarskaya-Smirnova. 2011. *Ideologii professionalizma i sotsial'noye gosudarstvo: Antropologiya professiy, ili postoronnim vkhod razreshen* [Ideologies of Professionalism and the Social State: Anthropology of Professions, or Intruders Welcome]. Moscow: OOO Variant; TsSPGI.

Rose, N. 2001. *The Politics of Life Itself: Biomedicine, Power, and Subjectivity in the Twenty-First Century.* Princeton, N.J.: Princeton University Press.

———. 2009. "Normality and Pathology in a Biomedical Age." *Sociological Review* 57 (2): 66–83.

Rose, N., and C. Novas. 2005. "Biological Citizenship." In *Global Assemblages: Technology, Politics, and Ethics as Anthropological Problems*, edited by Aihwa Ong and Stephen J. Collier. Malden, Mass.: Blackwell.

Rosenthal, B. 1997. *The Occult in Russian and Soviet Culture.* Ithaca, N.Y.: Cornell University Press.

Ross, C., and R. Turovsky 2015. "Centralized but Fragmented: The Regional Dimension of Russia's 'Party of Power.'" *Demokratizatsiya* 23 (2): 205–23.

Ruggie, M. 2004. *Marginal to Mainstream: Alternative Medicine in America.* Cambridge: Cambridge University Press.

"Russia's Registry of Medicinal Substances" [Gosudarstvennyy reyestr lekarstvennykh sredstv]. 2008. In *Federal'naya sluzhba po nadzoru v sfere zdravookhraneniya i sotsial'nogo razvitiya.* Moscow: Nauch. tsentr ekspertizy sredstv med. primeneniya.

Sablin, I. 2019. "Tibetan Medicine and Buddhism in the Soviet Union: Research, Repression, and Revival, 1922–1991." In *Healers and Empires in Global History.* Cham, Switzerland: Palgrave Macmillan.

Said, E. W. 1978. *Orientalism*. New York: Vintage.

Samuel, G. 1993. *Civilized Shamans: Buddhism in Tibetan Societies*. Washington, D.C.: Smithsonian Institution Press.

———. 2006. "Tibetan Medicine and Biomedicine: Epistemological Conflicts, Practical Solutions." *Asian Medicine* 2 (1): 72–85.

Sanzhin, B. B. 2010. "Formirovaniye i razvitiye turisticheskogo klastera v respublike Buryatiya na osnove gosudarstvenno-chastnogo partnerstva" [The Formation and Development of the Tourism Cluster in the Republic Buryatia on the Basis of a State-Private Partnership]. *Ekonomicheskoye vozrozhdeniye Rossii* 26 (4): 133–42.

Saunders, B. 2008. *CT Suite: The Work of Diagnosis in the Age of Noninvasive Cutting*. Durham, N.C. Duke University Press.

Saxer, M. 2004. "Journeys with Tibetan Medicine: How Tibetan Medicine Came to the West; The Story of the Badmayev Family." Ph.D. diss. Oxford University.

———. 2013. *Manufacturing Tibetan Medicine: The Creation of an Industry and the Moral Economy of Tibetanness*. Vol. 12. Brooklyn, N.Y.: Berghahn.

Scheid, V. 2002. *Chinese Medicine in Contemporary China: Plurality and Synthesis*. Durham, N.C.: Duke University Press.

Scheid, V., and H. MacPherson. 2012. *Integrating East Asian Medicine into Contemporary Healthcare*. Edinburgh and New York: Churchill Livingstone Elsevier.

Scheper-Hughes, N. 1990. "Three Propositions for a Critically Applied Medical Anthropology." *Social Science & Medicine* 30 (2): 189–97.

———. 1992. "Nervoso: Medicine, Sickness, and Human Needs." In *Death without Weeping: The Violence of Everyday Life in Brazil*. Berkeley: University of California Press.

Semashko, N. A. 1934. *Health Protection in the USSR*. London: Victor Gollancz.

Semichov, B. 1932. "Tibetskaya Meditsina v BMASSR" [Tibetan Medicine in the BMASSR]. *Sovetskaya Etnografiya* 5–6:216–28.

Sergeeva, M. S. 2015. "'Physiological Collectivism': The Origins of the Institute of Blood Transfusion's Ideas and Their Practical Realization." *History of Medicine* 2 (4): 420–30.

Sharp, L. 2006. *Strange Harvest: Organ Transplants, Denatured Bodies, and the Transformed Self*. Berkeley: University of California Press.

Shastina, N. P. 2003. "A. M. Pozdneev." *Mongolica* 6:7–18.

Shkinder, N. L. 2009. "Reformy Zdravookhraneniya i Gumanizatsiya Meditsinskogo Vuza" [Healthcare Reforms and the Humanization of the Medical University]. In *Sbornik statey i tezisov dokladov uchastnikov vtoroy Mezhregional'noy nauchno-prakticheskoy konferentsii*. Yekaterinburg: UGMA.

Sidorov, S. 2008. *Rassvet beskonechnoy zhizni: Uchebnik tibetskoy meditsiny* [The Dawn of Eternal Life: Manual of Tibetan Medicine]. Moscow: Zolotoye Secheniye.

Silverstein, M., and G. Urban. 1996. *Natural Histories of Discourse*. Chicago: University of Chicago Press.

Slezkine, Y. 1994. "The USSR as a Communal Apartment, or How a Socialist State Promoted Ethnic Particularism." *Slavic Review* 53 (2): 414–52.

Smirnov, E. 2009. "Slozhnaya Situatsiya s Lekarstvennymi Rasteniyami v Mire Otrazitsya Na Rossiyskoy Farmotrasli" [The Complex World Situation with Medicinal Plants Will Impact Russian Pharma]. *Farmatsevticheskiy Vestnik* 5 (537) https://pharmvestnik.ru/articles/12027.html.

Snelling, J. 1993. *Buddhism in Russia: The Story of Agvan Dorzhiev, Lhasa's Emissary to the Tzar*. Shaftesbury, Dorset and Rockport, Mass.: Element.

Soaeifer, V. 1994. *Lysenko and the Tragedy of Soviet Science*. New Brunswick, N.J.: Rutgers University Press.

Sobo, E. J. 2015. Social Cultivation of Vaccine Refusal and Delay among Waldorf (Steiner) School Parents. *Medical Anthropology Quarterly* 29 (3): 381–99.

Sokoloff, D. D., S. A. Balandin, I. A. Gubanov, C. E. Jarvis, S. R. Majorov, and S. S. Simonov. 2002. "The History of Botany in Moscow and Russia in the 18th and Early 19th Centuries in the Context of the Linnaean Collection at Moscow University (MW)." *Huntia: A Yearbook of Botanical and Horticultural Bibliography* 11 (2): 129–91.

Sokolov, A. 1974. "Dzhud-Shi Otrkyvaet Sekrety" [Dzhud-Shi Reveals Secrets]. *Pravda* (159), June 8.

St. 50. Federal'nyy zakon ot 21 noyabrya 2011 N 323 "Ob osnovakh okhrany zdorov'ya grazhdan v Rossiyskoy Federatsii" [Article 50. Federal Law from 21 November 2011 N 323 "On the Foundations of Health Protection of the Citizens of the Russian Federation."]

Stalin, J. 1929. *The National Question and Leninism*. New York: International Publishers.

Star, S. L. 2010. "This Is Not a Boundary Object: Reflections on the Origin of a Concept." *Science, Technology & Human Values* 35 (5): 601–17.

Star, S. L., and J. Griesemer. 1989. "Institutional Ecology, Translations, and Boundary Objects: Amateurs and Professionals in Berkeley's Museum of Vertebrate Zoology, 1907–39." *Social Studies of Science* 19 (3): 387–420.

Starks, T. 2008. *The Body Soviet: Propaganda, Hygiene, and the Revolutionary State*. Madison: University of Wisconsin Press.

Stengers, I. 2000. *The Invention of Modern Science*. Vol. 19. Minneapolis: University of Minnesota Press.

———. 2003. "The Doctor and the Charlatan." *Cultural Studies Review* 9 (2): 11–36.

———. 2005. "The Cosmopolitical Proposal." In *Making Things Public: Atmospheres of Democracy*, edited by B. Latour and P. Weibel. Cambridge Mass: MIT Press.

———. 2011. *Cosmopolitics II*. Minneapolis: University of Minnesota Press.

Stevenson, L. 2012. "The Psychic Life of Biopolitics: Survival, Cooperation, and Inuit Community. *American Ethnologist* 39 (3): 592–613.

———. 2014. *Life Beside Itself: Imagining Care in the Canadian Arctic*. Oakland: University of California Press.

Stewart, K. 2012. "Precarity's Forms." *Cultural Anthropology* 27 (3): 518–25.

Studentsov, E. P., S. M. Ramsh, N. G. Kazurova, O.V. Neporozhneva, A.V. Garabadzhiu, T. A. Kochina, M. G. Voronkov, V. A. Kuznetsov, and D. V. Krivorotov. 2013. "Adaptogeny i rodstvennyye gruppy lekarstvennykh preparatov-50 let poiskov" [Adaptogens and Related Groups of Medicinal Products—50 Years of Research]. *Obzory po klinicheskoy farmakologii i lekarstvennoy terapii* 11 (4): 3–43.

Sukachev, V. N., ed. 1964. *Osnovy Lesnoy Biogeotsenologii* [Foundations of Forest Biogeocenology]. Moscow: Nauka.

Sulakshin, S. S., V. N. Leksin, A. N. Shvetsov, L. A. Reymer, and A. S. Malchinov. 2013. *Regional'noye izmereniye gosudarstvennoy ekonomicheskoy politiki Rossii* [Regional Measurements of Russia's State Economic Policy]. Moscow: Nauchnyy Ekspert.

Sunder Rajan, K. 2006. *Biocapital: The Constitution of Postgenomic Life*. Durham, N.C.: Duke University Press.

Tambiah, S. J. 1976. *World Conqueror and World Renouncer: A Study of Buddhism and Polity in Thailand against a Historical Background*. Cambridge: Cambridge University Press.

Taussig, M. 2010. *The Devil and Commodity Fetishism in South America*. Chapel Hill: University of North Carolina Press.

Thrift, N. J. 2005. *Knowing Capitalism*. London: Sage.

Todorova, M. 2009. *Bones of Contention: The Living Archive of Vasil Levski and the Making of Bulgaria's National Hero*. Budapest: Central European University Press.

Tolz, V. 2005. "Orientalism, Nationalism, and Ethnic Diversity in Late Imperial Russia." *Historical Journal* 48 (1): 127–50.

Trotsky, L. 2005. *Literature and Revolution*. Chicago: Haymarket.

Tsing, A. 2005. *Friction: An Ethnography of Global Connection*. Princeton, N.J.: Princeton University Press.

———. 2015. *The Mushroom at the End of the World: On the Possibility of Life in Capitalist Ruins*. Princeton, N.J.: Princeton University Press.

Tsydypov, Ch. Ts. 1988. "Kanony vostochnoy pul'sodiagnostiki i problemy eye ob"yektivizatsii" [Canons of Eastern Pulse Diagnosis and the Problem of Its Objectivization]. In *Pul'sovaya diagnostika tibetskoy meditsiny*. Novosibirsk: Izdatel'stvo Nauka.

Tsyrempilov, N. 2012. "'Alien' Lamas: Russian Policy towards Foreign Buddhist Clergy in the Eighteenth to Early Twentieth Centuries." *Inner Asia* 14 (2): 245–55.

Tumanov, I. I. 1979. *Fiziologiya zakalivaniya i morozostoykosti rasteniy* [The Physiology of Tempering and the Cold Resistance of Plants]. Moscow: Nauka.

Twigg, J., and K. Schecter. 2003. *Social Capital and Social Cohesion in Post-Soviet Russia*. Armonk, N.Y.: M. E. Sharpe.

Vasylyev, A. V., and T. P. Poloz. 2000. "Lekarstvennyye rasteniya Rossii—neissyakayemyy istochnik dlya sozdaniya novykh vysokoeffektivnykh lechebno-profilakticheskikh preparatov i biologicheski aktivnykh pishchevykh dobavok" [Medicinal Plants of Russia—A Bottomless Source for the Creation of Medical-Prophylactic Drugs and Biologically Active Supplements]. *Voprosy meditsinskoy khimii* 2:101–9.

Velminski, W. 2017. *Homo Sovieticus: Brain Waves, Mind Control, and Telepathic Destiny*. Cambridge, Mass.: MIT Press.

Venuti, L. 2000. "Translation, Community, Utopia." In *The Translation Studies Reader*, edited by Lawrence Venuti. London and New York: Routledge.

Verdery, K. 1999. *The Political Lives of Dead Bodies: Reburial and Postsocialist Change*. New York: Columbia University Press.

Verkovenskyi, A. 2011. "Evolyutsiya postsovetskogo dvizheniya russkikh natsionalistov." [The Evolution of the Post-Soviet Russian Nationalist Movement]. *Vestnik Obshchestvennogo Mneniya* 107 (1): 11–35.

Vetitnev, A.M., and L. B. Zhuravleva. 2006. *Kurortnoye delo* [Health Resort Practice]. Moscow: Knorus.

Vishnevsky, A.G., Y. I. Kuzminov, V. I. Shevskyi, I. M. Sheyman, and L. I. Shishin. 2006. *Rossiyskoye zdravookhraneniye: Kak vyyti iz krizisa* [Russian Healthcare: How to Get Out of the Crisis]. Moscow: GU VSHE.

Vitvitsky, N. 1933. *The Case of N. P. Vitvitsky, V. A. Gussev . . . : Heard Before the Supreme Court of the USSR in Moscow, April 12–19, 1933*. Vol. 1. Moscow: State Law Publishing House.

Vlasov, S. 1982. "Eksperiment Dlinnoy v Pol Veka" [An Experiment That Lasted Half a Century]. *Ogonek* 8.

Voice of America. 2011. "Russia Boasts More Faith Healers Than Physicians." June 21, 2011. https://www.voanews.com/europe/russia-boasts-more-faith-healers-real-physicians.

Vostkokov, V. 1998. *Tayny Tibetskoy Meditsiny* [Secrets of Tibetan Medicine]. Donetsk: Stalker.

"V Rossii tselitel'stvo prinosit $50–60 millionov v god" [Russia Folk Healing Brings $50–60 Millions a Year]. *Argumenty i Fakty*, November 4, 2009. http://www.aif.ru/health/article/30582.

Vyalkov, A. I., A. N. Razumov, and I. P. Bobrovnitzky. 2003. "Vosstanovitel'naya meditsina kak novoye napravleniye v nauke i praktike zdravookhraneniya" [Restorative Medicine as a New Direction in the Science and Practice of Healthcare]. *Diagnosticheskiye i ozdorovitel'nyye tekhnologii vosstanovitel'noy meditsiny: spravochnik* 1:16–22.

Walters, P. 2001. "Religion in Tuva: Restoration or Innovation?" *Religion, State & Society* 29 (1): 23–38.

Waugh, L. R. 1982. "Marked and Unmarked: A Choice between Unequals in Semiotic Structure." *Semiotica* 38 (3–4): 299–318.

Wood, F. 2010. "Occult Innovations in Higher Education: Corporate Magic and the Mysteries of Managerialism." *Prometheus* 28 (3): 227–44.

Yakovlev, N. N. 1986. *Zhivoye i sreda: Molekulyarnyye i funktsional'nyye osnovy prisposobleniya organizma k usloviyam sredy* [Living and Environment: Molecular and Functional Bases of the Organism's Adaptation to Environmental Conditions). Leningrad: Nauka.

Yegorov, I. 2009. "Post-Soviet Science: Difficulties in the Transformation of the R&D Systems in Russia and Ukraine." *Research Policy* 38 (4): 600–609.

Yermenko, K. V. 2007 *Optimal'noye sostoyaniye organizma i adaptogeny* [Optimal State of the Body and Adaptogens]. St. Petersburg: Elbi.

Yurchak, A. 2008. "Necro-Utopia." *Current Anthropology* 49 (2): 199–224.

Zabrodin, A. 2005. "Kontseptsiya N. V. Lazareva Ob Adaptogenakh v Aspekte Ucheniya o Nervnoy Trofike" [N. V. Lazarev's Concept of Adaptogens from the Perspective of the Teachings on Nervous Trophic]. *Psikhofarmakologiya i Biologicheskaya Narkologiya* 5 (4): 1108–12.

Zhambalova, S. G. 1997. *Atlas Tibetskoy Meditsiny—Sokrovishche Buryatii* [The Atlas of Tibetan Medicine—a Buryat Treasure]. Ulan-Ude: Buryatskoye knizhnoye Izdatel'stvo.

Zhamsuev, B. B., and C. P. Banchinova. 2008. *Zemlya Vadzhrapani: Buddizm v Zabaykal'ye* [The Land of Vajrapani: Buddhism in the Trans-Baikal Region]. Moscow: Izdatel'stvo Dizayn. Informatsiya. Kartografiya.

Zhan, M. 2009. *Other-Worldly: Making Chinese Medicine through Transnational Frames*. Durham, N.C. Duke University Press.

Zhukovskaya, N. L. 1998. "Atlas tibetskoy meditsiny na perekrestke religii i politiki" [The Atlas of Tibetan Medicine at the Crossroads of Religion and Politics]. In *Mir traditsionnoy mongol'skoy kul'tury*. Lewiston, Queenston: Edwin Mellen.

INDEX

attention: and ecology, 256; Ivanov and, 225; and medicinal substances, 236, 251; and methodology, 18–21; patients and, 177–85; peripheral, 18–21; and pulse diagnosis, 100–1; therapeutic, 14

Atzagat Buddhist monastery, 52–53, 53*f*, 54, 56, 65

authority. *See* legitimacy

Automated Pulse Diagnostic Complex (APDC), 70–73; body of, 87; calibration of, 102; design of, 90–91; development of, 81–87, 93; issues with, 99–102; ownership, 97–98; patent for, 86; sensors of, 87

Ayuna (pediatrician), 147–48

Ayuna (practitioner), 256–57

Ayur (researcher), 95–99, 105

Ayurveda, 203

Babu Lama (Buddhist lama), 151–53

badan, 154

Badaraev (physician), 148–50

badgan, 30, 232, 286n3

Badmaev, Aleksandr, 39–40

Badmaev, D. D., 63

Badmaev, Nikolai, 55, 57–59, 61

Badmaev, Pyotr, 39–48

Bakhtin, Mikhail, 269

Baldanzhapov, P. B., 63

balneology, 54, 210. *See also* resort medicine

Barnaulov, O. D., 253

Bartol, Vladimir, 267

BAS. *See* biologically active substances

Bassin, Mark, 286n5

"Battle of the Psychics," 267–70

Bayar Badmaevich (*emchi*), 204–11, 263

bear bile, 235

bendazol, 170

Benjamin, Walter, 40

Bergenia root, 154, 291n14

Bering, Jonassen, 37

bile, 30–31. *See also* shara

biofield, term, 83

biogeocenosis, 253; term, 293n6

biologically active substances (BAS), 248

biomedicine, 19; Babu Lama on, 152–53; Bayar Badmaevich on, 208–9; and bodies, 76; East-West Medical Center and, 159; Erden Lama on, 227; history in Russia, 143; as *krysha,* 203; legitimacy of, 195–96; patients on, 190; rhetoric of, 124; and root causes, 188; Soviet Union and, 51; term, 16; Tsyrenma and, 33; Vladimir Viktorovich and, 112, 114. *See also* critiques of Russian healthcare models

biopolitics: of integrative medicine, 10–18; limits of, 15; national health and, 200; and Russia's medical markets, 113

biosociality, term, 174

biosphere, Vernadsky on, 165

biotic communities, 252–54

The Blue Beryl, 64

Blue Beryl Medical Center, 231–34, 261

body(ies): alienation of, 181–85; biomedical practice and, 76; Buryatia and, 122; East-West Medical Center and, 173–78; Foucault on, 276–77; and information, 84; theorizations of, 17; Mariana on, 211–12; plants and, 236; post-socialist, 161–64, 277; potential of, 163, 225; and preparation of medicines, 249; and pulse diagnosis, 100–1; Soviet project and, 272

bones, uses in medicine, 231–37, 260

botanical life-forms, 20, 229–62; Badmaev and, 59–60; collecting, 238–39, 257–58; exploitation of, 154–55;

Gammerman and, 61; identification of, Pozdneev and, 49; preparation of, 212–17, 243–52; regulation of, 212–14; Soviet Union and, 55, 289n17. *See also* herbal medicines; medicinal substances

Botkin, Sergei, 159, 165, 167–68, 291n2

boundar(ies): body and, 138, 173; botanical ingredients and, 242–43; and *emchi* practice, 145; epistemological, 29, 72, 148; institutional, 21; of kinds of medicines, 196; object, 243; pulsometer and, 93

brand of Buryatia, 65; Buryat Atlas and, 68; center-periphery models and, 125–34; "The Convention of World Mongols" on, 147, 149

Brekhman, Israel, 170–72, 292n3

Brezhnev, Leonid, 82

Buck-Morss, Susan, 139, 197, 287n11

Buddhism, 3, 5; Bayar Badmaevich and, 204; and brand of Buryatia, 133; and center-periphery models, 127; concepts in Tibetan medicine, 32–33; and eclecticism, 151–52; and ethics, 14, 58, 152–53; and herbal medicines, 245–46; history in Siberia, 34, 38–39; and integrative medicine, 143; Irina and, 233; as *krysha,* 203; Roerich and, 164–65; Soviet Union and, 52, 54–56, 288n13; temples, 37–39, 52–53, 53*f,* 54, 56, 65, 204

Bulgakov, Mikhail, 263, 271–72

bureaucracy, personalized medicine and, 185

Bureau for the Study of Oriental Medicine, 55

burning-bush root, 233

Buryat Atlas, 64–68

Buryat people: *emchi* conceptualizations of bodies and, 227; ethnicity, 34–35; land rights, and, 45; Pan-Mongol world and, 149; Russian empire and, 35–36; Soviet nationality policy and, 50–51

Buryat Research Center, Institute of Biologically Active Substances, 244

Buryat Science Center, 63; and pulsometer, 78, 88, 90

Buryatia, 1–3, 107*f;* Badmaev and, 45; brand of, 65, 68, 125–34, 147, 149; characteristics of, 4; and ecology, 124–25, 130, 132, 254–62; Empire and, 39–49; national anthem of, 291n11; and regional politics, 126–31; Soviet Union and, 50–51; and Tibetan medicine, 106–56

calcination, 215–16, 291n12

calcite, taming, 249

capitalism, and esoterica, 273. *See also* markets

care itineraries, 178–79, 186–87, 189–91

care practices: Buddhist ethics and, 14; and translation, 29

Castaneda, Carlos, 273

center-periphery models, 122–25; and Buryatia's brand, 125–34; critiques of, 13–14, 17, 127

Chadha, A., 77

children, treatment of, 191–92, 234–35

Chinese medicine, 203; and acupuncture, 62; and athletes, 138; and pulse, 74, 78, 86; Vladimir Viktorovich and, 111

Choedrak, Tenzin, 70–71

cholera, 167

chronic illnesses, 173; as disadaptation, 191–93; East-West Medical Center and, 173–77, 179, 181–82; Erden Lama on, 220–22; herbal medicines and, 188

insurance system, 109, 159, 210, 264; Vladimir Viktorovich on, 116

integrative medicine: Bayar Badmaevich on, 206–9; biopolitics of, 10–18; and brand of Buryatia, 134; Buryatia and, 122–25; critique of, 220–28; difficulties with, 264–66; East-West Medical Center and, 157–60, 162–64; geographical specificity and, 106–56; Gregoryi Mikhaylovich on, 113; resistance to, 146–54; term, 10, 194–95; terminology and, 140–41; Vladimir Viktorovich on, 111–15, 121–22

International Academy of Traditional Tibetan Medicine, 7

invisibility: administrative, 206–7; of labor on herbal medicines, 216; of traditional medicine, 20, 266. *See also* visibility

Irina (patient), 231–34

Irkutsk, 131

Iroltuev, Choyzon Dorzhi, 49, 52

Istok, 86

Ivanov, Porfiry Korneevich, 223–27

Jambaldorje, 240

Kagarlitsky, Boris, 128

Kalmykia, 5

Kaminsky, G. N., 61

Kashkadamov, V. P., 57–58

Katerina (patient), 174, 179, 187, 190–91

Keane, Webb, 91

Khamchikhin, Aleksandr, 291n8

khi, 30. *See also* wind

Khrushchev, Nikita, 226

Kleinman, Arthur, 162

knowledge production, 196–97; cybernetics and, 82; pulse diagnosis and, 100–1; pulsometer and, 79, 88, 90;

Soviet Union and, 49; translation and, 28; Western, 207

Kogan, Genokh, 60

Kokorev, A. V., 48

krysha, 203–4

kumyz therapy, 259–60

labor, and mixing medicines, 14–15, 145, 214–16, 230, 250–51

laboratory science: Badmaev and, 59–60; Botkin and, 165

Lake Baikal, 131–32

landscape, 258–59; and foraging, 275

language: of conventionality, 217–20; cyberspeak, 82; and medicinal substances, 237–43; and pulse diagnosis, 75, 92; and Tibetan medicine, 46, 108, 140–46. *See also* translation

Latour, Bruno, 196

Lazarev, Nikolai, 170

learning Tibetan medicine, 28; "The Convention of World Mongols" and, 150–51; *Gyüshi* and, 26–27; history of, 37; medicinal substances and, 237–43; pulsometer and, 103–5

leech therapy, 202, 210

legality: and ephedra, 213–14, 241; and nutritional supplements, 244; and supplies, 215–16; and traditional medicine, 198–204

legitimacy: of biomedicine, 195–96; *Gyüshi* translations and, 27; *krysha* and, 203–4; of Moscow traditional clinics, 118; of phytotherapy, 245; of Pro-Culture, 66; of pulsometer, 88–93, 105, 290n4; Soviet Union and, 57–59; of Tibetan medicine, 198–204; Tsyrenma on, 103

Lenin, V. I., 49–50, 278

Leslie, Charles, 162

LGBTQ community, and terminology, 218

licensing, and traditional healing, 202–3

life: Foucault on, 12, 113; and nonlife, 235–36, 277

lifestyle: East-West Medical Center and, 176; Erden Lama on, 220–22; and herbal medicine regime, 247; Soviet medicine and, 171

Lillia (patient), 189–90

listening, to pulse, 75, 92

liveliness, of medicinal substances, 243–53

Liza (PR representative), 217

Lobsan-Galsan, 48

localization, 19; of bodies and medicine, 194–228; East-West Medical Center and, 162–64; Erden Lama on, 227; and herbal medicines, 246–47, 252–54; and pulse diagnosis, 76, 87; Tibetan medicine in Buryatia, 106–56

Logvinov, V. S., 92

loss, translation and, 29

LotusMed, 110–20

Luzhkov, Yuri, 129

Lydia (mathematician), 99

Lyudmila (pharmacist), 212

magic, post-socialist Russia and, 200–1, 263–79

magnetic imaging, 77, 83, 86

mahabhuta, 31

making live, Foucault on, 12, 113

Maksim (worker), 261

Malakhov, Genady, 226

Mandala model, 127

manual therapy, 202

Maramba, Choy, 38

marginality, Buryatia and, 127

margins: as "center-periphery" spatializations, 108, 124, 126–27, 131–32, 138, 174; of embodiment, 227, 277; as marginalization, 146, 225; overview of, 10–13; of error, 98, 119

Mariana (pharmacist), 211

Marianna Vladimirovna (curator), 67–68

markets, of nonbiomedical therapies, 7, 19; and healthcare, 12–18, 24, 111, 115–17, 119, 123, 170, 199, 231, 243–44, 266, 272; and neoliberalism, 273, 275, 279; and regional branding, 130

Martin, Terry, 288n11

Marxism, 49, 58; and emplacement, 168; Ivanov on, 223, 225

massage, medical, 120, 136, 141, 176, 202

materia medica. See medicinal substances

media: and Badmaev, 46–47, 61; and Buryat Atlas, 66, 68; and Buryatia, 126, 130; and paranormal, 82; and Tibetan medicine, 7, 56

medicinal substances, 158f, 229–62, 230f; attention and, 236; Badmaev on, 42–43; Pozdneev and, 48; preparation of, 145, 212–17, 243–52; scarcity/abundance and, 248; Semichov and, 56; state registry of, 213, 241–42. *See also* botanical life-forms; herbal medicines

medicine, classification of, 143, 198–99, 202

Medvedev, Dmitry, 274–75, 290n7

Men Tsee Khang, 86

metabolism, Brekhman on, 171

methodology, attention and, 18–21

Michaels, Paula, 51

minerals, 229. *See also* calcite

mkhris, 30. *See also* culprits

Mobius, Karl, 253

personalized medicine: challenges in, 173; East-West Medical Center and, 159, 161, 164–69; and paperwork, 185; patients on, 182

Petryna, Adriana, 174

pharmacology, Soviet: and Tibetan medicine, 49–64. *See also* pills

phlegm, 30–31. See also *badgan*

phytotherapy, 154, 202, 219, 241; classification of, 206; Eastern versus Western, 207–8; term, 245; theory of, 252

pills: and anxiety, 188; Bayar Badmaevich on, 208–11; costs of, 209; effects of, 209; versus herbal medicines, 245; Mariana on, 211; patients on, 181; rhetoric of, 124; self-medicating with, 187; Vladimir Viktorovich on, 116

placebo effect, 84

place spirits, 106, 212, 257

plants. *See* botanical life-forms

pluralism, therapeutic, 3, 18, 195–96, 200; East-West Medical Center and, 162–64

politics: Badmaev on, 43; "The Convention of World Mongols" on, 147, 149 ; and geopolitical imaginaries, 108, 127, 131, 149, 269; and regional identity, 37

pollution, 256

polyarthritis, 181

Pomerantsev, Peter, 267

Poslepova, M. L., 253

post-socialist Russia: and bodily alienation, 181–85; East-West Medical Center and, 161–64; and extraction, 229–62; and health, 17, 108–22; landscape of, 258–59; and magic, 200–1, 263–79; nonbiomedical healing in, 3; and pensioners, 178; and

Tibetan medicine, 64–69; Vladimir Viktorovich on, 117–18

Potapov, Leonid, 65–66

potential of bodies: tempering and, 225; traditional medicine and, 163

powders, Tibetan. *See* herbal medicines

power relations: and medicinal substances, 242–43; and translation, 29, 41

Pozdneev, Aleksei, 39, 47–49, 287n10

prayer wheels, 221*f*

precarity, 264, 275–76. *See also* uncertainty

prevention, Soviet medicine and, 168. *See also* dispenserization

Pro-Culture, 66

progress, Soviet ideology and, 197

prosthesis: pulsometer as, 72, 92, 104–5; Vladimir Viktorovich on, 120

public health, 114–15; Badaraev on, 150; "The Convention of World Mongols" on, 147; restorative medicine and, 137; Soviet Union and, 168

pulse diagnosis, 2, 70–105; attention and, 100–1; Godik on, 85; language in, 92; texts on, 75–76

pulse wave, 94; factors affecting, 92

pulsometer: challenges with, 101–2; development of, 70–73, 81–87, 97; legitimacy of, 88–93; mechanism of, 93–102; as unreliable witness, 73–80

Pupyshev, Viktor, 88

purification, 196

purity, Buryatia and, 132, 254–61

Putin, Vladimir, 95, 128, 138, 189

qigong, 84

Rabinow, Paul, 174

radiation medicine, 170

senses, translating between, 92, 97

sensors, of APDC, 87, 94

serfdom, abolition of, 36, 167

Sergei (practitioner), 97–98, 100, 102, 194–96

shara, 30. *See also* culprits

Siberia: Empire and, 34–39; image of, 286n5

Sibkursan, 54

Slezkine, Yuri, 50

sliz', 30. *See also* culprits

smoker's foot, 83–84

socialism. *See* post-socialist Russia; Soviet Union

Solomon, Gross, 168

Soviet Academy of Scientists, Siberian Branch, 157

Soviet Union: and adaptation, 170–73; and bodily ideologies, 220–23; and center-periphery model, 13; and emplacement, 168–69; and health definitions, 17; and imaging projects, 81–87; and medicine, 196; and paranormal, 81; and progress, 197; and pulse diagnosis, 72, 77–78; and supply chains, 212; and Tibetan medicine, 9, 49–64, 289n17; and time, 139; and uncanny, 270; Vladimir Viktorovich and, 115

Sowa Rigpa. *See* Tibetan medicine

space, 31

space medicine, 136–40

Special Economic Zone, Buryatia as, 130

specificity: geographical, 106–56; and Tibetan medicine, 27

sports medicine, 138

Speranskii, Mikhail, 35

srolo 6, 214–15

Stalin, J., 49–50, 288n11

state: and Buddhism, 5; and Buryatia, 45, 108; and medicine, changes in, 200; and pensioners, 174, 191; Putin and, 128; and Tibetan medicine, 4–5, 7–8, 135–36, 198–204. *See also* critiques of Russian healthcare models

State Registry of Medicinal Substances, 213, 241–42

State University, Ulan-Ude, 78

Stengers, Isabelle, 78, 198, 276

Steppe Dumas, 35–36

Stewart, Kathleen, 275

stocking up on health, 186–91, 266. *See also* collection

students, pulsometer and, 94–99

subaltern therapeutics, term, 200

suffering: Badmaev on, 44; collectivity and, 177; Irina on, 233; Ivanov on, 223–24; and medical concepts, 14–15

Sukachev, V. N., 254

sundress radio, 20, 244

suppliers, 145, 212, 215–16

surgery, Irina on, 234

surreal, 263–79

swine flu, 175

symptoms, treating, 119–20

synthetic pharmaceuticals. *See* pills

syrye: term, 229. *See also* medicinal substances

systematicity, 142; and categories of medicine, 143, 199; Godik and, 84–85; Tibetan medicine and, 144–46, 197; Vladimir Viktorovich on, 114

Taban Arshan, 213

Tamara Anatolyevna (research biologist), 5–6

Tambiah, Stanley, 127

teas, medicinal, 211

technology: Badaraev on, 150; East-West Medical Center and, 160; Erden Lama on, 227; pulsometer, 70–105; Tibetan medicine and, 134–40

tempering, 220–27

Tenzin Gyatso, 67

terminology: botanical, 237–43; of center-periphery models, 126–27; in Tibetan medicine, 108, 140–46, 200, 286n3; of unconventionality, 217–20

Territorially Compulsory Insurance Funds (TFOMS), 109

texts: and medicinal substances, 239; on pulse diagnosis, 75–76; and pulsometer, 89, 91; and translation, 25–34

theosophical movement, 165

third state, Brekhman on, 172

Thubpten Gyatso, 65

Tibetan medicine, 1–24; and adaptability, 172–73; and brand of Buryatia, 133–34; in Buryatia, 106–56; for children, 191–92; contact with Tibet, 35; and healthcare system, 200; history of, 6–9, 25–69; images of, changes in, 124–25; and infectious disease, 42–44; as innovative technology, 134–40; Irina on, 233; issues in, 6; Moscow clinics and, 108–22; pulse diagnosis in, 70–105; Roerich and, 166; Soviet Union and, 49–64, 289n17; symptom interview in, 183–84; terminology in, 108, 140–46, 200, 286n3

Tibetan medicines. *See* medicinal substances

time: Dashi and, 269; pulsometer and, 80; Soviet imaginaries and, 139, 197

tinctures, 250

Tolz, Vera, 287n7

tourism: Buryatia and, 130, 155, 256; Tibetan medicine and, 87

toxic substances, 242

tradition, term, 218–19

traditional Chinese medicine. *See* Chinese medicine

traditional medicine, 1–2, 143; accumulation of, 210–11; and adaptability, 172–73; adaptation of, 123–24; East-West Medical Center and, 161, 164–69; and ethnic identity, 118; globalization of, 122–23; invisibility of, 20; legal issues and, 198–204; and modern, 18–19, 194–228; rhetoric of, 124; Soviet Union and, 51; state healthcare and, 109; term, 16, 198; types of, 203; Vladimir Viktorovich and, 111

Transbaikal territories, 34; Badmaev and, 45

translation, 25–29, 39–49, 278; Badmaev and, 59; Benjamin and, 40; code breaking and, 77; formularies and, 37–38; and medical concepts, 30–34; and medicinal substances, 213–18, 237–43; Mongol scholars and, 48; othering, 40; and pulsometer, 79–80, 91–92; Roerich and, 166

travnik, term, 245

Trotsky, Leon, 274

Tsing, Anna, 275

Tsydypov, Chimit Tsyrenovich, 81, 85–86, 89–91

Tsyrempilov, Nikolai, 35

Tsyrenma (*emchi*), 256; on *Gyüshi*, 25–26; on labor, 214–16; and language issues, 33; on legitimacy, 103; on pulse diagnosis, 74, 101; and

Tatiana Chudakova is Assistant Professor of Anthropology at Tufts University. Her work has appeared in *American Ethnologist*, *Medical Anthropology Quarterly*, and *Comparative Studies in Society and History*. She is the recipient of the General Anthropology Division Prize for Exemplary Cross-Field Scholarship (2018).

9 780823 294305